Dietetic and Nutrition Case Studies

This book is dedicated to Pat Judd (1947–2015), inspirational dietitian and educator.

Dietetic and Nutrition Case Studies

EDITED BY

Judy Lawrence

Registered Dietitian, the Research Officer for the BDA, and Visiting Researcher, Nutrition and Dietetics, King's College London, England

Pauline Douglas

Registered Dietitian, a Senior Lecturer and Clinical Dietetic Facilitator, Northern Ireland Centre for Food and Health (NICHE), Ulster University, Northern Ireland

Joan Gandy

Registered Dietitian, a Freelance Dietitian and Visiting Researcher in Nutrition and Dietetics, University of Hertfordshire, England

WILEY Blackwell

Registered office: John Wiley & Sons, Ltd, The Atrium, Southern Gate, Chichester, West Sussex, PO19 8SQ, UK

Editorial offices: 9600 Garsington Road, Oxford, OX4 2DQ, UK
The Atrium, Southern Gate, Chichester, West Sussex, PO19 8SQ, UK
111 River Street, Hoboken, NJ 07030-5774, USA

For details of our global editorial offices, for customer services and for information about how to apply for permission to reuse the copyright material in this book please see our website at www.wiley.com/wiley-blackwell

Library of Congress Cataloging-in-Publication Data

Names: Lawrence, Judy, 1960- , editor. | Gandy, Joan, editor. | Douglas, Pauline, 1961- , editor.
Title: Dietetic and nutrition case studies / edited by Judy Lawrence, Joan Gandy, Pauline Douglas.
Description: Chichester, West Sussex ; Hoboken, NJ : John Wiley & Sons, 2016. | Complemented by: Manual of dietetic practice / edited by Joan Gandy in conjunction with the British Dietetic Association. Fifth edition. 2014. | Includes bibliographical references and index.
Identifiers: LCCN 2015040817 (print) | LCCN 2015042999 (ebook) | ISBN 9781118897102 (pbk.) | ISBN 9781118898239 (pdf) | ISBN 9781118898246 (epub)
Subjects: | MESH: Dietetics. | Nutritional Physiological Phenomena. | Diet Therapy. | Problem-Based Learning.
Classification: LCC RM216 (print) | LCC RM216 (ebook) | NLM WB 400 | DDC 615.8/54–dc23
LC record available at http://lccn.loc.gov/2015040817

A catalogue record for this book is available from the British Library.

Wiley also publishes its books in a variety of electronic formats. Some content that appears in print may not be available in electronic books.

Set in 9/12pt, MeridienLTStd by SPi Global, Chennai, India.

1 2016

Dietetic and Nutrition Case Studies

EDITED BY

Judy Lawrence

Registered Dietitian, the Research Officer for the BDA, and Visiting Researcher, Nutrition and Dietetics, King's College London, England

Pauline Douglas

Registered Dietitian, a Senior Lecturer and Clinical Dietetic Facilitator, Northern Ireland Centre for Food and Health (NICHE), Ulster University, Northern Ireland

Joan Gandy

Registered Dietitian, a Freelance Dietitian and Visiting Researcher in Nutrition and Dietetics, University of Hertfordshire, England

WILEY Blackwell

This edition first published 2016 © 2016 by John Wiley & Sons, Ltd

Registered office: John Wiley & Sons, Ltd, The Atrium, Southern Gate, Chichester, West Sussex, PO19 8SQ, UK

Editorial offices: 9600 Garsington Road, Oxford, OX4 2DQ, UK
The Atrium, Southern Gate, Chichester, West Sussex, PO19 8SQ, UK
111 River Street, Hoboken, NJ 07030-5774, USA

For details of our global editorial offices, for customer services and for information about how to apply for permission to reuse the copyright material in this book please see our website at www.wiley.com/wiley-blackwell

Library of Congress Cataloging-in-Publication Data

Names: Lawrence, Judy, 1960- , editor. | Gandy, Joan, editor. | Douglas, Pauline, 1961- , editor.
Title: Dietetic and nutrition case studies / edited by Judy Lawrence, Joan Gandy, Pauline Douglas.
Description: Chichester, West Sussex ; Hoboken, NJ : John Wiley & Sons, 2016. | Complemented by: Manual of dietetic practice / edited by Joan Gandy in conjunction with the British Dietetic Association. Fifth edition. 2014. | Includes bibliographical references and index.
Identifiers: LCCN 2015040817 (print) | LCCN 2015042999 (ebook) | ISBN 9781118897102 (pbk.) | ISBN 9781118898239 (pdf) | ISBN 9781118898246 (epub)
Subjects: | MESH: Dietetics. | Nutritional Physiological Phenomena. | Diet Therapy. | Problem-Based Learning.
Classification: LCC RM216 (print) | LCC RM216 (ebook) | NLM WB 400 | DDC 615.8/54–dc23
LC record available at http://lccn.loc.gov/2015040817

A catalogue record for this book is available from the British Library.

Wiley also publishes its books in a variety of electronic formats. Some content that appears in print may not be available in electronic books.

Set in 9/12pt, MeridienLTStd by SPi Global, Chennai, India.

1 2016

Contents

Appendices

List of contributors

Ellie Allen
Clinical Lead Dietitian, University College London Hospitals NHS Foundation Trust, London, United Kingdom

Barbara Martini Arora
Freelance Registered Dietitian, Bromley, United Kingdom

Eleanor Baldwin
Advanced Dietitian – Adult Refsums Disease and Bariatrics, Chelsea and Westminster NHS Foundation Trust, London, United Kingdom

Julie Beckerson
Haemato-Oncology Specialist, Imperial College Healthcare NHS Trust, London, United Kingdom

Kathleen Beggs
Clinical Tutor, The University of British Columbia, Vancouver, BC, Canada

Helen Bennewith
Professional Lead for Addiction and Mental Health Dietetics, NHS Greater Glasgow and Clyde, Glasgow, Scotland, United Kingdom

Sarah Bowyer
PhD Research Student in Rural Health, University of the Highlands and Islands, Inverness, Scotland, United Kingdom

Rachael Brandreth
Children's Weight Management Dietitian, Royal Cornwall Hospital Trust, Cornwall, United Kingdom

Elaine Cawadias
Clinical Instructor, Faculty of Land and Food Systems, The University of British Columbia, Vancouver, BC, Canada

Alison Culkin
Research Dietitian, London North West Healthcare NHS Trust, London, United Kingdom

Rachael Donnelly
Acting Clinical Lead Dietitian, Guy's and St Thomas' NHS Foundation Trust, London, United Kingdom

Pauline Douglas
Senior Lecturer and Clinical Dietetic Facilitator, Northern Ireland Centre for Food and Health (NICHE), University of Ulster, Londonderry, Northern Ireland, United Kingdom

Hilary Du Cane
Freelance Dietitian and Marketeer, United Kingdom

Alastair Duncan
Lead Dietitian, NIHR Clinical Doctoral Research Fellow, Guy's and St. Thomas' NHS Foundation Trust, London, United Kingdom

Mary Flynn
Chief Specialist Public Health Nutrition, Food Safety Authority of Ireland, Dublin, Ireland; Visiting Professor, University of Ulster, Coleraine, Northern Ireland, United Kingdom

Caroline Foster
Specialist Dietitian, Leeds and York Partnership NHS Foundation Trust, Leeds, United Kingdom

Lisa Gaff
Specialist Dietitian, Addenbrookes Hospital, Cambridge University Hospitals NHS Foundation Trust, Cambridge, United Kingdom

Joan Gandy
Freelance Dietitian and Visiting Researcher, Nutrition and Dietetics, University of Hertfordshire, Hatfield, United Kingdom

Elaine Gardner
Freelance Dietitian, London, United Kingdom

Susie Hamlin
Senior Specialist Dietitian Liver Transplantation, Hepatology and Critical Care, St James's University Hospital, Leeds Teaching Hospitals NHS Trust, Leeds, United Kingdom

Nicola Henderson
AHP Team Lead, NHS Forth Valley, Larbert, United Kingdom

Sandra Hood
Diabetes Dietitian, The Diabetes Centre, Dorset County Hospital NHS Foundation Trust, Dorchester, Dorset, United Kingdom

Nicola Howle
Mental Health Dietitian, South Staffordshire and Shropshire Healthcare NHS Foundation Trust, Lichfield, United Kingdom

Bushra Jafri
Human Nutrition and Dietetics, London Metropolitan University, London, United Kingdom

Yvonne Jeanes
Senior Lecturer in Clinical Nutrition, University of Roehampton, London, United Kingdom

Sema Jethwa
Senior Diabetes Specialist Dietitian, University College London Hospital NHS Trust, London, United Kingdom; Freelance Dietitian, Hertfordshire, United Kingdom

Susanna Johnson
Community Paediatric Dietitian, Wembley Centre for Health and Care, Central London Community Healthcare NHS Trust, London, United Kingdom

Natasha Jones
Advanced Specialist Haematology/TYA dietitian, Addenbrookes Hospital, Cambridge University Hospitals NHS Foundation Trust, Cambridge, United Kingdom

Ruth Kander
Senior Dietitian and Consultant Dietitian, Imperial College Healthcare NHS Trust, London, United Kingdom and Consultant East Kent Dietitian.

Joanna Lamming
Specialist Weight Management Dietitian, East, Kent, United Kingdom

Anne Laverty
Specialist Dietitian, Learning Disabilities, Northern Health and Social Care Trust, Coleraine, Northern Ireland, United Kingdom

Judy Lawrence
Research Officer BDA and Visiting Researcher, King's College London, London, United Kingdom

Julie Leaper
Senior Specialist Dietitian (Liver/ICU) St James's Hospital, Leeds Teaching Hospitals NHS Trust, Leeds, United Kingdom

Sian Lewis
Macmillan Clinical Lead Dietitian, Chair of BDA Specialist Oncology Group, Velindre Cancer Centre, Wales, United Kingdom

Sherly X. Li
PhD Candidate, MRC Epidemiology Unit, University of Cambridge, Cambridge, United Kingdom

Seema Lodhia
HCA Healthcare, London, United Kingdom

Julie Lovegrove
Head of the Hugh Sinclair Unit of Human Nutrition, University of Reading, Reading, United Kingdom

Marjorie Macleod
Specialist Dietitian, Learning Disabilities Service, NHS Lothian, Edinburgh, Scotland, United Kingdom

Paul McArdle
Lead Clinical Dietitian and Deputy Head of Dietetics, NIHR Clinical Doctoral Research Fellow and Freelance Dietitian, Birmingham Community Healthcare NHS Trust, Birmingham, United Kingdom

Angela McComb
Health and Social Wellbeing Improvement Manager, Northern Health and Social Care Trust, Londonderry, Northern Ireland, United Kingdom

Caoimhe McDonald
Research Dietitian, Mercers Institute for Research on Ageing, St. James Hospital, Dublin, Ireland

Jennifer McIntosh
Clinical Lead Dietitian, Leeds and York Partnership NHS Foundation Trust, Leeds, United Kingdom

Yvonne McKenzie
Specialist in Gastrointestinal Nutrition, Clinical Lead in IBS for the Gastroenterology Specialist Group of the British Dietetic Association, Birmingham, United Kingdom

Kirsty-Anna McLaughlin
Community Nutrition Support Dietitian, Wiltshire Primary Care Trust, Wiltshire, United Kingdom

Kassandra Montanheiro
Macmillan Senior Specialist Dietitian, University College London Hospitals NHS Foundation Trust, London, United Kingdom

Eileen Murray
Specialist Mental Health Dietitian, NHS Greater Glasgow and Clyde Directorate of Forensic Mental Health and Learning Disabilities, Glasgow, Scotland, United Kingdom

Mary O'Kane
Consultant Dietitian (Adult Obesity), Leeds Teaching Hospitals NHS Trust, Leeds, United Kingdom

Sian O'Shea
Head of Nutrition and Dietetics for Learning Disabilities, Aberkenfig Health Board, Bridgend, United Kingdom

Sue Perry
Deputy Head of Dietetics, Hull Royal Infirmary, Hull and East Yorkshire Hospitals NHS Trust, Hull, United Kingdom

Gail Pinnock
Specialist Bariatric Surgery Dietitian, Homerton University Hospital NHS Foundation Trust, London, United Kingdom

Vicki Pout
Deputy Acute Dietetic Manager, Queen Elizabeth the Queen Mother Hospital, Kent Community Health NHS Foundation Trust, Margate, Kent, United Kingdom

Louise Robertson
Specialist Dietian, Inherited Metabolic Diseases, University Hospitals Birmingham NHS Foundation Trust, Birmingham, United Kingdom

Juneeshree S. Sangani
Freelance Dietitian, United Kingdom

Nicola Scott
Senior Specialist Haematology Dietitian, St James's University Hospital, Leeds Teaching Hospital NHS Trust, Leeds, United Kingdom

Ella Segaran
Specialist Dietitian for Critical Care, Chair of Dietitians in Critical Care Specialist Group of the BDA, St Mary's Hospital, Imperial College Healthcare NHS Trust, London, United Kingdom

Reena Shaunak
Diabetes Specialist Dietitian, West Middlesex University Hospital NHS Trust, Isleworth, United Kingdom

Bushra Siddiqui
Renal Dietitian, Queen Elizabeth Hospital Birmingham, University Hospitals Birmingham NHS Foundation Trust, Birmingham, United Kingdom

Isabel Skypala
Consultant Allergy Dietitian and Clinical Lead for Food Allergy, Royal Brompton and Harefield NHS Foundation Trust, London, United Kingdom

Alison Smith
Prescribing Support Dietitian, Aylesbury Vale Clinical Commissioning Group and Chiltern Clinical Commissioning Group, Aylesbury, United Kingdom

Chris Smith
Specialist Paediatric Dietitian, Royal Alexandra Hospital, Brighton, United Kingdom

Clare Stradling
NIHR Doctoral Research Fellow, Birmingham Heartlands Hospital, University of Birmingham, Birmingham, United Kingdom

Carolyn Taylor
Specialist Dietitian, Northern General Hospital, Sheffield Teaching Hospitals NHS Foundation Trust, Sheffield, United Kingdom

Lucy Turnbull
Clinical Lead for Chronic Disease and Weight Management Services, Central London Community Healthcare, London, United Kingdom

Evelyn Volders
Senior Lecturer Nutrition and Dietetics, Monash University, Melbourne, Victoria, Australia

Kirsten Whitehead
Assistant Professor, Division of Nutritional Sciences, University of Nottingham, Nottingham, United Kingdom

Kate Williams
Head of Nutrition and Dietetics, South London and Maudsley NHS Foundation Trust, London, United Kingdom

E. Mark Windle
Specialist Dietitian, Burns and Intensive Care, Mid Yorkshire Hospitals NHS Trust, Wakefield, United Kingdom

Preface

Problem-based learning (PBL) is increasingly becoming the preferred method of teaching in health care. There is currently a dearth of appropriately written case studies. This book takes a PBL approach to dietetics and nutrition and aims to address this gap. It has been written to complement the *Manual of Dietetic Practice* (MDP) (5th edition), and the case studies are cross-referenced accordingly. Uniquely, the case studies are written and peer reviewed by registered dietitians, drawing on their own experiences and specialist knowledge. This book has been written and edited with many readers in mind. Lecturers and staff in universities with courses in dietetics and nutrition will undoubtedly find it relevant although it will be useful to many other health care students and professionals. The case studies are also aimed at qualified dietitians and nutritionists as a tool to enhance their continuing professional development. Readers will be able to work through the case studies individually and in groups in different settings including dietetic departments. It will also help dietetic students and dietitians to identify further areas of practice that may be of interest to them.

Each case study follows the Process for Nutrition and Dietetic Practice (PNDP) that was published by the British Dietetic Association (BDA) in 2012. While throughout the world there are slight variations in nutrition and dietetic models and processes, the case studies can be successfully used alongside these. In addition, the Nutrition Care Process Terminology (NCPT), formally known as International Dietetics and Nutrition Terminology (IDNT), is used throughout the case studies – a feature practitioners worldwide will find useful.

Each case study starts with a scenario, which will enable the reader to identify the need for a nutritional intervention. This is followed by the assessment step of the PNDP and is standardised by the use the ABCDE format in most cases. Questions are posed about the assessment, the intervention and evaluation and monitoring steps. Some case studies also include further questions to stretch more newly qualified and more experienced practitioners. The PNDP is central to all areas of practice although it may be easier to identify each step in clinical areas than in other areas such as public health. This book includes real life case studies in public health, an increasingly important area of practice, and although they may be more detailed by carefully working through the case study and answers, it is possible to identify each and every step of PNDP. Questions on ethical issues are included in some case studies; however, ethics should always be of prime importance to any health care professional and is central to practice.

The book is split into two parts; firstly to reinforce keys areas of practice pertinent to this book it starts with the following introductory chapters:

- Model and process for dietetic practice
- Nutrition care process terminology
- Documentation and record keeping
- Assessment – including the ABCDE assessment process

This is followed by the case studies and separate answers. To avoid duplication the references for both the case studies and the answers are given at the end of each case study regardless of where they are cited. For completeness and to aid readers, many appendices from the *Manual of Dietetic Practice* are reproduced in the book. They include dietary reference values, weight and measures, dietary data, anthropometric data, energy prediction equations and so on and clinical chemistry.

Many of the case studies also have a link to a relevant PEN, Practice Based Evidence in Nutrition (PEN), practice question or resource. Dietitians in Australia, Canada, the United Kingdom and Ireland will be familiar with this global resource for nutrition practice.

We hope that readers enjoy using this book as much as we have enjoyed compiling it. Finally, we would like to thank the contributors and reviewers who have been invaluable when compiling this book.

Judy Lawrence
Pauline Douglas
Joan Gandy

Online resources

Additional resources, which may be of interest to readers of this book, can be found on the companion website for the *Manual of Dietetic Practice*, 5th Edition, edited by Joan Gandy.

http://www.manualofdieteticpractice.com/

The website includes

- Case study summaries (PDF)
- An alphabetical list of web resources
- Appendices from the book (PDF)
- Reference lists with CrossRef links
- Tables from the *Manual of Dietetic Practice* (PDF)
- Figures from the *Manual of Dietetic Practice* (PPT)
- Updates

PART I

CHAPTER 1

Model and process for nutrition and dietetic practice

Judy Lawrence

The nutrition care process and model was first conceived by the Academy of Nutrition and Dietetics (Lacey & Pritchett, 2003). Since then it has evolved and been adapted and is now used by dietitians and nutritionists worldwide. The case studies in this book are written with the nutrition and dietetic care process in mind. The process can be used in any setting including clinical dietetics and public health. Although case studies in this book are based around the British Dietetic Association's (BDA) (2012) model and process (Figure 1.1) used by dietitians in the United Kingdom, they can be used alongside other versions of the process and model as well. The model starts with the identification of nutritional need, followed by six stages, namely, assessment, identification of the nutrition and dietetic diagnosis, planning the nutrition and dietetic intervention, implementing the intervention, monitoring and reviewing the intervention and finally evaluating the intervention.

The case studies use the ABCDE approach (Gandy, 2014), were A is for anthropometry, B stands for biochemical and haematological markers, C for clinical, D for dietary and E is used to include economic, environmental and social issues that may be relevant. Information collected during the assessment is used to make the nutrition and dietetic diagnosis. More details of the assessment can be found in Chapter 4.

Identifying the nutrition and dietetic diagnosis

The nutrition and dietetic diagnosis is the nutritional problem that is assessed using the dietitian's clinical reasoning skills and resolved or improved by dietetic intervention. The nutrition and dietetic diagnosis is a key part of the care process, and once the correct diagnosis has been made the intervention and the most appropriate outcomes to monitor will fall into place. The nutrition and dietetic diagnosis is written as a structured sentence known as the PASS statement, where P is the problem, A the aetiology and SS the signs and symptoms. The PASS statement should describe the 'Problem' related to 'Aetiology' as characterised by 'Signs/Symptoms', for example; inadequate energy intake (problem) related to an overly restrictive gluten free diet (aetiology) as characterised by weight loss of 4 kg and anxiety regarding appropriate food choices

Dietetic and Nutrition Case Studies, First Edition.
Edited by Judy Lawrence, Pauline Douglas, and Joan Gandy.

Companion Website: http://www.manualofdieteticpractice.com/

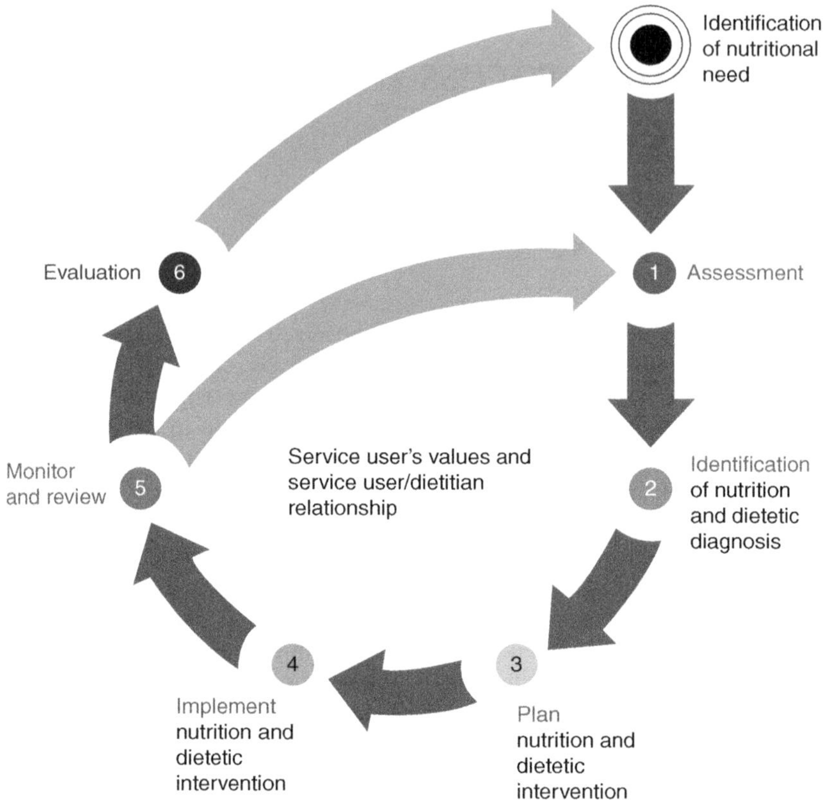

Figure 1.1 Nutrition and dietetic process (BDA (2012), p. 7. Reproduced with permission of British Dietetis Association).

(signs and symptoms). A well-written PASS statement is one where the dietitian or nutritionist can improve or resolve the problem, the intervention addresses the aetiology and the signs and symptoms can be monitored and improved. The nutrition and dietetic diagnosis can be broken down into the three steps; problem, aetiology and signs and symptoms.

Problem

This is the nutritional (dietetic) problem not the medical problem; it is the problem that can be addressed by dietetic intervention. In these case studies, the problems are expressed using the diagnosis terms as approved by the BDA. More details about the terminology can be found in Chapter 2 on international language and terminology. The problem is the change in the nutrition state that is described by adjectives such as decreased/increased, excessive/inadequate, restricted and imbalanced. In the United Kingdom, nutrition and dietetic diagnosis terms fall into one of the following seven categories:

- Energy balance;
- Oral or nutritional support;
- Nutrient intake;

- Function, for example, swallowing;
- Biochemical;
- Weight; and
- Behavioural/environmental.

There may be more than one problem, so a number of nutritional and dietetic diagnoses may be possible but these can often be consolidated into one diagnosis or one diagnosis may be prioritised, using clinical judgement and the client's wishes. Some nutrition and dietetic diagnosis may be more appropriate than others; practice and experience will hone this skill.

Aetiology

The aetiology is the cause of the nutritional problem. Causes may be related to behavioural issues such as food choices, environmental issues such as food availability, knowledge such as not knowing which foods are gluten free, physical such as inability to chew food, or cultural such as beliefs about foods. There may be more than one cause for the problem that a client has but the dietitian should be able to identify the basis of the problem using the information gained during the assessment process. For example, a client may have an incomplete knowledge of their gluten-free diet and this may be caused by:

- Missing a dietetic appointment;
- Not appreciating that all gluten-containing foods need to avoided;
- A misconception that the diet was not important; and
- A lack of awareness of the gluten content of many manufactured foods.

It is also important that the aetiology identified in the PASS statement is one that the dietitian can influence because the aetiology forms the basis of the intervention. It may be difficult to identify the cause of the problem and in such circumstances the pragmatic approach may be to identify the contributing factors. Once identified, the aetiology may be linked to the problem using the phrase 'related to'.

Signs and symptoms

Signs are the objective evidence that the problem exists; they may be from anthropometric measurements, biochemical or haematological results. Symptoms are subjective: they may be things that the patient/client has talked about such as tiredness, clothes being too tight or loose, difficulty swallowing and lack of understanding. Signs and symptoms gathered during the assessment process can be used to quantify the problem and indicate its severity. Signs and symptoms may be linked to the aetiology using the phrase 'characterised by'. It is not necessary to have both signs and symptoms in the diagnostic statement; one or the other is adequate.

Alternative diagnoses may be made when answering the questions in the case studies. It does not necessarily mean that your statement is incorrect; it may be a reasonable alternative or less of a priority. Check that your PASS statement describes a problem that can be altered by dietetic intervention and that the evidence collected during the assessment process suggests that it is important. The signs and symptoms should ideally be ones that can be measures to help advance the progress in alleviating the problem.

Nutrition intervention

The nutrition intervention is the action taken by the dietitian to address the diagnosis. Ideally, the intervention should be aimed at the cause of the problem, the aetiology, but if this is not possible then the intervention should address the signs and symptoms of the problem. In some cases, the intervention may be to maintain a current situation, for example, adult PKU. The intervention may involve the dietitian in delegating or co-ordinating the nutrition care done by others. The intervention has two stages: planning and implementation. For each PASS statement it is necessary to establish a goal based on the signs and symptoms (planning) and an appropriate intervention based on the aetiology (implementation). The intervention should of course be evidence based. Interventions may involve recommending, implementing, ordering, teaching or referring to other professionals.

Planning

Planning the intervention may involve collecting more information from the patient or from other sources. Planning should involve the patient/client/carer or group in agreeing and prioritising the necessary steps, to ensure that the care is patient centred.

Implementation

Implementing the intervention is the phase of the nutrition and dietetic care process, which involves taking action. The intervention may involve the dietitian in training someone else to take action, or in supporting the patient/client to make behavioural changes. The dietitian may facilitate change through others, for example a dietetic assistant, nurse, care assistant, carer or teacher. The implementation may be something that is done to an unconscious patient such as the delivery of a prescribed total parenteral nutrition feeding regimen. Alternatively, the intervention may involve a community or group, for example a school meals project or lipid lowering group.

Monitoring and review

Monitoring focuses on changes in the signs and symptoms that were identified in the initial assessment to see if progress is being achieved and goals are met. The goals should be SMART:

S – specific
M – measurable
A – achievable
R – realistic
T – timely

SMART goals should make the monitoring process easier. Monitoring should be ongoing or carried out at planned intervals so that the results of the monitoring process can be used to review the intervention and modify it, if necessary. This may involve a new assessment and a new nutrition and dietetic diagnosis, which will in turn lead to new goals and additional monitoring. Some of the case studies in this book involve more than one nutrition and dietetic diagnosis.

Evaluation

Evaluation takes place at the end of the process. It involves collecting data about the current situation and comparing it with data from the assessment, with a reference standard such as BMI indicators of obesity or HbA1c measures of diabetes, or with goals that were established early in the planning process. The effectiveness of the evaluation can be judged by changes in the signs and symptoms identified in the nutrition and dietetic diagnosis.

The nutrition and dietetic care process may be an ongoing process where an individual patient is seen many times over a number of years for a chronic condition such as diabetes or it may be a short episode of care.

References

BDA (2012) *Process and model for nutrition and dietetic practice.* URL https://www.bda.uk.com/professional/practice/process [accessed on 27 May 2015].

Gandy, J. (2014) Assessment of nutritional status. In: Gandy, J. (ed), *Manual of Dietetic Practice,* 5th edn. Wiley Blackwell, Oxford.

Lacey, K. & Pritchett, E. (2003) Nutrition care process and model: ADA adopts road map to quality care and outcomes management. *J Am Diet Assoc,* **103** (**8**), 1061–1072.

Resource

Qureshi, N. *et al.* (2014) Professional practice. In: Gandy, J. (ed), *Manual of Dietetic Practice,* 5th edn. Wiley Blackwell, Oxford.

CHAPTER 2
Nutrition care process terminology (NCPT)

Pauline Douglas

The challenges for the nutrition and dietetic practitioner are to prevent and reduce the burden of nutrition related health problems for individuals or groups of people. Dietitians and nutritionists must advance practice from experience based to evidence based and demonstrate quality practice and optimise nutritional outcomes. To do this they must have a common language that they can benchmark their practice with other dietitians. They must demonstrate practice through the acquisition and use of complex systems of communication. This allows them to convey meaningful information to others. In addition:

- It provides supporting documentation for the reimbursement of dietetic services provided.
- It engages dietitians from academia through to practice to provide a profession fit for purpose and competent to practice.

With an increasing mobility of heath care professionals around the world the language needs to be standardised to convey meaningful information in a uniform way. This allows for the comparison of like messages in a logical process to facilitate the production of evidence-based practice. Also service users are travelling within countries and across borders for treatment and expect a consistent quality of care.

Using standard terminology:

- Promotes consistency and continuity of care;
- Structures communication
  - Within and across professions;
  - Within and across nations;
- Allows evaluation of the quality of care;
- Facilitates research and building of a professional knowledge base (e.g. Practice-Based Evidence in Nutrition developed by Dietitians of Canada. There is now a PEN global dietetic partnership of associations of Australia, Canada, Ireland, New Zealand, South Africa and the UK, Evidence Analysis Library of Academy of Nutrition and Dietetics);
- Facilitates professional development; and
- Improves professional image, credibility, accountability of dietitians.

Dietetic and Nutrition Case Studies, First Edition.
Edited by Judy Lawrence, Pauline Douglas, and Joan Gandy.

Companion Website: http://www.manualofdieteticpractice.com/

Why is standardised language important?

It provides a common means of communication for healthcare professionals. Other healthcare professions, for example, nurses, physiotherapists, occupational therapists and so on have shown the benefits of having a standardised language. Making nursing practice count (Beyea, 1999) ensures that when a nurse talks about a stage three pressure area, another nurse fully understands what the first nurse is describing. An example from dietetics is that there are differing definitions and understanding of what is meant by nutritional support. In some countries this relates to enteral and parenteral nutrition and in others this also includes food fortification and oral nutritional supplementation.

A standardised language is complementary to a nutrition and dietetic process. It ensures that there is comparability in the terms used to describe diagnoses, interventions and outcomes of nutritional care. It is important to stress that this still ensures the dietitian provides individualised nutritional care for the patient or the population ensuring the patient/service user is at the centre of all care by taking into account their needs, values and culture.

Dietitians do not work alone. They are integral members of the inter-professional health team. As such communication of their work needs to be accessible to other healthcare professionals, commissioners of service or those reimbursing them for their services. The World Health Organization uses the International Classification of Diseases (ICD) as the standard diagnostic tool for epidemiology, health management and clinical purposes. It is used to monitor the incidence and prevalence disease for general health and populations. Similarly the International Classification of Functioning, Disability and Health (ICF) is the WHO framework for measuring health and disability at both individual and population levels.

In 2003 the Academy of Nutrition and Dietetics (AND) published the concepts of a nutrition care process and model. Other professional bodies have now modified this to best meet the needs of their members and their healthcare provision, for example, BDA (2012). In 2008, AND defined the language to complement the process. This was called International Dietetic and Nutrition Terminology (IDNT) now known as the Nutrition Care Process Terminology (NCPT). In Europe, the Dutch Dietetic Association were also developing another dietetic language. This was modelled on the International Classification of Function (ICF) and is now recognised as the ICF – Dietetique. Now as the work of the National Dietetic Associations from across the world is being published, working groups are being established to facilitate international collaboration to further develop dietetic practice in this area.

The International Health Terminology Standards Development Organization (IHTSDO) is a not for profit organisation based in Europe. This organisation owns and administers the rights to health terminologies and related standards including Systematised Nomenclature of Medicine – Clinical Terms (SNOMED – CT). SNOMED – CT is a comprehensive medical terminology incorporating several terminologies from various healthcare disciplines. While being of international scope it can be adapted to each countries requirements. This international dietetic working group has been working closely to incorporate NCPT as an integral element of SNOMED.

The WHO and IHTSDO have agreed to try to harmonise WHO classifications and SNOMED – CT terminologies to develop common terms used by both organisations. This has the potential to support further integration of different dietetic languages and thus enhance dietetic practice.

In Europe a key priority is *'to support Member States in developing common identification and authentication measures to facilitate transferability of data across border healthcare' (European Parliament and Council, 2011)*. As a result NCPT developments have facilitated eNCPT being available in several languages, for example, English, French, Italian, Spanish and Swedish again supporting international standards for dietetic practice and facilitating working across borders.

Nutrition care process terminology

The NCPT is used alongside the Nutrition and Dietetic Care Process. In the diagnosis the PASS statement (problem, aetiology, signs and symptoms) the problem is the change in nutrition state that is described by adjectives such as decreased/increased, excessive/inadequate, restricted and imbalanced. In addition nutrition and dietetic diagnosis terms fall into one of seven categories:

- Energy balance;
- Oral or nutritional support;
- Nutrient intake;
- Function, for example, swallowing;
- Biochemical;
- Weight; and
- Behavioural/environmental.

The descriptors used in the different countries can challenge the dietitian to define the problem in a way that their service users may find acceptable. The interested professional bodies are collaborating on this to gain appropriate, relevant country specific additions and alternatives. Dietetic professional bodies need to continue to work collaboratively to ensure deititians have a standardised language.

It is important that the dietetic profession continue to engage with and use the NCPT. It should become an integral element of academic training, further developed within practice placement settings and then fully embraced by dietitians throughout their professional practice.

Acknowledgements

The Professional Practice Committee of the European Federation of Associations of Dietitians especially Constantina Papoutsakis, Ylva Orrevall, Lene Thorensen, Naomi Trostler, Remijnse Wineke and Claudia Bolleurs for their insight and knowledge.

References

BDA (2012) *Model and Process for Dietetic Practice*. BDA, Birmingham.

Beyea, S.C. (1999) Standardised language – making nursing practice count. *AORN Journal*, **70**, 831–832, 834, 837–838.

European Parliament and Council. (2011) Directive 2011/24/EU of the European Parliament and of the Council of 9 March 2011, on the application of patients' rights in cross-border healthcare, Article 14, *Official Journal of the European Union*, **L 88**, 45.

Resources

AND Evidence Analysis Library. www.andeal.org.

BDA Diagnosis Terms. www.bda.uk.com/professional/practice/terminology.

Practice Based Evidence in Nutrition (PEN). www.pennutrition.com/index.aspx.

CHAPTER 3
Record keeping

Judy Lawrence

In the UK the Health and Care Professions Council (HCPC) (2013) requires that dietitians '*make reasoned decisions*' and '*record the decisions and reasoning appropriately*' as part of their Standards of Proficiency. There is also a specific record keeping standard of proficiency; standard 10 which is '*be able to maintain records appropriately*', this is expanded in points 10.1 and 10.2 which outline the need for records to be in line with relevant protocols, guidelines and legal requirements. This chapter discusses these guidelines and legal requirements. Dietitians from outside the UK should check with their own regulatory body and employer to ensure that their record keeping meets the required standard.

Legislation

In the UK there are a number of pieces of legislation that relate to records and record keeping.

The Data Protection Act 1998

The Act relates to the protection of personal data (e.g. medical notes) about a living individual, such as data held by a public authority (e.g. NHS). This includes patient record cards kept by a dietitian, medical records to which a dietitian may contribute and electronic records. Data is said to be identifiable even if the information is recorded against a number that can then be matched to a person by accessing a different piece of information. The Act also regulates the processing of personal data. The term processing includes the storage, use, disclosure and the destruction of the data. The Act has six principles, they are that data should be processed fairly and lawfully, that data collected for a specific purpose or purposes should not be further processed for any purpose that is incompatible with the original purpose, that data collection should not be excessive in relation to the purpose, data should be accurate and where necessary up to date, data should not be kept for longer than is necessary and finally data should be processed in accordance with the rights of the individual. These principles may be subject to interpretation by an employer, and there will be

Dietetic and Nutrition Case Studies, First Edition.
Edited by Judy Lawrence, Pauline Douglas, and Joan Gandy.

Companion Website: http://www.manualofdieteticpractice.com/

local policies relating to them, for example a patient has the right to request access to information about themselves. A patient can ask to see what you have written during a consultation and comment on what has been written. If a patient or carer writes requesting to see the notes it is necessary to conform to local policy requirements first, for example, an employer may require certain information as proof of identity from the patient or carer. All records are owned by the employing authority and requests for medical notes or electronic records should be dealt with by the clinical governance team. With regard to information being accurate, an opinion about a patient's nutritional condition that you believe to be accurate but that the individual disagrees with or believes to be inaccurate may be expressed. For example an anorexic patient may regard the statement that they are underweight as inaccurate. It is still legally possible to make this statement in their notes although a record that the patient disagrees with the assessment should be noted. The assessment should be backed by recording a weight and relevant BMI range.

Freedom of Information Act 2000

The Freedom of Information Act covers information held by public bodies in England, Wales and Northern Ireland, information in Scotland is covered by Scotland's 2002 Freedom of Information Act. The Freedom of Information Act is about removing unnecessary secrecy; it allows members of the public to request information from public authorities. The NHS and state schools are public authorities, but not all charities that receive public money would necessarily be covered by the Act. The Act does not cover patient's access to health records; this process is covered by the Data Protection Act as discussed above. A dietitian employed by the NHS and working in private practice would only have to disclose information about their NHS work under the Act. The Act only covers information that is recorded, it is not necessary to write information down specifically to disclose it if it is not already recorded. Minutes of meetings and continuing professional development (CPD) portfolios are regarded as records. Private information on a work computer such as a private email does not have to be disclosed, but it would be necessary to disclose work related emails if requested. Organisations should have policies or guidelines in place to help employees comply with the Act. The Act does not interfere with copyright laws or intellectual property rights. Therefore someone can request copies of diet sheets that but they cannot use this information to produce copies if the work is subject to copyright.

If a patient makes a request for information it is necessary to respond within 20 working days so it is important to contact the appropriate person in the organisation as soon as possible so that the request can be dealt with promptly. If a patient verbally asks for information they should be helped to put the request in writing and sent by post, email, a request on the organisation's Facebook page or Twitter feed, to the appropriate person. Any information that can be shared easily such as clinic times or numbers of people working in a department should not be subject to formal procedures. The Data Protection Act may prohibit the release of data that has been requested; the clinical governance team or appropriate person, should be consulted for advice. Clinical records should only be released by a person specified to do so within the organisation.

Access to Health Records Act 1990

This Act gives people the right to request access to the health records of a deceased person.

Guidelines

There are a number of guidelines available. The NHS has an information governance toolkit (https://www.igt.hscic.gov.uk/) that aims to help individuals and organisations to handle information properly. Each NHS organisation should have an individual appointed as a Caldicott Guardian, it is their responsibility to ensure that the organisation respects patient confidentiality and service user information.

The BDA (2008) has guidance on record keeping although it is important to recognise that the nutrition and dietetic care process should guide the content of record keeping, for example, assessment, diagnosis, intervention and so on. The Royal College of Physicians (2013) has also produced record keeping standards covering electronic health records that have been endorsed by the BDA. The case studies in this book have questions about recording information and these guidelines may be helpful, but individual employer's guidelines should be followed first.

The introduction of electronic records should improve accuracy in health care records by improving legibility and access. The use of common language and SNOMED terms should also improve communication and understanding between the various health professionals using the health record. For more information about the nutrition and dietetic terms in SNOMED, see Chapter 2.

Good record keeping should include the following points:

- Records should be made at the time of the event or as near as possible to that time.
- Records should be complete, accurate and fit for purpose.
- A complete record should include details of an assessment, what care has been provided or is planned, and any action that has been taken or shared with other health professionals.
- Handwriting on paper records should be legible and in black ink.
- Records should be dated and signed with a name and designation.
- Records should be clear, terms such as 'ate well' should be avoided.
- Records should be relevant and opinions justified if possible.
- Records should be in electronic format wherever possible.
- Always log off an unattended computer.

Social media

Records can be in a variety of formats that includes social media, telephone messages and videos. The BDA (2013) and the Dietitians Association of Australia (2011) both have useful publications to help get the most out of social media whilst avoiding some of the pitfalls. In essence it is essential to think before posting and don't make comments that would not be said a in person in a professional meeting. Don't reveal information that could identify a patient or client either directly or indirectly and don't repeat anything that is confidential.

References

BDA. (2008) *Guidance for dietitians for records and record keeping*. www.bda.uk.com/publications/professional/record_keeping [accessed on 22 September 2015].

BDA. (2013) *Professional guidance document. Making sense of social media*. www.bda.uk.com/professional/practice/professionalism/social_media [accessed on 22 September 2015].

Dietitians Association of Australia. (2011) *Dialling into the digital age. Guidance on social media for DAA members*. http://www.pennutrition.com/KnowledgePathway.aspx?kpid=3728&trid=22864&trcatid=33 [accessed on 8 October 2015].

Health and Care Professions Council (HCPC). (2013) *Standards of proficiency*. www.hpc-uk.org/assets/documents/10000050CStandards_of_Proficiency_Dietitians.pdf [accessed on 22 September 2015].

Royal College of Physicians. (2013) *Standards for the clinical structure and content of patient records*. https://www.rcplondon.ac.uk/resources/standards-clinical-structure-and-content-patient-records [accessed on 22 September 2015].

Resources

Health and Social Care Information Centre Guide to confidentiality in health and social care. (2013) *Treating confidential information with respect*. http://www.hscic.gov.uk/media/12822/Guide-to-confidentiality-in-health-and-social-care/pdf/HSCIC-guide-to-confidentiality.pdf [accessed on 22 September 2015].

Information Commission Office. *The guide to data protection*. https://ico.org.uk/for-organisations/guide-to-data-protection/ [accessed on 22 September 2015].

Information Commission Office. *The guide to freedom of information*. https://ico.org.uk/media/for-organisations/documents/1642/guide_to_freedom_of_information.pdf [accessed on 22 September 2015].

NHS England. (2014) *Documents and record management policy*. http://www.england.nhs.uk/wp-content/uploads/2014/02/rec-man-pol.pdf [accessed on 22 September 2015].

Qureshi, N. *et al*. (2014) Professional practice. In: Gandy, J. (ed), *Manual of Dietetic Practice*, 5th edn. Wiley Blackwell, Oxford.

CHAPTER 4
Assessment

Joan Gandy

Assessment is fundamental to dietetic and nutrition practice and an essential step in the nutrition and dietetic process (see Chapter 1). The BDA (2012) defined assessment as '*... a systematic process of collecting and interpreting information in order to make decisions about the nature and cause of nutrition related health issues that affect an individual, a group or a population*'. It forms the basis of the nutrition and dietetic diagnosis and intervention and is key in establishing outcome measures in order to evaluate and monitor the intervention.

The ABCDE format, as described by Gandy (2014) has been developed to structure and standardise dietetic and nutrition assessment. This format is used throughout this book and often summarised in a table. Table 4.1 gives details of the five domains used in this format.

The information collected during assessment and the tools used to collect this information will vary depending on the setting, for example, individual, group, community, and population.

Domains

Anthropometry, body composition and function

Anthropometry is often used in nutrition and dietetic assessments with height and weight being used most frequently. Since the introduction of easily available equipment body composition and functional assessments, for example, bioelectrical impedance analysis (BIA) and dynamometry, are increasingly being used by dietitians and nutritionists in a variety of settings.

Anthropometry

Anthropometry is defined as the external measurement of the human body. It is affected by nutritional and health status and other factors including ethnicity, age and gender. Anthropometric measurements are often used in prediction equations, for example, body mass index (BMI), or compared with standards. It is essential that standards that are appropriate to the age, ethnic or gender group be used. All equipment must be serviced regularly, for example, weighing scales, or replaced as appropriate

Dietetic and Nutrition Case Studies, First Edition.
Edited by Judy Lawrence, Pauline Douglas, and Joan Gandy.

Companion Website: http://www.manualofdieteticpractice.com/

Table 4.1 **Nutritional assessment domains.**

Domain	Example procedure for individuals
Anthropometry, body composition and functional	Weight, height, body mass index, skinfold thickness, waist circumference Bioelectrical impedance analysis Grip strength dynamometry Physical activity questionnaires
Biochemical and haematological	Vitamin status tests Lipid status Iron status – haemoglobin, ferritin and so on
Clinical	Physical appearance, blood pressure, medication, indirect calorimetry
Diet	24 h recall, food frequency questionnaire (FFQ)
Environmental, behavioural and social	Shopping habits, housing, cooking facilities, education

Source: Gandy (2014), Table 2.2.1, p. 48. Reproduced with permission from Wiley Blackwell.

for example tape measures will stretch over time. Anthropometry requires training and experience to produce reliable and reproducible results. It is essential to establish what, if any, standards are used within the local context, for example, NHS guidance.

Body weight

Weighing scales must be maintained and calibrated regularly and should be Class III or above. Body weight is affected by many factors including fluid retention (oedema, ascites), dehydration, accuracy of the scales, amputations, splints, casts and replacement joints. A weight adjustment table for amputations is shown in Appendix A5. If weight cannot be obtained self reported weight, estimated weight made by carers, relatives, dietitians or other health care professionals may be used. Specialist weighing equipment, for example, weighing beds and chairs are available in some clinical settings, for example, spinal cord injury, obesity clinics.

Height

Height is usually measured using a stadiometer. When height cannot be measured, for example, bed bound patients, or is unreliable, for example, scoliosis it can be estimated using alternative methods such as ulna length, knee height or demispan (Appendix A5).

Body mass index

BMI is a weight for height indicator that may be used to classify overweight and obesity and is calculated as weight (kg)/height (m^2). A ready reckoner and the WHO classifications of BMI for overweight and obesity are shown in Appendix A4. BMI does not give an indication of adipose distribution and therefore is being superseded as the preferred measure of non-communicable disease risk by waist circumference. It is affected by ethnicity, setting, age and body composition. If height is not available in the elderly (over 64 years) demiquet or mindex can be used for men and women respectively (Appendix A4).

Waist circumference

Waist circumference assesses visceral adiposity and is therefore increasing used to assess obesity related morbidity risk. NICE (2006) recommend the use of both BMI and waist circumference to assess health risks. Appendix A5 shows the WHO waist circumference classifications for health risks (WHO, 2008). It is measured at the halfway point between the lowest rib and the iliac crest in the midaxillary line.

Mid upper arm circumference

When neither weight nor height can be measured, the BMI can be estimated using the mid upper arm circumference (MUAC), or mid arm circumference (MAC). Appendix A5 shows reference data derived from an American population; UK data is not available.

Skinfold thickness

Calipers are used to take skinfold measurements at specific sites to estimate percentage body fat by substitution into prediction formulae, for example, Durnin & Womersley (1974). Triceps skinfold thickness (TSF) is used in bed bound patients to estimate endogenous fat stores (see Appendix A5). It can be combined with MUAC to evaluate body composition and is especially useful in patients with peripheral oedema or ascites

Mid arm muscle circumference (MAMC)

Mid arm muscle circumference (MAMC) is derived from TSF and MUAC as an indicator of muscle mass and therefore protein stores. The formulae used to derive MAMC and standards are shown in Appendix A5.

Body composition

Dietitians frequently use skinfold thicknesses to evaluate body composition however increasing other techniques such as BIA are being used.

Functional assessment

An example of this is hand grip strength (HGS) dynamometry (Appendix A5). Impaired HGS is associated with poor postoperative recovery (Griffiths & Clark, 1984) and related to loss of independence in the elderly. Increasingly dietitians assess physical activity levels; questionnaires are frequently used although other tools, for example, accelerometers are available.

Biochemical and haematological markers

Biochemical and haematological parameters are an important part of assessment and as outcome measures used in evaluation of the intervention. These markers are essential when monitoring many clinical conditions, e.g. diabetes mellitus, renal disease and in assessing the status of some nutrients, for example, iron status in anaemia.

Appendix A7 gives examples of reference ranges for some parameters; it is essential to recognise that normal ranges and standards will vary between laboratories and that reference ranges from the local setting must be used.

Clinical

The clinical assessment will include physical appearance, medical history, test results and current medication; both prescribed and obtained without prescription. These details can usually be collated from the nursing or medical notes or family or carers. When collating information on medication it is important to consider drug nutrient interactions. The medical history and test results are vital elements of the assessment giving essential information for developing the intervention. Physical observations are vital indicators of nutritional status and should not be overlooked. For example loose clothing may indicate weight loss, breathlessness may indicate anaemia or other clinical conditions.

Dietary assessment

Establishing the extent to which nutritional needs are being met is core to the nutrition and dietetic assessment. It is usually important to assess current food and beverage intake, changes (duration and severity) in appetite and factors that affect intake. In clinical situations may also be important to consider recent changes in meal patterns, food choice and consistency.

The choice of dietary assessment method will depend on many factors including setting, population, age, literacy, assessor training and experience, cost, nutrients to be assessed, etc (Welch, 2014). An understanding of the limitations and applications of each method is essential in clinical and other settings to ensure the most appropriate method. Assessment can be either respective or current. Table 4.2 describes the characteristics of the most frequently used dietary assessment methods. It is important to quantify foods and drinks consumed either by weighing or estimations. Photographs, models and standard size serving vessels may be used to aid quantification. Dietary data can be used qualitatively, for example, to assess food preferences or meal patterns however in clinical practice it is most frequently used quantitatively. The energy and nutrient content of the diet are calculated using food composition data. A software programme is most frequently used to facilitate these calculations. However an understanding of the limitations of food composition data is essential (Landais & Holdsworth, 2014). The results of any dietary assessment need to be interpreted in the context of the individual or population's requirements. This is usually done by comparison with dietary reference values such as those published by the Department of Health (1991) and SACN (2011) or dietary recommendations (SACN, 2008) or the Institute of Medicine. However it is important to consider the limitations of any dietary reference value (Gandy, 2014).

Environmental, behavioural and social assessment

These factors can have a significant impact on nutritional status. Relevant factors include psychological status, for example, depression, ability to buy, prepare and cook

Table 4.2 **Characteristics of dietary assessment methods.**

Method	Advantages	Limitations
Retrospective methods		
24 h recall (24 HR) (single or multiple days)	Not reliant on long-term memory; interview length 20–45 min	Single 24 HR can be used for group assessments but not for estimating intake of individuals
Diet history	Respondent literacy not required	Report of past intake is influenced by current diet; trained interviewers required
Food frequency questionnaire (FFQ) (if portion estimates included termed semi quantitative FFQ)	Useful for large sample sizes; relatively straightforward to complete	Need to be developed for specific population group to ensure important food items are covered and requires updating to accommodate changes to supply of foods; responses governed by cognitive, numeric, and literacy abilities of respondents also by length and complexity of the food list Not easy to develop for clinical practice since specific computer programs need to be developed
Short frequency questionnaires	Targeted to specific food types, administration simpler and easier than long questionnaires	Need to be developed for specific population group to ensure questions are relevant
Current methods		
Weighed food record (weighed inventory technique)	No requirement for memory retrieval as it records current intake; food intake weighed so estimates of quantity consumed not required	Literate, cooperative respondents required as burden is high; possible that respondents change usual eating patterns to simplify the record; high data entry costs
Food record with estimated weights	No requirement for memory retrieval as it records current intake	Literate, cooperative respondents required as burden is high; possible that respondents change usual eating patterns to simplify the record
Duplicate analysis	Greater accuracy	Very labour intensive; requires laboratory to do food composition analysis
Records using electronic equipment, for example, mobile phones, digital cameras	Visual records of foods. Avoids need for paper records. Data can be sent to investigators electronically	Currently involves labour intensive programmes to convert to usable data, that is, quantities and types of foods, although systems are in development to deal with this; limited use in older people who experience difficulties with using newer technology

Source: Gandy (2014), Table 2.3.1, p. 62. Reproduced with permission from Wiley Blackwell.

food and social factors religious and cultural beliefs, income, education and addiction, for example, alcoholism.

References

BDA (2012). *Process and model for nutrition and dietetic practice.* www.bda.uk.com/professional/practice/process [accessed on 27 May 2015].

Department of Health (DH) (1991) *Dietary reference values for food energy and nutrients for the United Kingdom.* Report of the Panel on dietary reference values of the Committee on Medical Aspects of Food Policy. *Report on Health and Social Subjects 41.* HMSO, London.

Durnin, J.V.G.A. & Womersley, J. (1974) Body fat assessed from total body density and its estimation from skinfold thickness: measurements on 481 men and women aged from 16 to 72 years. *British Journal of Nutrition,* **32**, 77–97.

Gandy, J. (2014) Assessment of nutritional status. In: Gandy, J. (ed), *Manual of Dietetic Practice,* 5th edn. Wiley Blackwell, Oxford.

Griffith, C.D.M. & Clark, R.G. (1984) A comparison of the 'Sheffield' prognostic index with forearm muscle dynamometry in patients from Sheffield undergoing major abdominal and urological surgery. *Clinical Nutrition,* **3**, 147–151.

Landais, E. & Holdsworth, M. (2014) Food composition tables and databases. In: Gandy, J. (ed), *Manual of Dietetic Practice,* 5th edn. Wiley Blackwell, Oxford.

National Institute for Health and Clinical Excellence (NICE) (2006) *Obesity Guidance on the Prevention, Identification, Assessment and Management of Overweight and Obesity in Adults and Children. Clinical Guideline 43.* NICE, London.

Scientific Advisory Committee on Nutrition (2008) *Dietary Reference Values for Energy TSO London.* www.sacn.gov.uk [accessed on 25 September 2015].

Scientific Advisory Committee on Nutrition (2011) *The nutritional wellbeing of the British population TSO London.* www.sacn.gov.uk [accessed on 25 September 2015].

Welch, A. (2014) Dietary assessment. In: Gandy, J. (ed), *Manual of Dietetic Practice,* 5th edn. Wiley Blackwell, Oxford.

World Health Organization (2008) *Waist circumference and waist–hip ratio.* Report of a WHO expert consultation. www.who.int [last accessed 16 February 2013].

Resources

Gandy, J. (2014) Assessment of nutritional status. In: Gandy, J. (ed), *Manual of Dietetic Practice,* 5th edn. Wiley Blackwell, Oxford.

Gandy, J. (2014) Dietary reference values. In: Gandy, J. (ed), *Manual of Dietetic Practice,* 5th edn. Wiley Blackwell, Oxford.

Gibson, R.S. (2005) *Principles of Nutritional Assessment,* 2nd edn. Oxford University Press, Oxford.

Landais, E. & Holdsworth, M. (2014) Food composition tables and databases. In: Gandy, J. (ed), *Manual of Dietetic Practice,* 5th edn. Wiley Blackwell, Oxford.

PEN: Practice Based Evidence in Nutrition-*Nutrition assessment.* http://www.pennutrition.com/KnowledgePathway.aspx?kpid=16177&trid=16444&trcatid=42 [accessed on 25 September 2015].

UK Food Databanks. http://www.ifr.ac.uk/fooddatabanks/nutrients.htm [accessed on 25 September 2015].

Welch, A. (2014) Dietary assessment. In: Gandy, J. (ed), *Manual of Dietetic Practice,* 5th edn. Wiley Blackwell, Oxford.

PART II

CASE STUDY 1
Veganism

Sandra Hood

Wendy is 32 years old, a single mother with a 6-year-old daughter. She has a law degree and works part time in a legal practice. Wendy has recently changed from a vegetarian diet, which she followed for the previous 10 years, to a vegan diet. Wendy is very active, walking her daughter to and from school daily, which is 3 miles away, making a total of 12 miles a day. She also attends ballet classes once a week. At her own request, she has been referred by her GP, following a recent diagnosis of rheumatoid arthritis (RA).

Assessment

Domain	
Anthropometry, body composition and functional	Weight 43 kg Height 1.49 m
Biochemical and haematological markers	None
Clinical	No medical history of note documented
Diet	*Breakfast* Banana (100 g) or avocado (145 g) *Lunch* Salad sandwich (140 g) followed by dried fruit (60 g) and sunflower seeds (15 g) *Dinner (main meal)* Wholemeal rice (180 g) or other grain with salad (250 g) or stir fried vegetables (180 g) *Snacks* – fresh fruit *Drinks* – water Prior to changing to a vegan diet, was very reliant on cheese
Environmental, behavioural and social	Very active

Dietetic and Nutrition Case Studies, First Edition.
Edited by Judy Lawrence, Pauline Douglas, and Joan Gandy.

Companion Website: http://www.manualofdieteticpractice.com/

She suffered from anorexia when she was 16 years old but is in remission and managing well although she remains anxious about her weight.

Questions

1. What is the definition of a vegan diet?
2. What other information do you need?
3. What is the nutrition and dietetic diagnosis? Write it as a PASS statement.
4. Which nutrients in particular should be considered when assessing a vegan diet?
5. What is Wendy's body mass index (BMI), and is this cause for concern?
6. Wendy has been self-referred via her GP. Do you need to inform the GP of your discussions with Wendy?

Further questions

7. Fish oil supplements rich in $n-3$ PUFAs have been found to ameliorate pain and symptoms of RA (Goldberg & Katz, 2007). Are there any plant-based alternatives?
8. Wendy is considering a further pregnancy. What would be your concerns?
9. What are the ethical implications of accepting a referral from Wendy when your clinical service is overstretched?

References

Appleby, P., Roddam, A., Allen, N. *et al.* (2007) Comparative fracture risk in vegetarians and non-vegetarians in EPIC Oxford. *European Journal of Clinical Nutrition*, **61** (**12**), 1400–1406.

Carter, J.P., Furman, T. & Hutcheson, H.R. (1987) Preeclampsia and reproductive performance in a community of vegans. *Southern Medical Journal*, **80** (**6**), 692–697.

Craig, W.J. & Mangels, A.R. (2009) Position of the American Dietetic Association: vegetarian diets. *Journal of the American Dietetic Association*, **109** (**7**), 1266–1282.

Crowe, F.L., Steur, M., Allen, N.E. *et al.* (2011) Plasma concentrations of 25-hydroxy vitamin D in meat eaters, fish eaters, vegetarians and vegans: results from the EPIC Oxford study. *Public Health and Nutrition*, **14** (**2**), 340–346.

Davis, B.C. & Kris-Etherton, P.M. (2003) Achieving optimal essential fatty acid status in vegetarians: current knowledge and practical implications. *American Journal of Clinical Nutrition*, **78** (**Suppl. 3**), 640S–646S.

De Bortoli, M.C. & Cozzolino, S.M. (2009) Zinc and selenium nutritional status in vegetarians. *Biological Trace Element Research*, **127** (**3**), 228–233.

Erdeve, O., Arsan, S., Atasay, B. *et al.* (2009) A breast-fed newborn with megaloblastic anaemia-treated with vitamin B12 supplementation of the mother. *Journal of Pediatric Hematology and Oncology*, **31** (**10**), 763–765.

Gibson, R.S. (1994) Content and bioavailability of trace elements in vegetarian diets. *American Journal of Clinical Nutrition*, **59** (**Suppl. 5**), 1223S–1232S.

Goldberg, R.J. & Katz, J. (2007) A meta-analysis of the analgesic effects of omega-3 polyunsaturated fatty acid supplementation for inflammatory joint pain. *Pain*, **129**, 210–223.

Institute of Medicine, Food and Nutrition Board (2001) *Dietary Reference Intakes for Vitamin A, Vitamin K, Arsenic, Boron, Chromium, Copper, Iodine, Iron, Manganese, Molybdenum, Nickel, Silicon, Vanadium, and Zinc*. National Academy Press, Washington, DC.

Kniskern, M.A. & Johnston, C.S. (2011) Protein dietary reference intakes may be inadequate for vegetarians if low amounts of animal protein are consumed. *Nutrition*, **27** (**6**), 727–730.

Kornsteiner, M., Singer, I. & Elmadfa, I. (2008) Very low $n-3$ long chain polyunsaturated fatty acid status in Austrian vegetarians and vegans. *Annals of Nutrition and Metabolism*, **52** (**1**), 37–47.

Leung, A.M., Lamar, A., He, X. *et al.* (2011) Iodine status and thyroid function of Boston-area vegetarians and vegans. *Journal of Clinical Endocrinology and Metabolism*, **96** (**8**), E1303–E1307.

Mangels, R., Messina, V. & Messina, M. (2010) *The Dietitian's Guide to Vegetarian Diets*, 3rd edn. Jones and Bartlett, Sudbury, MA, pp. 530–535.

Mariani, A., Chalies, S., Jeziorski, E. *et al.* (2009) Consequences of exclusive breast feeding in vegan mother newborn – case report. *Archives of Pediatrics*, **16** (**11**), 1461–1463.

Mathey, C., Di Marco, N., Poujol, A. *et al.* (2007) Failure to thrive and psychomotor regression revealing vitamin B12 deficiency in 3 infants. *Archives of Pediatrics*, **14** (**5**), 467–471.

Outilia, T.A., Karkkainen, M.U., Seppanen, R.H. *et al.* (2000) Dietary intake of vitamin D in premenopausal healthy vegans was insufficient to maintain concentrations of 25-hydroxyvitamin D and intact parathyroid hormone within normal ranges during the winter in Finland. *Journal of the American Dietetic Association*, **100** (**4**), 434–441.

Roed, C., Skovby, F. & Lund, A.M. (2009) Severe vitamin B12 deficiency in infants breastfed by vegans. *Ugeskr Laeger*, **171** (**43**), 3099–3101.

Rosell, M.S., Lloyd-Wright, Z., Appleby, P.N. *et al.* (2005) Long chain $n-3$ polyunsaturated fatty acids in plasma in British meat-eating, vegetarian and vegan men. *American Journal of Clinical Nutrition*, **82** (**2**), 327–334.

Sanders, T.A. (2009) DHA status of vegetarians. *Prostaglandins, Leukotrienes and Essential Fatty Acids*, **81** (**2–3**), 137–141.

Simpoulous, A.P. (2009) Omega-6/omega-3 essential fatty acids: biological effects. In: A.P. Simpoulous & N.G. Bazan (eds) Omega-3 fatty acids the brain and retina. *World Review of Nutrition and Dietetics*, **99**, 1–16.

Smolka, V., Bekarek, V., Hlidova, E. *et al.* (2001) Metabolic complications and neurologic manifestations of vitamin B12 deficiency in children of vegetarian mothers. *Journal of Czech Physicians*, **140** (**23**), 732–735.

Weiss, R., Fogelman, Y. & Bennett, M. (2004) Severe vitamin B12 deficiency in an infant associated with a maternal deficiency and a strict vegetarian diet. *Journal of Pediatric Hematolgy and Oncology*, **26** (**4**), 270–271.

Welch, A.A., Shakya-Shrestha, S., Lentjes, M.A. *et al.* (2010) Dietary intake and status of $n-3$ polyunsaturated fatty acids in a population of fish-eating and non-fish-eating meat-eaters, vegetarians and vegans and the product-precursor ratio [corrected] of alpha-linolenic acid to long-chain polyunsaturated fatty acids: results from the EPIC-Norfolk cohort. *American Journal of Clinical Nutrition*, **92** (**5**), 1040–1051.

Resources

Gardener, E. (2014) Vegetarianism and vegan diets. In: J. Gandy (ed), *Manual of Dietetic Practice*, 5th edn. Wiley Blackwell, Oxford.

PEN: Practice Based Evidence in Nutrition. *Do individuals with rheumatoid arthritis who follow a vegan diet have improvement in their arthritic symptoms compared to individuals with rheumatoid arthritis who follow a non-vegetarian diet?*. http://www.pennutrition.com/KnowledgePathway.aspx?kpid=978&pqcatid=146&pqid=7876.

CASE STUDY 2

Older person – ethical dilemma

Nicola Howle*

Rose is currently an inpatient at the mental health hospital; she is 93 years old. Her only family is her sister, who she lived with prior to admission. She often appears confused and has limited engagement in conversations. Rose is bedbound and hoisted for all transfers. She has been in hospital for 4 months; she was originally admitted to the acute hospital following a fall at home and was treated in the elderly assessment ward for a urinary tract infection. She was then discharged to a community hospital for assessment of her care needs and rehabilitation. During this time she refused to eat and drink, and underwent a period of naso-gastric (NG) feeding. She pulled the NG tube out twice and continued to refuse to eat and drink. The ward doctors felt she was depressed, so Rose was admitted to an older peoples assessment ward at the mental health hospital. At this time she was referred to the dietetic service for urgent provision of an NG feeding regimen to help build her up prior to commencing electroconvulsive therapy (ECT).

On attending the ward, the doctor and nursing staff are very concerned about Rose. She has been assessed by a second opinion doctor who states that Rose is unlikely to survive ECT. The ward staff are unconvinced that she is depressed as Rose has limited communication and they are unable to complete the assessments for depression. The ward staff and doctor feel that she is at the end of her life and should be kept comfortable. However, the consultant has asked for NG feeding for 2 weeks and to go ahead with ECT later that week. IV fluids have been prescribed as her oral intake is very poor.

*On behalf of the BDA Older People Specialist Group.

Dietetic and Nutrition Case Studies, First Edition.
Edited by Judy Lawrence, Pauline Douglas, and Joan Gandy.

Companion Website: http://www.manualofdieteticpractice.com/

Assessment

Domain	
Anthropometry, body composition and functional	Current weight on referral estimated to be <30 kg, ward unable to weigh due to poor skin integrity 1 month ago 30 kg 2 months ago 33 kg 3 months ago 35 kg 4 months ago 40 kg Height 1.66 m
Biochemical and haematological	On admission: Sodium 152 mmol/L Potassium 2.9 mmol/L C reactive protein (CRP) 70 mg/L Urea 4.4 mmol/L Creatinine 37 mmol/L Estimated glomerular filtration rate (eGRF) >90 mL/min
Clinical	Pressure areas intact, although Rose is at high risk of skin breakdown, continence pads leave red marks to her skin Speech and language therapy recommendations: syrup thickened fluids and pureed diet
Diet	Food and fluid chart *Breakfast* 3 tsp cereal, 60 mL tea (with semi-skimmed milk) *Mid-morning* Sip of juice *Lunch* 5 tsp fish in parsley sauce, sips of juice, 2 tsp of custard *Mid-afternoon* Declined drink *Evening meal* 2 tsp soup, declined main course, 3 tsp pureed pudding, sips pineapple juice
Environmental, behavioural and social	Communication problems Bedbound

Rose is very frail and at high risk of refeeding syndrome, and therefore a request was made to prescribe refeeding vitamins and minerals. Blood electrolytes were requested to be corrected. After a discussion with ward staff a feeding regimen was provided, in case an NG was placed. Staff were to encourage oral intake, including nourishing drinks with the aim to offer these hourly. Monitoring of tolerance, oral intake, bloods and bowels was requested.

Rose was reviewed regularly. Naso-jejunal (NJ) feeding was commenced alongside encouragement of oral intake, whilst she had ECT. NJ feeding was selected as it was safer to manage in a non-acute environment. Feeding was stopped after 2 weeks as no beneficial effect was seen from the feed or ECT. The consultant made the decision that she was for no further treatment. Rose was given tender loving care until she died 5 days later.

Questions

1. What was the initial nutrition and dietetic diagnosis, when Rose was first referred to the dietetic team? Write it as a PASS statement.
2. What would be the nutrition and dietetic diagnosis at the end of life?
3. What are the current national and local policy recommendations for prevention of refeeding syndrome?
4. Do you think that refeeding syndrome was a real issue for Rose?
5. From the biochemistry results provided which electrolytes need correcting? How could this be done?
6. Discuss the ethical implications of commencing NG feeding for Rose.
7. Devise a NJ feeding regimen for Rose.
8. Discuss the ethical implications of withdrawing NJ feeding after 2 weeks, when oral intake remains poor.
9. NJ feeding was selected as it was deemed safer to manage in a non-acute environment. Do you agree with this or could NG have been used?
10. Discuss the flow of patients through health care settings, Rose was in at least three wards, what affect could this have had on her?
11. Discuss the role of advanced care directives/living wills – what difference could it have made if staff and family had known what Rose's wishes would have been?

References

British National Formulary (2015) *RCPCH Publications Ltd and the Royal Pharmaceutical Society of Great Britain*. London.

NICE (2006) *Nutrition support in adults (CG 32)*. http://www.nice.org.uk/guidance/cg32 [accessed on 9 February 2015].

Resources

Eldridge, I. & Power, J. (2014) Palliative care and terminal illness. In: J. Gandy (ed), *Manual of Dietetic Practice*, 5th edn. Wiley Blackwell, Oxford.

Pout, V. (2014) Older adults. In: Gandy, J. (ed), *Manual of Dietetic Practice*, 5th edn. Wiley Blackwell, Oxford.

CASE STUDY 3

Older person

Vicki Pout*

Vinnie is a retired gentleman who has lived in his own home for the past 65 years after marrying his wife Jean. He was widowed 15 months ago. Vinnie has two children who live over 100 miles away and three grandchildren. He has no other remaining family. His children and grandchildren visit on average once every 6 weeks but have busy lives and he does not like to admit to them that he is lonely. Although he is the longest resident in the neighbourhood, he does not know many of his neighbours. Vinnie worked as a bank clerk until he retired at the age of 65; he has few hobbies. Although he has little significant medical history, Vinnie feels tired and run down as he has had several falls recently. He has had two admissions to hospital with urinary tract infections over the past 12 months. Falls screening and MUST on his last admission to hospital showed unintentional weight loss. The hospital dietitian gave him advice on improving his oral intake using high protein and energy foods. At this point he reported that he was eating fine but did admit to skipping meals as there was little point in preparing a meal for one and in the past Jean had always been the cook.

The dietitian who saw him in hospital had concerns about how much he was eating at home. Vinnie reported that he understood the implications of not meeting his nutritional requirements and agreed to community dietetic follow up. Vinnie was discharged with ongoing input from the community rehabilitation team and transferred to the dietitian within the team. Vinnie was seen for 6 weeks on a daily basis by the community rehabilitation team. Within the first 2 weeks Vinnie had another fall and was diagnosed with depression. When the dietitian saw him he reported that he still regularly missed meals but felt that it was natural for older people not to have a big appetite.

*On behalf of the BDA Older People Specialist Group.

Dietetic and Nutrition Case Studies, First Edition.
Edited by Judy Lawrence, Pauline Douglas, and Joan Gandy.

Companion Website: http://www.manualofdieteticpractice.com/

Assessment

Domain	
Anthropometry, body composition and functional	Weight Current 77 kg 3 months ago 81 kg 6 months ago 87 kg 9 months ago 92 kg Height Stooped posture so unable to measure height with stadiometer Reported height 1.8 m
Biochemical and haematological	None relevant
Clinical	Previous UTI × 2 Recent fall Depression
Diet	Diet history *Breakfast* Cup of tea (190 g), full fat milk (25 g) and one sugar (5 g), slice of toast (27 g) with butter (10 g) and marmalade (15 g) *Mid-morning* Cup of tea, as above *Lunch* Either sandwich (2 × 36 g bread + 2 × 10 g butter) with ham (23 g) or cheese (30 g) or bowl of tinned soup (190 g) with a slice of bread (36 g) Tinned fruit in syrup (120 g), cup of tea at end of meal (as above), water with meal *Mid-afternoon* Sometimes has a piece of cake (40 g) or a biscuit (13 g) with a cup of tea (as above) *Evening* As for lunch
Environmental, behavioural and social	Lives alone Lonely

The community dietitian visited Vinnie and talked through the principles of maximising nutritional intake using suitable choices and having small frequent meals and snacks. Vinnie stated that he was following the advice given to him in hospital and could not understand why he was not gaining weight. The dietitian talked about the effect of low mood on food intake and asked what meals Vinnie liked and how he liked to have his food. Vinnie felt that he was doing everything he could to improve his intake.

When the dietitian next visited Vinnie she noticed that there was very little food in the house. She continued to build rapport with Vinnie and they reminisced about food when he was younger and meals with his wife Jean and their children. Vinnie explained to the dietitian that he was indeed very lonely and did not enjoy eating alone. He also explained that as he had gone out to work he did not play a part in the cooking of the family meals and did not have very good cooking skills. The dietitian talked with Vinnie and explored options to improve his cookery skills and also find ways to make some meals more sociable. Vinnie was able to join a lunch club and enjoyed meeting people who lived in the area.

Questions

1. What is the nutrition and dietetic diagnosis? Write it as a PASS statement.
2. Discuss the impact the ageing process has on anthropometric measurements.
3. How may the location of a dietetic consultation affect the care planning process?
4. If Vinnie was under the care of your community services what options would there be in terms of meal provision and social interaction services?
5. What are the common misconceptions that are held around nutrition and older life?
6. Discuss the links between falls and nutrition in older life.
7. How can a holistic approach be used in care planning with older people?
8. What precautions should be taken when using dietetic notes in the community?

Resources

PEN: Practice Based Evidence in Nutrition *Gerontology*. www.pennutrition.com/KnowledgePathway.aspx?kpid=2541&trid=2570&trcatid=38.

Pout, V. (2014) Older adults. In: J. Gandy (ed), *Manual of Dietetic Practice*, 5th edn. Wiley Blackwell, Oxford.

CASE STUDY 4

Learning disabilities: Prader–Willi syndrome

Sian O'Shea, Marjorie Macleod & Anne Laverty

John was 35 years old with Prader–Willi syndrome (PWS) when he moved into a large community care home when his mother (main carer) died. John was later referred by his key worker to the specialist learning disability (LD) service, as he was about to move from the large controlled environment of a staffed care home to a shared flat in the community that did not have the same degree of supervision. His weight had been steadily increasing and the carers raised concerns that with less supervision and more opportunities for John to enjoy social eating within his local community, his weight would get out of control.

John's welfare was a fundamental issue; it was vital that the required care plan be clearly understood before any decision regarding accommodation was made. A formal risk assessment had to be conducted, which would help in clarifying his requirements. In John's case, offering a food choice intensified his anxieties resulting in outburst of behaviour, such as wrecking the room or frightening workers/public by his lashing out. It was recommended that to meet his future needs he required:

- Long-term structure and routine in relation to food and behaviour;
- Structured approach;
- Consistent staff team;
- Fully inclusive supervision;
- Adequate support measures for staff;
- A detailed menu plan outlining clear expectations, clear messages, clear boundaries leaving NO room for interpretation;
- Safe environment;
- A team trained in the management of PWS;
- Suitable day activities which minimise the opportunities to access food; and
- Suitable accommodation where access to food could be controlled; sharing a flat might prove problematic due to conflict of interests regarding access to foods/fluids.

This approach is in contrast to the prevailing social care ethic that favours choice. Staff can find this difficult as they often feel that it is an infringement of a person's human rights and totally unacceptable. However, understanding of this is a core element in managing a patient's care. They should have the opportunity to explore and

Dietetic and Nutrition Case Studies, First Edition.
Edited by Judy Lawrence, Pauline Douglas, and Joan Gandy.

Companion Website: http://www.manualofdieteticpractice.com/

discuss this significant change in their work practice. It is essential that all staff realise the importance of all of them keeping to the agreed plans.

Patient history and care plan

6–15 years ago

John moved into a shared flat in a sheltered housing complex, managed by social care staff. He was matched to share with an elderly man with LD, who had also been a resident in the residential unit. His meals at home were supervised and he was helped with his daily living tasks. Day care was provided 5 days/week at a local day centre.

The new diet plan was implemented. All day care and residential staff were fully trained in PWS management, which included his diet plan. Effectiveness was monitored by regular weight checks. During this time, there were frequent food challenges and outbursts. The turnover of staff created additional challenges in care management. The LD team continued to provide on-going training to staff to help sustain the package. At one point the day care and residential staff were in open dispute with each other as how best to manage the diet. A simple summary sheet was prepared to help carers understand PWS as the constant requirement to train staff was a drain on service resources. The care staff indicted that they required additional support from the LD team to help maintain the package. Six weekly support meetings were set up with the dietitian/psychologist and speech and language therapist (SLT).

The diet plan, which included a daily food menu of breakfast/lunch/evening meal and snack choices that John could understand. The plan was laid out in simple, clear language, which was supported with pictures. The SLT did further assessments and established that John had very slow processing and had difficulty with short-term memory. He performed well on formal testing with good understanding of grammatical forms and vocabulary. However, on speaking to him, it was found that his verbal comprehension was extremely poor. Visual enforcers were used to aid his comprehension, along with constant reinforcement by staff to remind him of his treatment plan. For particularly difficult situations such as going out to parties, social stories were provided along with pictorial dietary agreements. They found that it was essential to give John a copy of the agreements at least 14 days earlier to enable him to absorb the information thus minimising any challenging behaviour and allowing him to keep his anxieties under control so as to enable him to enjoy the occasions. The dietitian was paramount in the management of this. Despite all of these efforts, the placement eventually broke down. Although weight during this episode fluctuated greatly, it was subsequently reduced to 65 kg.

Six years ago to present

A new placement was identified with a younger flat mate. Core to the new placement was an agreement that only core staff should be employed for his management; only in a crisis would agency staff be used. Again, the staff team were provided training by the dietitian, on PWS and the food plan. Agreement was reached that any changes in the diet plan would be made only by the specialist dietitian. A review of his energy requirements was completed as the team had been successful in slowly reducing his weight to a normal BMI. His weight was very successfully managed at a normal BMI of 21.5–23 kg/m^2, which was a weight of 42–45 kg. More importantly, he sustained his weight in this range for a period of over 2 years with no major fluctuations.

The specialist dietitian continues to monitor John's weight and be available for the challenges relating to foods. Menus have been revised but this has been a gradual process because of John's resistance to change and the anxiety that change creates. The transition from the high-fat menu to more healthy options has taken several years and has been beneficial as it allows him larger portions. Although the team support continues, it is noticeable that recent involvement has been minimised. Specialist dietitians continue to be available to help resolve any breaches in adherence. The dietitian's current assessment is shown below.

Assessment

Domain	
Anthropometry, body composition and functional	Initial weight 75 kg Current weight range 42–45 kg Height 1.4 m
Biochemical and haematological	Lipid and glucose profile currently within normal ranges
Clinical	Constipation (bowel protocol in place) Poor muscle tone *Medication* Calcium, vitamin D Testosterone Lactulose prn
Diet	Daily – 600 mL of skimmed milk for use in drinks and breakfast cereal *Breakfast* Bowl of cereal (50 g), granule artificial sweetener if required (no sugar) Cup of tea (190 mL), sweetener if required, 1 slice of toast (27 g) low fat spread (10 g), marmalade (15 g) *Mid-morning* Cup of tea (190 mL), or sugar free drink 1 piece of fruit *Lunch* Cheese and pickle sandwich (185 g) or ham and cheese sandwich (180 g); 25 g crisps or other foods, for example, 10 g small bar chocolate are offered twice a week as a treat Low fat (diet) yoghurt (125 mL) Sugar free fruit squash (50 mL diluted with 130 mL water) with meal

Assessment *(continued)*

Domain	
	Mid-afternoon Cup of tea (190 mL), artificial sweetener if required Choice from a biscuit cake list based on 150 calories per portion *Evening meal* – varies examples include: Lasagne (420 g) or Chicken (170 g) with potatoes (mashed (120 g) or boiled (220 g)) and vegetables (boiled carrots 85 g, cabbage 120 g or runner beans 120 g), gravy (120 g) or Stir fry (350 g) and rice (290 g) or Fish whiting (240 g)) 1/7 with potatoes (220 g) and peas (100 g) Choice of dessert – low fat (diet) yoghurt or 1 portion fruit or 1 jelly pot (5/7) *Evening* Cheese (30 g) and biscuits (4 × 13 g) or 1 slice toast (27 g)
Environmental, behavioural and social	Housing, cooking facilities/abilities, education/staff training/MDT working/activities/risk assessment. No food choice, as it leads to behavioural outbursts. Does have choice in relation to clothes/books/TV program/outings and day activities Poor cognitive skills, challenging behaviour

Questions

1. What is PWS?
2. PWS is a learning disability; summarise the other factors you may consider when assessing the nutritional requirements of an adult with a learning disability.
3. What are the nutritional consequences of PWS?
4. Calculate John's energy requirements for weight maintenance and weight loss. What else should you consider when prescribing a weight reduction diet for an adult with PWS?
5. What is the nutrition and dietetic diagnosis? Write as a PASS statement.
6. What is the aim of your intervention plan? What outcome measures would you use to monitor John?
7. What steps would you take to involve John in goal setting?
8. How do you involve his carers?
9. What other services or heath care professionals should be involved in John's care?

Further question

10. Discuss capacity to consent in an adult with a learning disability.

References

Department of Health (DH) (2005) *Mental Capacity Act 2005: Code of Practice Department of Constitutional Affairs*. www.dca.gov.uk [accessed on 9 October 2015].

Department of Health, Social Services & Public Health (DHSSPS) (2003) *Seeking Consent: Working with people with learning disabilities*. Scotland. www.dhsspsni.gov.uk [accessed on 13 October 2015].

Hoffman, C.J., Aultman, D. & Pipes, P. (1992) A nutrition survey of and recommendations for individuals with Prader-Willi syndrome who live in group homes. *Journal of the American Dietetic Association*, **92** (**7**), 823–830, 833.

International Prader–Willi Association. (2010) *Dietary Management*. www.ipwso.org/dietary-management [accessed on 12 June 2015].

Lindmark, M., Trygg, K., Giltvedt, K. *et al.* (2010) Nutrient intake of young children with Prader–Willi syndrome. *Food and Nutrition Research*, **54**, 2112.

Prader–Willi Syndrome Association (2010) *A Prader–Willi food pyramid*. www103.ssldomain.com/pwsausa/syndrome/foodpyramid.htm [accessed on 12 June 2015].

Purtell, L., Viardot, A., Sze, L. *et al.* (2015) Postprandial metabolism in adults with Prader–Willi syndrome. *Obesity*, **23**, 1159–1165.

Scottish Parliament. (2000) *Adults with incapacity (Scotland) Act*. The Stationery Office, Edinburgh.

van Mil, E., Westerterp, K.R., Gerver, W.J. *et al.* (2001) Body composition in Prader–Willi syndrome compared with non-syndromal obesity: relationship to physical activity and growth hormone. *Journal of Pediatrics*, **139**, 708–714.

Resources

Burton, S., Laverty, A. & Macloed, M. (2014) Learning disabilities. In: J. Gandy (ed), *Manual of Dietetic Practice*, 5th edn. Wiley Blackwell, Oxford.

Prader–Willi Syndrome Association UK. www.pwsa.co.uk.

CASE STUDY 5

Freelance practice

Pizza goes to school

Hilary Du Cane

Pizza has long been a popular food on school menus. However, many pizzas include processed meats, salty toppings and fatty cheese, giving pizza in general a bad reputation for its nutritional attributes. The corporate client in this case supplies pizza components to schools and other outlets, along with recipes, menus, cooking and serving equipment, marketing templates and training.

School food standards in England have been radically changed several times since 2004 and the pizza supplier has needed specialist nutritional support throughout, to adapt to the changes and remain a leading supplier to schools. Demands for nutritional services ranged from detailed nutritional analysis of products and recipes to categorisation within the latest school food groups (Children's Food Trust, 2015) advice on portions, product development and additional specification covering sustainability issues (Food for Life Partnership, 2015). As a small firm, the pizza supplier had previously had little involvement with nutrition and could not justify employing a specialist. Therefore, they chose a freelance dietitian, among personnel with food industry experience as well as business and marketing skills, and continue to draw on their services as needed.

Questions

1. What are the basic principles of the Children's Food Trust's (2015) food-based standards?
2. What effect do you think the 2015 standards will have on freelance dietitians' workload?
3. Freelance dietetics is highly competitive, particularly in the corporate and organisational market. What can you do to ensure that you and your skills are in demand?
4. Like other areas of dietetics this type of work will follow the dietetic process/model. How would you assess the needs of a corporate client in a case like this?
5. Describe the dietetic intervention. What services would you offer the client?

Dietetic and Nutrition Case Studies, First Edition.
Edited by Judy Lawrence, Pauline Douglas, and Joan Gandy.

Companion Website: http://www.manualofdieteticpractice.com/

6. What support can a freelance dietitian draw on to complete this type of project?
7. How can these resources and experience be built up over time?
8. Who would pay for the freelancer's CPD?
9. To what extent do food industry managers determine the nutritional outputs they need when they call in a freelance dietitian?
10. How do corporate clients find a freelance dietitian?
11. How would you go about setting up a freelance practice?
12. Can a newly graduated dietitian freelance immediately after qualifying?
13. What are the pros and cons of starting out at a very low daily charge in order to get some work underway?
14. How can you ensure you get paid for your freelance work?

References

Children's Food Trust (2015) *School food standards*. www.childrensfoodtrust.org.uk/schools/the-standards [accessed on May 2015].

Food for Life Partnership (2015) *Criteria and guidance*. www.foodforlife.org.uk/school-awards/criteria-and-guidance [accessed on May 2015].

Resources

Gardner, E. (2015) Freelance dietetics. In: J. Gandy (ed), *Manual of Dietetic Practice*, 5th edn. Wiley Blackwell, Oxford.

Nutrition and Dietetic Resources (NDR). www.ndr-uk.org.

CASE STUDY 6

Public health – weight management

A multi-faceted approach

Sarah Bowyer, Kirsten Whitehead & Elaine Gardner

Delivering for Health (Scottish Executive, 2005) provided a national plan for Scotland, which focussed specifically on tackling health inequalities. For primary care services, an evolved *anticipatory care model* was developed to target geographic areas of greatest need as well as to concentrate on a multi-disciplinary approach for preventative and integrated care embedded in the communities. Developed as Keep Well Programmes in urban areas and Well North programmes in rural areas, initiatives were piloted to improve the health of Scottish residents, particularly in those aged between 45 and 64 years.

This case study concerns a pilot project that used individual and community approaches to address food access and opportunities for physical activity as two aspects of public health measures that can impact weight management. The NHS Highland Health Board's public health strategy to tackle weight management incorporated a Well North initiative. This was delivered, in conjunction with the Health Board wide service of the Counterweight Programme (http://www.counterweight.org), as part of a Healthy Weight Care Pathway, which overarched and supported these two treatment routes. Table 6.1 explains how planning, implementation and evaluation were combined to deliver within the 2-year project timescale.

The project aimed for co-design, and where possible, co-delivery of initiatives within the community, which were supported by the NHS, the local authority and the third sector, in a mutually supportive and coordinated way. It was undertaken in four neighbouring rural communities served by four medical practice teams and was aimed to target the whole community. There were 4641 people living in the area (General Register Office for Scotland, 2011) aged over 16 years and registered with a GP. Using national prevalence rates, it was estimated that this included 1860 (40%) overweight and 1120 (24%) obese individuals (Scottish Government, 2010a). The area is defined as *very remote rural* by the Scottish Government 8-fold urban/rural classification (Scottish Government, 2010b) and is a geographical region renowned for its outstanding natural beauty, resulting in tourism being a major source of local employment.

Dietetic and Nutrition Case Studies, First Edition.
Edited by Judy Lawrence, Pauline Douglas, and Joan Gandy.

Companion Website: http://www.manualofdieteticpractice.com/

Table 6.1 Timescale of key activities planned, implemented and evaluated

Time scale (Months)	Public health weight management programme			Collaborative actions and activities	Evaluation
	Weight management care pathway	**Counterweight programme**	**Well North programme**		
1–6	Meetings with medical practice teams	Training of NHS dietitian to deliver Counterweight training programme	Community survey Meetings with key community individuals and groups	Initial stakeholder meeting	Analysis of the community consultation
6–12	Refinement and development	Training and mentoring of community nursing staff to qualify as Counterweight practitioners	Community development worker recruitment. Subsequent work to develop schemes Food access survey Applications invited for small grants scheme	Bimonthly stakeholder and community members meeting Bimonthly newsletter collated by dietitian with contributions from participating agencies/organisations	*Two meetings cancelled due to inclement weather*

12–18	Pilot of weight management care pathway toolkit with medical practice teams	Nursing staff delivering Counterweight programme to patients	Implementing funded projects Provision of health behaviour change training courses Provision of walk-leader training by 'Step it Up Highland'		220 participants attending activities across 10 funded projects The main health improvements reported by participants related to improved self-esteem and reduced social isolation Number of referrals from medical practice teams into funded projects - unknown Number of patients referred to Counterweight programme – 225 for Community Health Partnership region (unknown for individual 4 medical practices)
18–23	Evaluation and refinement of care pathway toolkit	Nursing staff delivering Counterweight programme to patients	Implementing funded projects		
24			Bread making workshops	Showcase event celebrating local action	Qualitative evaluation of programme by outside agency

Scoping exercise for the Well North programme

A community consultation used an asset-based approach to discover local factors and potential issues around food access and participation in physical activities.

Results

At the initial meeting of members of the communities and invited local stakeholders, the results of the community survey and the food access survey were presented. Discussions began to consider interventions to improve dietary intake and physical activity levels.

Members representing each of the four communities selected an initial action that they agreed was most pertinent for their area, for example, cooking sessions (incorporating healthy eating guidelines and budget constraints), providing transport to local swimming pools and gym facilities located 26 miles (60 min drive) away.

Bi-monthly project meetings were initiated to provide project updates, ongoing evaluation and a focussed discussion on a relevant topic, which included: 'Safe and easy access for walking and cycling – where are we at? Where are we going? And how do we get there?' and 'Grow it, buy it, cook it, eat it' Table 6.1 illustrates how the actions were developed and rolled out as the project evolved.

Collaboration in the delivery of services and more 'joined up services'

Dietitians liaised with the medical practice teams to encourage collaborative working, for example, referral of patients into Well North local projects and using the medical centre as a community hub to advertise these local activities and events. The Weight Management Care Pathway was distributed to primary care teams in the case study area, along with a questionnaire to investigate its usability, practicality and overall opinions. Other targeted medical practices in NHS Highland were included in the consultation. Training of public, private and third sector employees and volunteers was provided to upskill local workers (Table 6.1).

In order to support and enhance local activity, a small grants scheme was made available to fund new or existing initiatives. Successful applications came from organisations such as lunch clubs, a higher education college, family support groups, a pony club and a social enterprise supporting mental health. These clearly demonstrated how their actions could help improve food intake and/or physical activity and how these would be sustained after completion of the 2-year period funded project. Terms and conditions of receiving an award included participation in the monthly stakeholder meetings, and carrying out regular evaluation. The Well North community development worker supported their activities, which included creation of allotments, community gardening, cookery classes, hosting circus skills workshops and delivering short, guided health walks.

As the initial community consultation generated ideas for a community bakery, a final activity and show case event was framed around bread making. A professional baker ran two bread-making workshops and gave a presentation about 'real' bread and community baking as part of an evening event, which also displayed the work of the groups who had received a small grant award.

Evaluation

Each component, stage and action of the whole public health weight management programme was evaluated as detailed in Table 6.1. A range of quantitative and qualitative measurements were made.

The wider Well North initiative commissioned an evaluation based on the *performance story* technique. Key stakeholders were identified for interviews and the posts included project lead, dietitian, local GP, community council and project participants. The evaluation used qualitative methods; all interviews were recorded and the transcripts were analysed using methods that triangulated significant themes against outputs and outcomes.

Reflection

- Co-produced health initiatives need to be embedded in the community to work in true collaboration.
- Community consultation can reveal ideas and interest but a significant amount of community development and engagement work needs to be undertaken to ensure that action and attendance are achieved.
- Referrals to the Well North activities were low from primary care teams highlighting the need for better collaboration in the design and delivery of services.
- The limited timescale proved to be an extra pressure when building trusting relationships between the programme staff and the community, and when embedding the new way of working into the community. Established key groups and key people in the community are vital links when short-term funding is available.
- The evaluation needs to include unexpected outcomes; although this project sought to improve diet and physical activity, the greatest reported gains were in reduced social isolation and improved self-efficacy; both of which are fundamental to sustaining health and wellbeing.
- This evaluation and the lessons learned from this project have been important levers in the development of long-term community development approaches to Healthy Weight in NHS Highland.

Acknowledgements

Fiona Clarke RD MPhil, Senior Health Improvement Specialist, NHS Highland.
NHS Highland Health Board.
The West Coast Communities of the Scottish Highlands.

Questions

1. How were the needs of this population assessed?
2. Is it appropriate to make a nutritional nutrition and dietetic diagnosis? If so, what might it be?
3. How is the prevalence of nutrition-related diseases potentially exacerbated in a rural area?
4. What evidence-based clinical weight management programmes are available through the NHS in your region?
5. What impact could tourism have on residents' health?
6. What other demographic knowledge would be useful in planning the programme?
7. What specific issues might you look for in rural areas with regards to food access?
8. What groups are working in the local area on initiatives to improve and/or support healthy eating or physical activity?
9. What is meant by the term third sector?
10. Who would you recommend the consultancy company speak to in order to undertake their evaluation?
11. What outcomes do you feel would be important?
12. Would reduced levels of obesity be a useful outcome measure?
13. How could you document any comments regarding how people felt about taking part?
14. What other participation methods could be used to engage the public?

Further questions

15. This case study is an example of a *community development approach*. Review the seven main principles of this approach (human dignity, participation, empowerment, ownership, learning, adaptiveness and relevance) (Macdowall *et al.*, 2006) and provide examples as to how these have been addressed.
16. Research the term *performance story technique* and state why this method was appropriate in this case study.

References

Dart, J.J. (2008) *Report on outcomes and get everyone involved: The Participatory Performance Story Reporting Technique*. www.clearhorizon.com.au/tag/performance-story-reporting/ [accessed on 18 September 2014].

Food Standards Agency (2008) *Accessing healthy food: a sentinel mapping study of healthy food retailing in Scotland [Online]*. http://www.fhascot.org.uk/Resource/accessing-healthy-food-a-sentinel-mapping-study-of-healthy-food-retailing-in-scotland-s04005 [accessed on 2 June 2014].

General Register Office for Scotland (2011) *Census 2011: detailed characteristics on Populations and Households in Scotland- Release 3E [Online]*. http://www.scotlandscensus.gov.uk/news/census-2011-detailed-characteristics-population-and-households-scotland-release-3e [accessed on 30 June 2014].

Macdowall, W., Bonnell, C. & Davies, M. (2006) *Health Promotion Practice*. Open University Press, Maidenhead.

Scottish Executive (2005) *Delivering for health [Online]*. http://www.scotland.gov.uk/Publications/2005/11/02102635/26356 [accessed on 2 June 2014].

The Scottish Government (2010a) *The Scottish Health Survey 2009, Volume1: Main Report [Online]*. http://www.scotland.gov.uk/Publications/2010/09/23154223/0. [accessed on 2 June 2014].

The Scottish Government (2010b) Scottish Government Urban/Rural Classification 2009–2010 [Online]. http://www.scotland.gov.uk/Publications/2010/08/2010UR [accessed on 12 June 2014].

Resource

Nelson, A. (2014) Public health nutrition. In: J. Gandy (ed), *Manual of Dietetic Practice*, 5th edn. Wiley Blackwell, Oxford.

CASE STUDY 7

Public health – learning disabilities

A community-based nutrition education programme for people with learning disabilities

Angela McComb* & Elaine Gardner*

The *Cook it!* programme (www.publichealth.hscni.net/publications/cook-it-fun-fast-food-less-community-nutrition-education-programme) was developed in Northern Ireland for use among the general population. It aims to increase people's knowledge and understanding of good nutrition and food hygiene, and to develop skills and confidence to cook healthy meals from scratch. The programme is delivered by trained facilitators within local communities over six 2-h sessions, which include discussion, activities (both written and practical) and hands-on cooking. In collaboration with a range of stakeholders, the Public Health Agency (Northern Ireland) has undertaken to adapt the programme to make it suitable for use with people who have learning disabilities.

Learning disability is defined as '*a significantly reduced ability to understand new or complex information, to learn new skills (impaired intelligence), with a reduced ability to cope independently (impaired social functioning), which started before adulthood, with a lasting effect on development*' (DH, 2010).

In Northern Ireland the prevalence rate for learning disability is reported to be 9.7 persons per 1000 although it has been suggested that actual prevalence may be higher than this as a large proportion of individuals with a learning disability do not present themselves to services (Slevin *et al.*, 2011). The Northern Ireland Learning Disability Service Framework (DHSSPS, 2012) recommends that '*people with a (learning) disability should be provided with healthy eating support and advice appropriate to their needs*'.

*On behalf of The Public Health Nutrition Network.

Dietetic and Nutrition Case Studies, First Edition.
Edited by Judy Lawrence, Pauline Douglas, and Joan Gandy.

Companion Website: http://www.manualofdieteticpractice.com/

The pilot phase

An advisory group was established to guide the development of the programme, including the content, resources and a pilot.

To take account of the challenges facing people with learning disabilities in learning new information and developing new skills, the number of sessions in the pilot programme was extended to eight weekly sessions, each lasting 2 h.

Most sessions included a practical cooking activity, and information was provided on a number of key issues, including:

- Food safety and food hygiene.
- An introduction to the food groups on the eatwell plate.
- The rescommended intake of fruit and vegetables.
- The importance of fibre, protein and calcium (over three sessions).
- How to ensure good dental health and prevent tooth decay.
- The importance of reducing intake of foods that are high in fats and sugars to manage weight.

The resources for the programme were developed following guidance from Mencap to ensure that they were easily accessible (Mencap, 2002). Examples of resources used include coloured recipe flip cards incorporating photographs of ingredients and cooking methods; 'spot the hygiene risk' cards and word searches.

The resources were used during the programme, and the clients took them home to serve as an *aide memoire* and to encourage and enable them to cook and adopt safe food hygiene practices in their own home.

Results of the pilot study

Results from the pilot indicated that learning disabled participants lacked food preparation and cooking skills and the draft programme was a useful tool to teach these practical skills to participants.

Overall, the pilot resources were found to be useful. However, the learning disabled people needed more time to absorb the new information and develop basic practical skills, and so it was impossible to cover all of the information in the session plans.

Although there was some evidence that participants gained new knowledge about healthy eating or food hygiene, variation in the use of the Talking Mats® tool by the facilitators made it difficult to be confident about this finding.

A number of recommendations were identified to guide further development of the programme. These included:

- Groups should be limited to 4–5 people to ensure that adequate support and supervision can be provided to individuals, whilst creating the environment for good group dynamics.
- Adequate time should be allocated to ensure that everyone can practice and develop basic food preparation skills, for example, peeling potatoes, chopping onions. This requires a flexible approach to the delivery of the sessions.

- Family members/carers of learning disabled participants should be engaged throughout and informed about the practical skills developed through the programme. They should also be given guidance on how they can support and encourage the learning disabled individual to practice their newly acquired skills within the home environment.
- A number of specific resources should be retained, including the flip chart-style recipe cards, 'Spot the hygiene risk' quiz, the food hygiene DVD (in a shortened format), eatwell mats and food models. Word searches should be omitted from the programme because of the limited reading ability reported among the groups.
- Recipes should be reviewed to ensure that methods are appropriately detailed and are balanced in terms of both preparation and cooking tasks, to ensure that the participants can make them within their home environment.
- If communication tools such as Talking Mats® are to be used within future evaluations, questions should be carefully developed, tested and revised with learning disabled individuals; be easily administered within the time restraints of the programme and be consistently delivered across by all facilitators.
- A forum for facilitators involved in programme delivery should be developed to allow the sharing of ideas and further enhance future programme development.

Questions

1. Do people with learning disabilities have any particular health problems? Are they more at risk of certain conditions/issues than the rest of the population?
2. What nutrition and dietetic diagnosis might prompt you to adapt Cook it for this community? Write it as a PASS statement.
3. Why would the *Cook it!* programme resources need to be adapted for people with learning disabilities? How would they need to be adapted?
4. What other factors, apart from literacy issues, would need to be considered when planning cooking sessions for those with a learning disability?
5. How and when would you evaluate this pilot programme?
6. Attendance at programmes that are delivered over consecutive weeks can be erratic for those with learning disabilities. Consider why this might be so, and suggest ways that attendance could be promoted.
7. If you wished to adapt the *Cook it*! programme for BME (Black, minority and ethnic) groups, what other points would need to be considered?

Further questions

8. When adapting the *Cook it!* programme for people with learning disabilities, what stakeholders should be involved?
9. Why was it beneficial to run a pilot? How do you feel about such a long list of recommendations? Does this mean it has not worked?
10. How would you take this programme forward? What recommendations would you prioritise?

References

Department of Health (2010) *Valuing people now: a three-year strategy for people with learning disabilities. England: DH.* http://webarchive.nationalarchives.gov.uk/20130107105354/http://www.dh.gov.uk/prod_consum_dh/groups/dh_digitalassets/documents/digitalasset/dh_093375.pdf [accessed on 25 September 2015].

Department of Health, Social Services and Public Safety (DHSSPS) (2012) *Service Framework for Learning Disability. Belfast: DHSSPS.* http://www.dhsspsni.gov.uk/sqsd_service_frameworks_learning_disability.

Emerson, E., Baines, S., Allerton, L. *et al.* (2011) *Health inequalities and people with learning disabilities in the UK: 2011. Improving health and lives: Learning Disability Observatory.* https://www.improvinghealthandlives.org.uk/publications/978/Health_Inequalities_&_People_with_Learning_Disabilities_in_the_UK:_2011.

Emerson, E. & Hatton, C. (2008) *People with Learning Disabilities in England. UK: Centre for Disability Research.* http://www.lancaster.ac.uk/staff/emersone/FASSWeb/Emerson_08_PWLDinEngland.pdf.

Mencap. (2002) *Am I making myself clear? Mencap's guidelines for accessible writing. United Kingdom: Mencap.* http://www.accessibleinfo.co.uk/pdfs/Making-Myself-Clear.pdf [accessed on 25 September 2015].

Slevin, E., Taggart, L., McConkey, R. *et al.* (2011) *A rapid review of literature relating to support for people with intellectual disabilities and their family carers when the person has behaviours that challenge and/or mental health problems. Belfast: University of Ulster.* http://www.publichealth.hscni.net/sites/default/files/Intellectual%20Disability.pdf [accessed on 25 September 2015].

Resources

BEMIS (Ethnic minorities in Scotland). http://bemis.org.uk [accessed on 25 September 2015].

Burton S, Laverty A, Macleod (2014) *People with learning disabilities.* In: Gandy, J. (ed), *Manual of Dietetic Practice*, 5th edn. Wiley Blackwell, Oxford.

National Council for Voluntary Organisations. www.ncvo.org.uk.

Northern Ireland Council for Minority Minorities. www.nicem.org.uk [accessed on 25 September 2015].

Voice4Change. www.voice4change-england.co.uk [accessed on 25 September 2015].

CASE STUDY 8

Public health – calorie labelling on menus

Putting calories on menus to create a healthier food environment

Mary Flynn

Spiralling rates of overweight and obesity show that the environment is obesogenic, that is, an environment where becoming overweight and obese is easy and where healthy eating and active living are difficult. In addition, over recent decades there has been an increase in people eating out and 'on-the-go'. When foods and drink are prepared outside of the home, consumers do not know their energy content. Many foods and drinks that may be perceived as healthy often are much higher in energy than consumers realise.

Calorie menu labelling may reverse some obesogenic characteristics of the food environment. Impressed by the potential of calories on menus in other countries, Ireland's Minister for Health at the time (Dr James Reilly) contacted all large international food chain outlets urging them to put calories on their menus. The Minister asked the Food Safety Authority Ireland (FSAI) to initiate action on this throughout the entire food service sector. This case study outlines the work of FSAI in this area.

The response from consumers to a national consultation was overwhelmingly in favour of calorie menu labelling with 96% wanting to see calories on menus to support their efforts at healthy eating and weight control. Most (83%) wanted to see calories displayed in all types of food outlets. Health professional stakeholders' views mirrored that of consumers with over 90% in support of calorie menu labelling as an obesity prevention strategy.

However, among food service businesses (FSBs), support for menu calorie labelling was just over 50% with stronger support evident among younger women. Many disagreed with best practice principles of calorie menu labelling where calories are displayed on all food items available in all places where consumers make food choices. The FSBs reported a complete lack of knowledge and skills to calculate the calorie content of their dishes as well as the necessary financial resources to implement and maintain this.

Dietetic and Nutrition Case Studies, First Edition.
Edited by Judy Lawrence, Pauline Douglas, and Joan Gandy.

Companion Website: http://www.manualofdieteticpractice.com/

The consultation and survey of FSBs identified the main reasons for their opposition to calorie menu labelling, which was the initial and on-going cost of calculating the calories in the dishes they serve. Given the crisis obesity posed for health services and the consumer demand for calorie information, the Minister called on all FSBs to voluntarily display calories on their menus. He asked the FSAI to support FSBs in this area and evaluate their voluntary participation within a year.

A year later, the evaluation of uptake of menu labelling found that 75% of large food chains had begun putting calories on their menus but only 20% of small-to-medium size food service outlets (SMEs) reported either having this in place (8%) or being in the process of implementing it (12%). However, 38% of the remaining SMEs reported 'wanting to put calories on their menus' mainly because this was what consumers clearly want. Not having the ability to calculate the calories themselves in a cost-effective way was the main reason given by the FSBs for not putting this information in place. Over a third (37%) of SMEs were not in favour of calorie menu labelling at all. Press releases of these evaluation findings and the subsequent media coverage, kept FSBs and consumers engaged in the initiative.

To address the main problem preventing calorie menu labelling by FSBs, the FSAI started developing a calorie calculator designed specifically to meet their needs. The goal was to enable FSBs with no nutritional background to calculate the calorie content of their dishes and amend these as they adjusted ingredients. As no suitable calorie calculator was available a team was recruited to develop this.

An innovative calorie calculator (MenuCal www.menucal.ie) designed to enable SMEs put calorie information on their menus was developed by the multidisciplinary team using a test re-test approach with end users (chefs, cooks and FSBs). The accuracy of calorie calculations by these end users (chefs, cooks and FSBs) using MenuCal was assessed. A special advanced feature to assess fat uptake during shallow and deep frying was developed and validated as a 'fat wizard' add-on after testing.

The MenuCal system ensures that all user data is kept confidential. However, the system can provide generic data provided by users on their business size, type, number of staff and geographic location. This is a valuable tool enabling on-going monitoring and review by FSAI.

Questions

1. Identify the two most significant stakeholder groups.
2. How would you collect information on the views of consumers and FSBs?
3. How would you increase feedback from FSBs?
4. What is the nutrition and dietetic problem for public health?
5. How would you evaluate uptake of calorie menu labelling amongst FSBs?
6. Who should be included in the team to develop the calorie calculator?
7. Briefly describe the training required in terms of what is appropriate and cost-effective.
8. How would you ensure ongoing engagement?

Resources

Courtney, L.M., Bennett, A.E., Douglas, F. *et al.* (2012) Technical aspects of calorie menu labelling in Ireland: stakeholder views. *Proceedings of the Nutrition Society*, **71**, E44. doi:10.1017/S0029665112001012.

Douglas, F.E., Bennett, A.E., Courtney, L. *et al.* (2012) Putting calories on menus in Ireland: what consumers want. *Proceedings of the Nutrition Society*, **71**, E42. doi:10.1017/S0029665112000997.

Douglas, F.E., Keaveney, É.P.S., Ní Bhriain, M. *et al.* (2014) Overcoming calorie calculation challenges for fried foods within MenuCal©. *Proceedings of the Nutrition Society*, **73**, E77. doi:10.1017/S0029665114001062.

Food Safety Authority of Ireland (2012) *Calories on Menus in Ireland – Report on a National Consultation*. FSAI,Dublin 1. http://www.fsai.ie/resources_publications.html.

Flynn, M.A.T., Douglas, F.E., Williams, S.J. *et al.* (2015) Developing MenuCal© - a system to enable food businesses to pt calories on their menus. *Proceedings of the Nutrition Society*, **74**, 303–312.

Flynn, M.A.T., Douglas, F.E., Williams, S.J. *et al.* (2014) Developing MenuCal© - a system to enable food businesses to pt calories on their menus. *Proceedings of the Nutrition Society*, **73 (2014)**, E92. doi:10.1017/S0029665114001232.

Kelly, S. M. *et al.* (2014) Putting calories on the menu in Ireland: evaluation of an online calorie calculator for food businesses. *Proceedings of the Nutrition Society*, **73** (**OCE2**), E59 http://journals.cambridge.org/download.php?file=%2FPNS%2FPNS73_OCE2%2FS0029665114000883a.pdf&code=ecab7b8d2de722bf3f42f347c677729f.

Kennelly, J.P. *et al.* (2013) Calorie menu labelling in Ireland: assessment of quality and accuracy. *Proceedings of the Nutrition Society*, **72** (**OCE3**) EI68. http://journals.cambridge.org/download.php?file=%2FPNS%2FPNS72_OCE3%2FS0029665113001912a.pdf&code=b829a9045e37d138799cf8f415584175.

Logue, D.M. *et al.* (2014) Calorie menu labelling in Ireland: a survey of food service businesses. *Proceedings of the Nutrition Society*, **72** (**OCE3**), E167. http://journals.cambridge.org/download.php?file=%2FPNS%2FPNS72_OCE3%2FS0029665113001900a.pdf&code=e7edcd911a0eb4e3a8274c4fdfabca59.

CASE STUDY 9

Genetics and hyperlipidaemia

Sherly X. Li & Julie Lovegrove

Hannah is a 30-year-old single mother with two young children. She is of Chinese descent and moved to the United Kingdom 6 years ago; she has a good level of English. Recently, her mother suffered a heart attack, which prompted Hannah's first visit to the general practitioner (GP). Meanwhile, Hannah performed a predictive genetic test independently through an online company, which showed an increased risk of developing cardiovascular disease (CVD); she has the ε4 variant of the *APOE* gene. The company has recommended a daily supplement as well as dietary changes. Blood tests showed raised blood lipids and her GP referred Hannah to a dietitian for lifestyle management. Hannah is very concerned and anxious about her health.

Assessment

Domain	
Anthropometry, body composition and functional	Weight 67.5 kg (stable for past year) Height 1.65 m Waist circumference 83 cm
Biochemistry and haematology	Fasting glucose 5.2 mmol/L Fasting lipids Total cholesterol (TC) 6.9 mmol/L Low density lipoproteins (LDL) cholesterol 5.4 mmol/L High density lipoproteins (HDL) cholesterol 1.5 mmol/L Triglycerides (TG) 2.2 mmol/L Liver function tests Albumin 36 g/L Protein 82 g/L Total bilirubin 5 μmol/L Gamma glutamyl transpeptidase (GGT) 60 U/L Alkaline phosphatase (ALP) 160 U/L Alanine aminotransferase (ALT) 60 U/L Aspartate aminotransferase (AST) 40 U/L

Dietetic and Nutrition Case Studies, First Edition.
Edited by Judy Lawrence, Pauline Douglas, and Joan Gandy.

Companion Website: http://www.manualofdieteticpractice.com/

Assessment *(continued)*

Domain	
Clinical	Past medical history – none Medication/supplementation – none Blood pressure (BP) 145/80 mmHg
Diet	Diet history *Breakfast* Chinese rice porridge made with soya milk (200 g) Chinese bun (plain wheat flour) (40 g) Pickled vegetables (75 g) *Mid-morning* Ryvita crackers (2 × 20 g) Kaya (coconut jam) (15 g) Fruit juice (190 mL) *Lunch (at local café)* Meat pie (150 g) or pasty (145 g) or battered fish (170 g) Chips (200 g) Strawberry milk shake (300 mL) *Afternoon snack* Biscuits (e.g. oat based or shortbread) (3 × 13 g) or cake, for example, chocolate/cream éclair (65 g) or cake slice (35 g) *Dinner – home cooked* White rice (180 g) Stir-fry (may be vegetables/ meat/ combination), uses oyster sauce and Chinese spices (360 g) Soup (mainly stock-based with tomatoes and egg) 1 bowl (180 g) Fruit (e.g. apple) – 1 piece (112 g) Ice cream (95 g) *Evening snack* Chocolate biscuits (2 × 18 g) Crisps (40 g) Chinese cake (2 × 40 g)
Environmental, behavioural and social	Chinese culture influences her cooking, shopping and food beliefs Her mother lives with her and helps in caring for her children. She attends Yum Cha once a week with her family. This is a popular Chinese style of eating brunch or morning/afternoon tea, which is composed of various small dishes of foods (similar to tapas or mezze) Yoga 3 times per week

Questions

1. Calculate Hannah's body mass index; what does it tell you? Comment on ethnicity and BMI cut offs.
2. What does her waist circumference tell you?
3. Why is it important to measure Hannah's fasting glucose and lipids?
4. What modifiable and non-modifiable risk factors for CVD does Hannah present with?
5. What other potential risk factors or characteristics should you clarify in the assessment? Tabulate your answers using the ABCDE format.
6. Define combined hyperlipidaemia. What are the modes of inheritance for combined hyperlipidaemia? Discuss the inheritance of these conditions and their characteristics. Consider if it is a monogenic or polygenic condition and the role of environmental versus genetic risk factors.
7. Assuming Hannah has acquired combined hyperlipidaemia (multifactorial condition), what is the dietetic diagnosis? Write this as a PASS statement. (NB: assume this mode of inheritance, until told otherwise.)
8. Comment on Hannah's current diet.
9. What are the aims of the dietetic intervention?
10. Describe the dietetic intervention.
11. What outcome measures would you use to monitor Hannah's progress?
12. What are the barriers to change? How can you help Hannah to overcome them?

Further questions

13. What dietary changes would you recommend for the following lipid abnormalities? Elevated total cholesterol and/or LDL-C, elevated TG and low HDL-C
14. What advice would you give Hannah on the online genetic test she has undertaken and their recommendation for supplementation?
15. Whilst speaking about what prompted her to take this test, Hannah reveals that she has a family history of CVD. Apart from her mother's recent heart attack, her father (56 years) has hypertension and hyperlipidaemia and is managed through medication. Her maternal deceased grandmother also had a premature heart attack at the age of 55. Her brother and maternal grandfather were healthy. She has two maternal aunts but is unsure about their health status. With this additional information, draw a pedigree focusing on hyperlipidaemia and CVD.
16. From the pedigree why would you suspect that Hannah may be at risk of the inherited condition familial combined hyperlipidaemia (FCH)?
17. If she was diagnosed with FCH, would your dietary recommendations change?
18. What will this mean for Hannah's family?

References

British Cardiac Society, British Hypertension Society, Diabetes UK, HEART UK, Primary Care Cardiovascular Society and T. S. Association (2005) JBS 2: Joint British Societies' guidelines on prevention of cardiovascular disease in clinical practice. *Heart,* **91** (**suppl. 5**), v1–v52.

Brouwers, M.C., van Greevenbroek, M.M., Stehouwer, C.D., de Graaf, J. & Stalenhoef, A.F. (2012) The genetics of familial combined hyperlipidaemia. *Nature Reviews Endocrinology,* **8** (**6**), 352–362.

Camp, K.M. & Trujillo, E. (2014) Position of the academy of nutrition and dietetics: nutritional genomics. *Journal of the Academy of Nutrition and Dietetics,* **114** (**2**), 299–312.

Gaddi, A., Cicero, A., Odoo, F. *et al.* (2007) Practical guidelines for familial combined hyperlipidemia diagnosis: an up-date. *Vascular Health and Risk Management,* **3** (**6**), 877–886.

Gandy, J. (2014) Drug nutrient interactions. In: J. Gandy (ed), *Manual of Dietetic Practice,* 5th edn. Wiley Blackwell, Oxford.

HeartUK. (2014) *Familial Combined Hyperlipidaemia (FCH) [Online].* http://heartuk.org.uk/health-and-high-cholesterol/what-causes-high-cholesterol/familial-combined-hyperlipidaemia-fch [accessed on 3 May 2014].

IDF (2005) *The IDF consensus worldwide definition of the metabolic syndrome [Online].* http://www.idf.org/webdata/docs/MetSyndrome_FINAL.pdf [accessed on 3 May 2014].

Lichtenstein, A.H., Appel, L.J., Brands, M. *et al.* (2006) Diet and lifestyle recommendations revision 2006: a scientific statement from the American Heart Association Nutrition Committee. *Circulation,* **114** (**1**), 82–96.

Lovegrove, J.A. & Gitau, R. (2008) Personalized nutrition for the prevention of cardiovascular disease: a future perspective. *Journal of Human Nutrition and Dietetics,* **21** (**4**), 306–316.

NICE (2013) *Assessing Body Mass Index and Waist Circumference Thresholds for Intervening to Prevent ill Health and Premature Death Among Adults from Black, Asian and Other Minority Ethnic Groups in the UK.* NICE, UK, pp. 1–50.

Reiner, Ž., Catapano, A.L., De Backer, G. *et al.* (2011) ESC/EAS Guidelines for the management of dyslipidaemias: The Task Force for the management of dyslipidaemias of the European Society of Cardiology (ESC) and the European Atherosclerosis Society (EAS). *European Heart Journal,* **32** (**14**), 1769–1818.

WHO (2004) Appropriate body-mass index for Asian populations and its implications for policy and intervention strategies. *The Lancet,* **363** (**9403**), 157–163.

Resources

Instone, J. & Whelan, K. (2014) Genetics and nutritional genomics. In: J. Gandy (ed), *Manual of Dietetic Practice,* 5th edn. Wiley Blackwell, Oxford.

National Coalition for Heath Professional Education in Genetics – Genetics and nutrition. www.nchpeg.org/nutrition.

National Genetics Education and Development Centre. www.geneticseducation.nhs.uk/index.aspx.

Nutrigenomics Organization (NuGO). http://www.nugo.org.

Thaker, A. (2014) Dietary patterns of Black and minority ethnic groups. In: J. Gandy (ed), *Manual of Dietetic Practice,* 5th edn. Wiley Blackwell, Oxford.

Thaker, A. & Barton, A. (2012) *Multicultural Handbook of Food. Nutrition and Dietetics.* Blackwell Science, Oxford.

CASE STUDY 10
Intestinal failure

Alison Culkin

Jack is a 44-year-old Caucasian man, who was referred for nutritional management of a high output jejunostomy following surgery 6 weeks earlier for ischaemic small bowel. He has 120 cm of jejunum to a stoma. He has started mobilising around the ward but spends most of the day in a chair or in bed. Jack was on parenteral nutrition via a peripherally inserted central catheter (PICC) but developed a central venous catheter infection; therefore, the PICC was removed 2 weeks ago. Since then he has been maintained on 2 L of intravenous (IV) fluids and electrolytes via a peripheral cannula whilst awaiting a permanent central venous catheter for home. He is eating and drinking freely and reports a good appetite. Oral fluid intake is 2 L/day, stoma output is 3 L/day and urine output is 1.5 L/day. Jack works as a mechanic and lives with his boyfriend. He is usually active and plays football twice a week and is keen to regain weight and strength.

Assessment

Domain	
Anthropometry, body composition and functional	Weight Current 66 kg 3 months ago 80 kg Height 1.8 m Mid upper arm circumference 27.3 cm Tricep skinfold thickness 5.2 mm Grip strength dynamometry 20 kg
Biochemical and haematological	Sodium 132 mmol/L Potassium 5.0 mmol/L Urea 8.8 mmol/L Creatinine 91 mmol/L Albumin 30 g/L Corrected calcium 2.52 mmol/L Phosphate 1.36 mmol/L

Dietetic and Nutrition Case Studies, First Edition.
Edited by Judy Lawrence, Pauline Douglas, and Joan Gandy.

Companion Website: http://www.manualofdieteticpractice.com/

Assessment (*continued*)

Domain	
	Magnesium 0.63 mmol/L Alkaline phosphatase 633 IU/L Bilirubin 20 µmol/L Alanine transaminase (ALT) 290 IU/L CRP 11 mg/L White cell count 10.4×10^9 L Haemoglobin (Hb) 104 g/L Vitamin B_{12} 700 pg/mL Ferritin 27 mg/L
Clinical	Looks dehydrated, eyes sunken, dry flaky skin, complaining of thirst, low blood pressure, muscle wasting *Medication* Omeprazole 20 mg od Codeine phosphate 30 mg qds Loperamide 6 mg qds 1 L oral rehydration solution
Diet	24 h recall and food record chart in hospital *Breakfast* Weetabix × 2 (2 × 20 g) with full fat milk (100 mL), banana (100 g), orange juice(125 mL), coffee with full fat milk (25 mL), 2 sugars (2 × 5 g) *Mid-morning* Tea with full fat milk (25 mL), 2 tsp sugar (2 × 5 g), 2 digestive biscuits (2 × 15 g) *Lunch* Cheese and tomato sandwich (185 g), full fat yoghurt (125 g), sports drink (500 mL) *Mid-afternoon* Tea with full fat milk (25 mL), 2 tsp sugar (2 × 5 g), a slice of sponge cake (40 g) *Evening meal* Shepherds pie (400 g) with carrots (60 g) and gravy (50 g), rice pudding (200 g), tea with full fat milk (25 mL), 2 tsp (2 × 5 g) sugar *Bedtime* Water
Environmental, behavioural and social	Jack goes to the supermarket once a week but his boyfriend does most of the cooking. He usually has a fry up for lunch at a café near the garage where he works

Questions

1. What is the nutrition and dietetic diagnosis? Write this as a PASS statement.
2. The doctors request that he starts on the intestinal failure regimen. What advice would you give to maximise his oral intake and reduce his stoma output?
3. What are the aims of the dietetic intervention plan?
4. What SMART goal(s) and outcome measures would you use to monitor the objectives?
5. How would you involve Jack in his dietetic goal setting?
6. Explain how you would implement the dietetic intervention?
7. How would you document Jack's care?
8. What aspects of Jack's care would require you to work collaboratively with other allied health professionals (AHPs)? List the AHPs and the aspects of care they manage.
9. What information would you need to collect to monitor and review Jack?
10. How would you obtain feedback from Jack on your service?

Further questions

11. What are the important biochemical results and how did you distinguish them from the other results provided?
12. What are the possible barriers to change?
13. How can you help overcome these barriers?

Reference

BDA (2008) *Guidance for dietitians for records and record keeping.* https://www.bda.uk.com/publications/professional/record_keeping [accessed on 28 November 2015].

Resources

Culkin, A. (2014). In: J. Gandy (ed), *Intestinal failure and resection. In Manual of Dietetic Practice,* 5th edn. Wiley Blackwell, Oxford.

Culkin, A. (2014) Intestinal failure and nutrition. In: M. Lomer (ed), *Advanced Nutrition and Dietetics in Gastroenterology*. Wiley-Blackwell, Oxford.

CASE STUDY 11

Irritable bowel syndrome

Yvonne McKenzie

Jackie is 35 years old. She did not have any problems with her health until 3 years ago but now she has heartburn, burping and bloating. She has had a gastroscopy, which showed a small hiatus hernia. Her symptoms settled down but in the following year she moved to another part of the country and her present problems, of vast abdominal bloating towards the end of the day, started, along with a tendency towards diarrhoea. Her weight remains steady.

Jackie had an appendicectomy when she was 11 years old. Her father had colorectal cancer and died in his sixties. The gastroenterologist has agreed with her GP that her symptoms are typical of bowel irritability but they seem to have come out of the blue. Colonoscopy and pelvic ultrasound showed no underlying pathology. He prescribed amitriptyline, 10 mg nocte, asking her to take it for at least 3 weeks, and refers her to the dietitian to see whether dietetic intervention might help her symptoms.

Assessment

Domain	
Anthropometry	Weight 66 kg Height 1.56 m BMI 27 kg/m^2
Biochemical and haematological	Normal
Clinical	Medication – amitriptyline 10 mg Current symptoms (scoring – impact on quality of life) Abdominal pain 6/10 Bloating with distension 10/10 Wind 10/10; Sense of urgency 10/10 Bowels open 2–3 × per day Bristol stool form type 5–7 Lactose intolerance

Dietetic and Nutrition Case Studies, First Edition.
Edited by Judy Lawrence, Pauline Douglas, and Joan Gandy.

Companion Website: http://www.manualofdieteticpractice.com/

Assessment (*continued*)

Domain	
Diet	Diet history *Breakfast* Porridge (30 g) with water and skimmed milk (50 g), honey (10 g), blueberries (50 g) or pomegranates (40 g) *Lunch* (From home, eaten quickly at desk while checking emails) Large bowl of salad – leaves, beetroot, tomato, cucumber, celery, radishes, coleslaw, potato salad (85 g), with ham (35 g), cottage cheese (112 g), salmon (100 g) or prawns (60 g) or soup (220 g) in winter *Evening meal* Meat (130 g) or fish (150 g), variety of vegetables, for example, cabbage (95 g), carrot (60 g), leek (160 g), broccoli (85 g); potato (175 g), no other starchy foods *Snacks* Fruit (2 pieces a day, e.g. apple (112 g), pear (170 g), plums (120 g), grapes (100 g)), low calorie wafer (15 g) or yoghurt (125 g), fromage frais (100 g) or jelly (115 g) *Drinks* Tea, coffee, water, fruit teas, for example, liquorice, fennel
Environmental behavioural and social	Attends a weekly community weight management class Walks a lot Shops online or at a large supermarket

Jackie wants to weigh 60 kg and has been struggling to lose weight for the past year. She tells you what foods seem to exacerbate symptoms. Cold milk on granola gives her abdominal cramping, urgency and looseness, but warm milk on porridge seems to be fine; cake and mushy peas give her wind. She gave up eating bread 8 months ago because it made her bloating worse. She recently went to an office party, where within an hour of eating her bloating was really bad.

Questions

1. What medical condition should have been excluded when presented with a patient with IBS and why? What might the patient be asked to ensure that her diet was appropriate for this diagnostic testing in primary care?
2. What is the nutrition and dietetic nutritional diagnosis? Write as a PASS statement.

3. Describe the intervention.
4. What healthy eating advice can you give her?
5. At her first consultation, to what extent should Jackie's desire to lose weight be considered?
6. Estimate her fibre intake and compare it with the amount recommended in the UK general healthy eating guideline. What is your evaluation?
7. To increase food variety, what starchy foods might be suggested that she includes? What are the barriers to this change?
8. Compare her calcium intake to normal requirements and if necessary, suggest how it can be increased if she follows a low lactose diet.
9. She has not taken the prescribed amitriptyline. How could this be discussed? What advice could be given?
10. Jackie asks whether she should take a probiotic. How do you respond?
11. What outcome measures relevant to IBS could you use to assess the success of the intervention?
12. What is the new nutrition and dietetic diagnosis? Write as a PASS statement.

Further questions

13. What are FODMAPs?
14. Which foods high in FODMAPs short-chain carbohydrates are most likely to be implicated in her diarrhoea and bloating?
15. Describe two mechanisms that underpin the restriction of short-chain carbohydrates in IBS?
16. How quickly might she respond positively to the dietary intervention?
17. For how long will you advise her to follow a diet restricted in short-chain carbohydrates?
18. How important and relevant is it for her to undertake planned, systematic re-introduction of foods high in short-chain carbohydrates?
19. If a diet restricted in short-chain carbohydrates is not successful, what dietary advice will you give her as treatment to improve her IBS symptoms? What else can you recommend or do to help her?

References

Ford (2014) Efficacy of prebiotics, probiotics, and synbiotics in irritable bowel syndrome and chronic idiopathic constipation: systematic review and meta-analysis. *American Journal of Gastroenterology*, **109** (**10**), 1547–1561. doi:10.1038/ajg.2014.202 Epub 2014 Jul 29.

Halmos, E.P., Christophersen, C.T., Bird, A.R. *et al.* (2014) Diets that differ in their FODMAP content alter the colonic luminal microenvironment. *Gut*, **0**, 1–8 Published Online First.

Ludvigsson, J.F., Bai, J.C., Biagi, F. *et al.* (2014) Diagnosis and management of adult coeliac disease: guidelines from the British Society of Gastroenterology. *Gut*, **63** (**8**), 1210–1228. doi:10.1136/gutjnl-2013-306578.

NICE (2009) *Coeliac disease: recognition and assessment of coeliac disease CG86*. www.nice.org.uk/guidance/cg86 [accessed on 5 March 2015].

NICE (2015) *Irritable bowel syndrome in adults: diagnosis and management of irritable bowel syndrome in primary care (CG61)*. www.nice.org.uk/guidance/cg61 [accessed on 6 March 2015].

Staudacher, H. *et al.* (2012) Fermentable carbohydrate restriction reduces luminal bifidobacteria and gastrointestinal symptoms in patients with irritable bowel syndrome. *Journal of Nutrition*, **142** (**8**), 1510–1518.

Resources

McKenzie, Y. (2014) Irritable bowel syndrome. In: J. Gandy (ed), *Manual of Dietetic Practice*, 5th edn. Wiley Blackwell, Oxford, pp. 460–465.

PEN: Practice Based Evidence in Nutrition. *Gastrointestinal Disease – Irritable Bowel Syndrome*. http://www.pennutrition.com/KnowledgePathway.aspx?kpid=3382&trid=19021&trcatid=38.

Staudacher, H.M. *et al.* (2014) Mechanisms and efficacy of dietary FODMAP restriction in IBS. *Nature Reviews Gastroenterology and Hepatology*, **11**, 256–266.

CASE STUDY 12
Liver disease

Susie Hamlin & Julie Leaper

Richard is a 48-year-old Caucasian male who lives with his wife and two children. Three months ago he visited his GP after noticing that he was jaundiced following a family wedding. He subsequently was diagnosed with decompensated liver disease due to previously undiagnosed liver cirrhosis secondary to alcohol.

He is not completely abstinent but has significantly cut down his alcohol intake from 48 units to 12 units per week. Due to his initial diagnosis of alcohol related liver disease (ARLD) Richard has not been well enough to return to work as an accountant and is currently on reduced sick pay. He has noticed he has lost a lot of his muscle mass and his weight has dropped from 84 kg to 70 kg. He has moderate ascites. His appetite is poor. His GP has referred him to dietetic services for assessment and advice.

Assessment

Domain	
Anthropometry, body composition and functional	Weight 70 kg with moderate ascites Height 1.80 m Handgrip strength 26 kg = 65% (Bishop *et al.*, 1981) Mid arm muscle circumference (MAMC) 18.3 cm = below 5th centile (Todorovic & Micklewright, 2011) Unable to walk his dog due to fatigue
Biochemical and haematological	Vitamin A 0.85 μmol/L Vitamin D (1,25 OHD) 48 nmol/L Vitamin E 8 μmol/L Prothombin time 23 s Sodium 134 mmol/L Hb 120 g/L Ascorbic acid 0.76 μmol/L

Dietetic and Nutrition Case Studies, First Edition.
Edited by Judy Lawrence, Pauline Douglas, and Joan Gandy.

Companion Website: http://www.manualofdieteticpractice.com/

Assessment *(continued)*

Domain	
Clinical	Occasional constipation, pale stools 6–7 L ascites drained via large volume paracentesis drain (LVP) every 3 weeks as an inpatient *Medication* Thiamine 300 mg and vitamin B Co strong, 2 tablets tds Calcium 1 g and vitamin D 800 IU/day Spironolactone 400 mg/day Furosemide 100 mg/day
Diet	24 h recall = 1490 kcal, 52 g protein, 4.1 g salt Dietary Intake declines as ascites accumulates and increases in the days following the drain
Environmental, behavioural and social	Wife does all the cooking and shopping, eats with family Home owner University educated

Questions

1. What is the nutrition and dietetic diagnosis? Write this as a PASS statement.
2. What other assessments do you suggest for this patient? Present your results in a table using the ABCDE format.
3. Which predictive equations would you use to estimate energy and protein requirements and why?
4. Calculate his requirements for energy and protein. Explain what weight you use and why.
5. How much salt would you recommend he has per day?
6. What is the aim of your dietetic intervention plan? Include SMART goals and outcome measures.
7. What kind of meal pattern would you recommend for Richard?
8. What information would you need to collect to monitor and review Richard?
9. What outcome measures would you use to monitor your objectives?
10. How would you document Richards's care?

Further questions

11. Is there any specialist consideration you may have when increasing protein in Richards's diet?
12. What pattern of protein intake may be beneficial?
13. Why is Richard on thiamine and vitamin B Co strong?
14. How appropriate is it to consider long term (+1 year) outcomes?
15. What biochemical abnormalities may you see while on diuretics that may require dietetic intervention?

References

Amodio, P., Bemeur, C., Butterworth, R. *et al.* (2013) The nutritional management of hepatic encephalopathy in patients with cirrhosis: International Society for Hepatic Encephalopathy and Nitrogen Metabolism Consensus. *Hepatology*, **58**, 325–336.

Angeli, P., Fasolato, S., Mazza, E. *et al.* (2010) Combined versus sequential diuretic treatment of ascites in non-azotaemic patients with cirrhosis: results of an open randomised clinical trial. *Gut*, **59** (**1**), 98–104.

Bishop, CM., Bowen, PF., Ritchley, SJ. (1981) Norms for nutritional assessment of American adults by upper arm anthropometry. *American Journal of Clinical Nutrition*, **34**,**11** 2590–2599.

Collier, J.D., Ninkovic, M. & Compston, J.E. (2002) Guidelines on the management of osteoporosis associated with chronic liver disease. *Gut*, **50** (**Suppl. 1**), i1–i9.

European Association for the Study of Liver (2010) EASL clinical practice guidelines on the management of ascites, spontaneous bacterial peritonitis, and hepatorenal syndrome in cirrhosis. *Journal of Hepatology*, **53**, 397–417.

Gauthier, A., Levy, V.G. & Quinton, A. (1986) Salt or not salt in the treatment of cirrhotic ascites: a randomized study. *Gut*, **27**, 705–709.

Guevara, M., Cárdenas, A., Uriz, J. *et al.* (2005) Prognosis in patients with cirhosis and ascites. In: *Ascites and Renal Dysfunction in Liver Disease: Pathogenesis, Diagnosis and Treatment*. Blackwell, Malden, pp. 260–270.

Guevara, M. & Gines, P. (2005) Hepatorenal syndrome. *Digestive Diseases*, **23** (**1**), 47–55.

Henry, C.J.K. (2005) Basal metabolic rate studies in humans: measurement and development of new equations. *Public Health Nutrition*, **8**, 1133–1152.

Kondrup, J. & Muller, M.J. (1997) Energy and protein requirements of patients with chronic liver disease. *Journal of Hepatology*, **27** (**1**), 239–247.

Moreau, R., Delegue, P., Pessione, F. *et al.* (2004) Clinical characteristics and outcome of patients with cirrhosis and refractory ascites. *Liver International*, **24**, 457–464.

NICE (2010) *Alcohol-Use Disorders*. National Institute for Clinical Excellence, NICE, London.

Plank, L.D., Gane, E.J., Peng, S. *et al.* (2008) Nocturnal nutritional supplementation improves total body protein status of patients with liver cirrhosis: a randomized 12-month trial. *Hepatology*, **48** (**2**), 557–566.

Plauth, M., Cabre, E., Riggio, O. *et al.* (2006) ESPEN guidelines on enteral nutrition: liver disease. *Clinical Nutrition*, **25** (**2**), 285–294.

Todorovic, V. & Micklewright, A. (2011) *A Pocket Guide To Clinical Nutrition*, 4th edn. Parenteral and Enteral Nutrition Group of the British Dietetic Association, BDA, Birmingham.

Tsien, C.D., McCullough, A.J. & Dasarathy, S. (2011) Late evening snack . exploiting a period of anabolic opportunity in cirrhosis. *Journal of Gastroenterology and Hepatology*, **27**, 430–441.

Tsuchiya, M., Sakaida, I., Okamoto, M. *et al.* (2005) The effect of a late evening snack in patients with liver cirrhosis. *Hepatology Research*, **31** (**2**), 95–103.

Yamanaka-Okumura, H., Nakamura, T., Takeuchi, H. *et al.* (2006) Effect of late evening snack with rice ball on energy metabolism in liver cirrhosis. *European Journal of Clinical Nutrition*, **60** (**9**), 1067–1072.

Resource

Hamlin, S. & Leaper, J. (2014) Liver and biliary disease. In: J. Gandy (ed), *Manual of Dietetic Practice*, 5th edition, Wiley Blackwell, Oxford.

CASE STUDY 13
Renal disease

Sue Perry

Martin is a 67-year-old retired married man who was diagnosed with stage 3 chronic kidney disease (CKD) 5 years ago. Martin went to see his GP a week ago, following recent onset of haematuria and lethargy. He was found to have proteinuria and a urinary tract infection (UTI) that was treated with antibiotics. Blood tests were also taken to check kidney function. Martin has been referred urgently because of his recent hyperkalaemia; as a result his Ramipril has been stopped. The GP also noted his recent weight loss.

Assessment

Domain				
Anthropometry, body composition and functional	Weight Current – 69 kg 3/12 ago – 75 kg Height 1.75 m Current BMI 22.5 kg/m^2			
Biochemistry and haematology		*Present*	*1/52 ago*	*3/12 ago*
	Urea (mmol/L)	21	26	18
	Creatinine (μmol/L)	205	214	178
	Sodium (mmol/L)	139	141	138
	Potassium (mmol/L)	6.0	6.2	4.5
	Bicarbonate (mmol/L)	20	19	25
	Albumin (g/L)	34	35	38
	eGFR mL/min	30	28	35
Clinical	Proteinuria UTI treated by antibiotics *Past medical history* Hypertension and hypercholesterolaemia *Medication* Amlodipine 10 mg od, Ramipril 5 mg od, Simvastatin 20 mg od			

Dietetic and Nutrition Case Studies, First Edition.
Edited by Judy Lawrence, Pauline Douglas, and Joan Gandy.

Companion Website: http://www.manualofdieteticpractice.com/

Assessment (*continued*)

Domain	
Diet	(24 h recall) *Breakfast* Cornflakes (30g) plus semi-skimmed milk (100g) (no sugar) 200 mL glass of orange juice Cup of tea (no sugar, 15g semi-skimmed milk) *Mid-morning* Mug of Complan (55g strawberry powder, 200 mL water) *Lunch* Small bowl of vegetable soup (150g) 1 slice of whole meal bread (25g) with polyunsaturated spread (7g) No longer having a banana Cup of coffee *Mid-afternoon* Cup of tea; 1 digestive biscuit *Evening meal* 2 small slices roast chicken (75g), 2 small roast potatoes (2×50g), gravy 1 tbsp carrots, 1 tbsp sprouts (steamed); Fruit yoghurt (125g) Cup of tea *Bedtime* Mug of Complan 1 digestive biscuit
Environmental, behavioural and social	None relevant

Martin attends the consultation with his wife. He states that he is recovering from the UTI but his appetite is still poor. His appetite started to reduce 6 weeks ago and his wife had bought him some over-the-counter supplement drinks to help.

Questions

1. What other assessments do you suggest and why? Present your results in the ABCDE format.
2. What is the nutrition and dietetic diagnosis? Write this as a PASS statement.
3. What is the aim of your dietetic intervention plan? Include SMART goal(s) and outcome measures.
4. How would you involve Martin in his dietetic goal setting?
5. How would you evaluate Martin's progress? Justify your choice of outcome measures.
6. How would you obtain feedback from Martin on your service?

7. What are the important biochemical results and how did you distinguish them from the other results provided?
8. What are the possible barriers to change?
9. Explain how you would implement the dietetic intervention.
10. What information would you need to collect to monitor and review Martin?

Further questions

11. What would your answer be if Martin asked what should he eat in order to help his kidney function once his appetite improves?
12. How else would you monitor nutritional status if Martin had oedema and his weight change was unreliable?
13. Should Martin have his nutritional status monitored regularly?
14. When should you refer on to specialist renal team?

References

Caggiula, A.W. & Milas, N.C. (1993) Approaches to successful nutritional intervention in renal disease. In: W.E. Mitch & S. Klahr (eds), *Nutrition and the Kidney*. pp. 365–387. Little, Brown and Company.

Cano, N., Fiaccadori, E., Tesinsky, P. *et al.* (2006) ESPEN guidelines on enteral nutrition: adult renal failure. *Clinical Nutrition*, **25**, 295–310.

Jones-Burton, C., Mishra, S.I., Fink, J.C. *et al.* (2006) An in-depth review of the evidence linking dietary salt intake and progression of chronic kidney disease. *American Journal of Nephrology*, **26**, 268–275.

Jones, C.H. (2001) Serum albumin – a marker of fluid overload in dialysis patients? *Journal of Renal Nutrition*, **11**, 59–56.

National Institute of Health and Clinical Excellence (NICE) (2008) *CG 73. Chronic kidney disease: early identification and management of chronic kidney disease in adults in primary and secondary care.* http://www.nice.org.uk/Guidance/CG73 [accessed on June 2014].

Perry, S. & Hartley, G. (2014) Acute and chronic kidney disease. In: J. Gandy (ed), *Manual of Dietetic Practice*, 5th edn. Wiley Blackwell, Oxford.

Pollock, C., Voss, D., Hodson, E. *et al.* (2005) Caring for Australasians with renal impairment (CARI). The CARI guidelines. Nutrition and growth in kidney disease. *Nephrology*, **10** (**S5**), S177–S230.

Scottish Intercollegiate Guidelines Network (SIGN) (2008) *Diagnosis and management of chronic kidney disease: a national clinical guideline.* www.sign.ac.uk/pdf/sign103.pdf [accessed on April 2011].

The Renal Association Guidelines (2010) *Nutrition in CKD.* http://www.renal.org/Clinical/GuidelinesSection/NutritionInCKD.aspx [accessed on June 2014].

The Renal Association Guidelines (2011) *Detection, monitoring and care of patients with CKD.* http://www.renal.org/Clinical/GuidelinesSection/Detection-Monitoring-and-Care-of-Patients-with-CKD.aspx [accessed on June 2014].

Resource

Perry, S. & Hartley, G. (2014) Acute and chronic kidney disease. In: J. Gandy (ed), *Manual of Dietetic Practice*, 5th edn. Wiley Blackwell, Oxford.

CASE STUDY 14

Renal – black and ethnic minority

Bushra Siddiqui & Bushra Jafri

Amina is a 70-year-old widow. She moved to the United Kingdom 50 years ago with her husband. They have two children who live nearby and help with their day-to-day activities. She is a retired sales assistant. While she can speak English she likes to speak in Urdu when possible. She always asks to see the same doctor and dietitian who are able to communicate in Urdu with her. As a Muslim, Amina has a Halal diet.

Assessment

Domain			
Anthropometry	Weight 73 kg Height 1.60 m BMI 29 kg/m^2		
Biochemistry and haematology		*Current*	*6/12 ago*
	Sodium (mmol/L)	143	140
	Potassium (mmol/L)	6.2	4.8
	Urea (mmol/L)	28.5	22.3
	Creatinine (mmol/L)	680	700
	Bicarbonate (mmol/L)	28	22
	Phosphate (mmol/L)	2.05	1.91
	Albumin (g/L)	32	29
Clinical	End-stage renal failure Transplant failed and accepted for haemodialysis Right brachio cephalic fistula created for haemodialysis *Medication* Alfacalcidol 0.75 μg od Allopurinol 100 mg od Bumetanide 3 mg od Calcichew bd with meals Doxazosin 8 mg tds Prednisolone 7.5 mg od Sodium bicarbonate 1 g tds		

Dietetic and Nutrition Case Studies, First Edition.
Edited by Judy Lawrence, Pauline Douglas, and Joan Gandy.

Companion Website: http://www.manualofdieteticpractice.com/

Assessment *(continued)*

Domain	
Diet	*Breakfast* Medium bowl semolina pudding (Suji ka halva) (200 g), oiled bread (140 g) (Parata) Or 1 fried egg (60 g), oiled bread (140 g) (parata) Or Small bowl of high bran flakes (20 g), full fat milk (100 g) Tea, full fat milk (25 g), 2 tsps sugar *Mid-morning* Tea, full fat milk (25 g), 2 tsps sugar 1–2 custard cream biscuits (11–22 g) *Lunch* 1–2 small chapattis (55–110 g) (roti) made of brown flour with potato and beef curry (260 g) (Aloo ghosh salaan) Or 1–2 small chapattis (55–110 g) (roti) with lentils (200 g) (masoor daal) *Mid-afternoon* 2 peaches (300 g) *Evening meal* Banana (125 g) sandwich made with two slices of wholemeal bread (160 g) Or Jacket potato (100 g) (small), cheese (20 g), kheer (200 g) (rice pudding made with whole milk), mithai *Evening snack* 2 small plums (110 g) 220 mL yoghurt drink (lassi) *Other snacks* Dried fruit raisins (30 g), banana chips (13 g), nuts – cashews (25 g), cake (70 g) rusks (10–20 g) and Bombay mix snack (30 g) *Alcohol* None
Environmental, behavioural and social	Physical activity Walking (30 min once a day) Non-smoker

Questions

1. Use Amina's biochemistry to make a nutrition and dietetic diagnosis, and write it as a PASS statement.
2. What diet would you prescribe for Amina, and considering her culture how would you address her nutritional goals?
3. What SMART goals would you hope to help Amina achieve in the short term?
4. What short-term changes would you make to her diet over the next few sessions you have with her in order to achieve these goals? Remember to consider her culture.
5. What are the key dietary considerations?
6. How would you negotiate/prioritise these changes with Amina?
7. What SMART goals would you hope to help Amina achieve in the long term?
8. What long-term changes would you suggest to help Amina achieve these goals?
9. Estimate Amina's dietary intake from the diet history and compare with her dietary requirements.
10. What are the potential cultural barriers to change?
11. What outcomes would you monitor in order to evaluate the success of the proposed changes?
12. Would Amina be expected to fast during Ramadan? What advice might you give?

Reference

Renal Association (2009) *Nutrition in CKD.* www.renal.org/guidelines/modules/nutrition-in-ckd#sthash.cQGMOGsH.dpbs [accessed on 24 November 2014].

Resources

Perry, S. & Hartley, G. (2014) Acute and chronic kidney disease. In: J. Gandy (ed), *Manual of Dietetic Practice*, 5th edn. Wiley Blackwell, Oxford.

Thaker, A. (2014) Dietary patterns of black and minority ethnic groups. In: J. Gandy (ed), *Manual of Dietetic Practice*, 5th edn. Wiley Blackwell, Oxford.

CASE STUDY 15

Motor neurone disease/amyotrophic lateral sclerosis

Elaine Cawadias & Kathleen Beggs

Peter is a 60-year-old newly retired, university lecturer; he is married with two adult children, and has a very supportive wife. He was diagnosed with motor neurone disease/amyotrophic lateral sclerosis (MND/ALS) a year ago, following an initial symptom of unexplained progressive weakness in his right arm. The neurologist who diagnosed MND/ALS referred him to a specialist clinic. He recently developed bulbar symptoms (difficulty with swallowing regular liquids and some foods). Peter has been referred for eating advice and when necessary a feeding regimen following placement of either a percutaneous endoscopic gastrostomy (PEG) or a radiologically inserted gastrostomy (RIG).

Assessment

Domain	
Anthropometry, body composition and functional	Weight Current 68.2 kg Previous 77.3 kg Height 1.78 m Physical activity questionnaires – very physically active (runner)
Biochemistry	Lab tests prior to PEG/RIG according to protocol
Clinical	Physical appearance – slim, clothes loose suggesting recent weight loss. *Medication* Rilutek, statin Pulmonary function tests – forced vital capacity (FVC) 98% predicted 62% Peak cough flow – decreased from 400 to 250 L/min

Dietetic and Nutrition Case Studies, First Edition.
Edited by Judy Lawrence, Pauline Douglas, and Joan Gandy.

Companion Website: http://www.manualofdieteticpractice.com/

Assessment *(continued)*

Domain	
Diet	Usual daily intake pattern – 3 meals and 2 snacks, adequate in most areas though often low in dairy. Had been following low cholesterol, low-saturated fat diet to control serum cholesterol
Environmental, behavioural and social	Wife does grocery shopping and most meal preparations although he was making his own breakfast and lunch until arm weakness made this tiring

Questions

1. What other assessments do you suggest?
2. What is the nutrition and dietetic diagnosis? Write this as a PASS statement.
3. What is the aim of your intervention plan? Include SMART goal(s) and outcome measures.
4. What outcome measures would you use to monitor the objectives?
5. How would you involve Peter in his dietetic goal setting?
6. Explain how you would implement the dietetic intervention?
7. How would you document Peter's care?
8. What aspects of Peter's care would require you to work collaboratively with other allied health professionals (AHPs)? List the AHPs and the aspects of care they manage.
9. What information would you need to collect to monitor and review Peter? Justify your choice of outcome measures.
10. How would you obtain feedback from Peter and his wife on your service?
11. Which predictive equation would you use to estimate energy requirements and why?
12. How would you involve Peter in his dietetic goal setting when he is unable to communicate verbally with you?
13. What are the possible barriers to change?

Further questions

14. Specify some strategies to address areas of concern with this patient?
15. At the first follow up visit 3 months after initial clinic visit, Peter's weight has dropped by 2.5 kg (5 lbs); he continues to run for stress management. At the 6-month visit weight is down an additional 2 kg (4 lbs) and meal time is longer partly due to the effort of self-feeding and taking time to be careful to avoid choking. What are your recommendations at each visit?

16. When would you initiate a discussion regarding enteral nutrition (PEG/RIG)?
17. What information should be included in a discussion and education regarding PEG/RIG?

References

ALS CNTF Treatment Study (ACTS) Phase I-II Study Group (1996) The Amyotrophic Lateral Sclerosis Functional Rating Scale. Assessment of activities of daily living in patients with Amyotrophic Lateral Sclerosis. *Archives of Neurology*, **53**, 141–147.

BDA (2008) *Guidance for dietitians for records and record keeping*. https://www.bda.uk.com/publications/professional/record_keeping [accessed on 26 March 2015]; Information for non BDA members available at www.bda.uk.com.

Kasarskis, E.J., Mendiondo, M.S., Matthews, D.E. *et al.* for the ALS Nutrition/NIPPV Study Group (2014) Estimating daily energy expenditure in individuals with amyotrophic lateral sclerosis. *American Journal of Clinical Nutrition*, **99**, 792–803.

Resource

Cawadias, E. & Rio, A. (2014) Motor neurone disease. In: J. Gandy (ed), *Manual of Dietetic Practice*, 5th edn. Wiley Blackwell, Oxford, pp. 555–563.

CASE STUDY 16

Chronic fatigue syndrome/myalgic encephalopathy

Caroline Foster & Jennifer McIntosh

Melissa is 25 years old and was diagnosed with moderate chronic fatigue syndrome/ myalgic encephalopathy (CFS/ME) 12 months ago. With the onset of CFS/ME she has struggled working and as a result recently resigned after a period of 3 months sick leave. In view of this, Melissa and her husband have been unable to pay their rent and recently moved in with Melissa's mother. Her family is very supportive but moving back into the childhood home has impacted on Melissa's independence, in particular food choices. Prior to CFS/ME Melissa had been very active taking part in long distance running with friends and finds it very frustrating she is now unable to take part in this.

Melissa's symptoms include headaches, eye pain, muscle and joint pain, poor sleep and concentration, sensitivity to light, palpitations and dizzy spells. Melissa was experiencing stomach pain, nausea and diarrhoea and as a result eliminated lactose and gluten from her diet, resulting in an improvement in the stomach pain and diarrhoea but not the nausea.

Melissa has been referred due to poor nutritional intake, reduced appetite and recent weight loss of 4 kg. She weighs 52 kg with a height of 1.69 m. The referral also states Melissa takes a combination of vitamins in large doses including magnesium and coenzyme Q10. Two years ago she had low ferritin levels. Melissa is prescribed a low dose of amitriptyline (10 mg).

When attending the GP clinic she reports she has been offered a test for coeliac disease but has declined. Melissa reported only eating one meal per day such as chicken stews or casseroles, roast chicken or fish with vegetables and potatoes, which she eats in the evening, with very little else eaten throughout the day. She reported eating only when hungry and often feels nauseous. Melissa drinks multiple cups of coffee daily, avoids alcohol and will often drink energy drinks when feeling low in energy.

Dietetic and Nutrition Case Studies, First Edition.
Edited by Judy Lawrence, Pauline Douglas, and Joan Gandy.

Companion Website: http://www.manualofdieteticpractice.com/

Questions

1. Gather the information above into an assessment using the ABCDE format. Use average portions to estimate weights of foods that Melissa has eaten.
2. What is the nutrition and dietetic diagnosis diagnosis? Write it as a PASS statement.
3. Are there any special diets for CFS/ME?
4. What is the aim and objectives of the dietary intervention?
5. What outcomes would be appropriate to monitor the success of the intervention?
6. What advice would you give regarding the use of energy drinks?
7. How is coeliac disease diagnosed? Why might Melissa have declined to have this?
8. What advice would you give regarding gluten and lactose elimination?
9. How would you encourage Melissa to eat more than one meal a day when she is feeling nauseous?

Further questions

10. What advice would you give in relation to vitamin intake?
11. What is amitriptyline and why might this be prescribed?
12. Melissa is considering seeing a homeopath, how would you advise her about alternative therapies?
13. You phone Mellissa with some follow up information but only get an answer phone message. What message would you leave?

References

Baumer, J.H. (2005) Management of chronic fatigue syndrome/myalgic encephalopathy (CFS/ME). *Archives of Disease in Childhood – Education and Practice Edition*, **90**, 46–50.

Berkovitz, S., Ambler, G., Jenkins, M. *et al.* (2009) Serum 25-hydroxy vitamin D levels in chronic fatigue syndrome: a retrospective survey. *International Journal for Vitamin and Nutrition Research*, **79** (**4**), 250.

Fraser-Mayall, H. (2014) Coeliac disease. In: J. Gandy (ed), *Manual of Dietetic Practice*, 5th edn. Wiley Blackwell, Oxford.

Gandy, J. (2014) Alternative and complementary therapies. In: J. Gandy (ed), *Manual of Dietetic Practice*, 5th edn. Wiley Blackwell, Oxford.

Luscombe, S. (2012) *Chronic Fatigue Syndrome/ME and Diet Food Facts Sheet*. British Dietetic Association, Birmingham.

McIntosh, J. (2014) Chronic fatigue syndrome/myalgic encephalopathy. In: J. Gandy (ed), *Manual of Dietetic Practice*, 5th edn. Wiley Blackwell, Oxford.

McKenzie, Y. (2014) Irritable bowel syndrome. In: J. Gandy (ed), *Manual of Dietetic Practice*, 5th edn. Wiley Blackwell, Oxford.

McKenzie, Y. A. et al. (2012) *UK evidence – based practice guidelines for the dietetic management of Irritable bowel syndrome (IBS) in adults*. IBS dietetic guideline development group BDA.

Morris, D.H. & Stare, F.J. (1993) Unproven diet therapies in the treatment of the chronic fatigue syndrome. *Archives of Family Medicine*, **2**, 181–186.

NICE (2007) *Clinical Guideline for the diagnosis and management of CFS/ME*. www.nice.org.uk/guidance/cg53 [accessed on 25 November 2014].

NICE (2008) *Irritable bowel syndrome in adults Diagnosis and management of irritable bowel syndrome in primary care*. https://www.nice.org.uk/guidance/cg61 [accessed on 25 December 2014].

NICE (2009) *Clinical guideline for the diagnosis and management of coeliac disease*. www.nice.org.uk/guidance/cg86 [accessed on 25 November 2014].

Skypala, I. & Ventner, C. (2014). In: J. Gandy (ed), *Manual of Dietetic Practice*, 5th edn. Wiley Blackwell, Oxford.

Resource

McIntosh, J. (2014) Chronic fatigue syndrome/myalgic encephalopathy. In: J. Gandy (ed), *Manual of Dietetic Practice*, 5th edn. Wiley Blackwell, Oxford.

CASE STUDY 17

Refsum's disease

Eleanor Baldwin

Alan is a 34-year-old married man who lives with his wife and three-year-old daughter. He works in human resources for a retail company. At 15 years of age he experienced visual problems and was diagnosed with retinitis pigmentosa. He is 1.75 m tall and weighs 76 kg; a weight he has maintained for several years. As a child his growth and development were normal apart from short third fingers on both hands. He has recently been complaining of numb feet, scaly, itchy skin and deteriorating vision. Alan's blood biochemistry is normal apart from a plasma phytanic acid level of 850 µmol/L. Following genetic testing, he has been diagnosed with adult Refsum's disease. He has not been prescribed medication. He has been referred for dietary advice and provides you with the following food record:

24 h recall

Breakfast – Branflakes with semi skimmed milk, orange juice, toast with high polyunsaturated fat spread and jam.
Mid-morning – Cappuccino from machine with sugar and chocolate chip cookies
Lunch – Cheese and ham toasted sandwich, can of coke, crisps and an apple
Evening meal – Spaghetti bolognaise with parmesan cheese, bananas and ice-cream
Supper – Cheese and crackers, can of lager

Food frequency

Sweets and chocolates – two or three times a week
Crisps and nuts – daily
Alcohol – 2–6 units three or four times a week
Cakes – once or twice a week, typically doughnuts or chocolate muffins
Biscuits – most days
Takeaways – weekly, usually Indian or Chinese

Dietetic and Nutrition Case Studies, First Edition.
Edited by Judy Lawrence, Pauline Douglas, and Joan Gandy.

Companion Website: http://www.manualofdieteticpractice.com/

Questions

1. Use the ABCDE format to construct a table detailing your assessment of Alan. Use average portion sizes to enter amounts of foods.
2. Use the assessment information to make a nutrition and dietetic diagnosis. Express this as a PASS statement.
3. Give details of the dietetic intervention.
4. What is phytanic acid? Identify foods in the food record that may contain phytanic acid and suggest suitable alternatives.
5. How will Alan's symptoms respond to a reduction in phytanic acid?
6. Comment on the meal pattern and describe why it is important for him to maintain a regular meal pattern and constant weight.
7. What follow up would you offer Alan? What outcome measures would you use to monitor progress?

Further questions

8. Describe the metabolism of phytanic acid and the abnormality that occurs in adult Refsum's disease giving details of the disease process.
9. Discuss the genetics of the condition; what is the risk of Alan's daughter developing the disease.

Reference

Jansen, G.A. *et al.* (2004) Molecular basis of Refsum disease: sequence variations in phytanoyl-CoA hydroxylase (PHYH) and the PTS2 receptor (PEX7). *Human Mutations*, **23** (**3**), 209–218.

Resource

Baldwin, E. (2014) Refsum's disease. In: J. Gandy (ed), *Manual of Dietetic Practice*, 5th edn. Wiley Blackwell, Oxford.

CASE STUDY 18

Adult phenylketonuria

Louise Robertson

The dietitian receives a phone call from a specialist metabolic dietitian (MeD) at the regional metabolic centre. A patient with phenylketonuria (PKU) is being admitted next week for a planned knee cartilage repair operation. Anne is 24 years old and has followed a life-long, low phenylalanine diet. She will be staying in hospital 2 days post-surgery and the MeD would like the dietitian to organise her low phenylalanine diet for her hospital admission. The following details are provided:

Assessment

Domain	
Anthropometry, body composition and functional	Weight 65 kg, no recent weight loss Height 1.62 m
Biochemical and haematological	Urea, electrolytes and nutritional bloods normal at last clinic appointment 6/12 ago Phenylalanine 650 µmol/L (3/12 ago)
Clinical	Nothing reported
Diet	Low phenylalanine diet, 10 exchanges (ex) per day, XP Maxamum 50 g tds. Twenty-four hour diet history from last clinic appointment *Breakfast* 50 g XP Maxamum Cornflakes (2 × 15 g)(2 ex) and low protein milk (100 g), low protein toast (30 g × 2) with margarine (2 × 5 g) and jam (2 × 15 g) *Lunch* One bowl of Pasta salad (230 g) (low protein pasta), sweet corn (35 g)(1 ex), peppers (50 g, onion(40 g) and mayonnaise (30 g), one packet French fries crisps (45 g)(1 ex), apple (125 g)

Dietetic and Nutrition Case Studies, First Edition.
Edited by Judy Lawrence, Pauline Douglas, and Joan Gandy.

Companion Website: http://www.manualofdieteticpractice.com/

Assessment (*continued*)

Domain	
	Mid-afternoon 50 g XP Maxamum *Evening meal* Jacket potato (240 g)(3 ex), ½ can of spaghetti hoops (200 g) (3 ex) and salad, low protein cake (65 g) *Evening* 50 g XP Maxamum and three low protein biscuits (30 g)
Environmental, behavioural and social	Lives with her parents and works as a secretary

Anne wishes to continue to follow her low phenylalanine diet while recovering in hospital.

Questions

1. What is the nutrition and dietetic diagnosis?
2. What are the aim and objectives of the dietetic intervention?
3. Explain how you would implement the dietetic intervention?
4. How would you explain to the ward staff and the hospital chefs what a low phenylalanine diet for PKU is?
5. Provide an example of a 2-day low phenylalanine diet with 10 exchanges that could be provided in hospital.
6. How would you document Anne's care?
7. What information would you need to collect to monitor and review Anne?
8. What outcome measures would you use to monitor objectives?
9. How would you involve Anne in her dietetic goal setting?
10. How would you obtain feedback from Anne on your service?

Further questions

11. What other protein substitute could the patient take and what are the advantages of these protein substitutes?
12. What range should an adult patient with PKU keep their blood phenylalanine concentrations and how often should they be monitored?
13. What other considerations should females with PKU of child-bearing age be aware of?

14. Discuss what you would do if the patient with PKU was not following a low phenylalanine diet, and what would you advise?
15. What effects will surgery have on phenylalanine levels? How would you manage this?

References

Anjema, K., van Rijn, M., Verkerk, P.H. *et al.* (2011) PKU: high plasma phenylalanine concentrations are associated with increased prevalence of mood swings. *Molecular Genetics and Metabolism*, **104** (**3**), 231–234.

Blau, N., van Spronsen, F. & Levy, H.L. (2010) Phenylketonuria. *Lancet*, **376**, 1417–1427.

Christ, S.E., Huijbregts, S.C., de Sonnerville, L.M. *et al.* (2010) Executive function in early treated phenylketonuria: profile and underlying mechanisms. *Molecular Genetics and Metabolism*, **99** (**Suppl 1**), S22–S32.

Das, A.M., Goedecke, K., Meyer, U. *et al.* (2013) Dietary habits and metabolic control in adolescences and young adults with phenylketonuria: self-imposed protein restriction may be harmful. *Journal of Inherited Metabolic Disease Reports* **2013** **13**:149-158.

Gentile, J.K., TenHoedt, A.E. & Bosch, A.M. (2010) Psychosocial aspects of PKU: hidden disabilities-a review. *Molecular Genetics and Metabolism*, **99** (**Suppl. 1**), S64–S67.

ten Hoedt, A.E., de Sonneville, L.M.J., Francois, B. *et al.* (2011) High phenylalanine levels directly affect mood and sustained attention in adults with phenylketonuria: a randomised, double-blind, placebo-controlled, crossover trial. *Journal of Inherited Metabolic Disease*, **34** (**1**), 165–171.

Maillot, F., Cook, P., Lilburn, M. *et al.* (2007) A practical approach to maternal phenylketonuria management. *Journal of Inherited Metabolic Disease*, **30**, 198–201.

Medical Research Council Working Party on Phenylketonuria (1993) Recommendations on the dietary management of phenylketonuria. *Archives of Disease in Childhood*, **68**, 426–427.

The National Society for Phenylketonuria (UK) (2004) *Management of PKU, A consensus document for the diagnosis and management of children, adolescents and adults with phenylketonuria.* http://www.nspku.org/sites/default/files/publications/Management%20of%20PKU.pdf [accessed on 24 November 2014].

The National Society for Phenylketonuria (UK) (2013) *Dietary Information for the Treatment of Phenylketonuria.* www.nspku.org/publications/publication/dietary-information-booklet [accessed on 24 November 2014].

Trefz F., Maillot F., Motzfeldt, K. *et al.* (2011) Adult phenylketonuria outcome and management. *Molecular Genetics and Metabolism*, 2011, **104 Suppl**, S26–S30.

Resource

Boocock, S., Le, R., Micciche, A. *et al.* (2014) Inherited metabolic disorders in adults. In: J. Gandy (ed), *Manual of Dietetic Pratcice*, 5th edn. Wiley Blackwell, Oxford.

CASE STUDY 19

Osteoporosis

Caoimhe McDonald

Mary is a 68-year-old lady, married with two children that are living abroad. She lives with her husband who does the shopping and cooking. Mary was a cleaner but had to stop work because of her difficulty in mobility and she takes little exercise. She attends the outpatient bone health and osteoporosis clinic in a large teaching hospital and has been referred to you for dietetic assessment and advice.

Assessment

Domain	

Anthropometry, body composition and functional	Current weight 42.5 kg
	Weight 4/12 ago 49 kg
	Stadiometer height 1.53 m
	Knee heel height 1.59 m
	Demispan (left arm) 1.58 m
	BMI
	  16.9 kg/m^2 using knee heel height
	  18.2 kg/m^2 using stadiometer height
	Tricep skinfold thickness 11.9 mm
	Mid upper arm circumference (left) 21.8 cm
	Mid arm muscle circumference (left) 18.1 cm
	Calf circumference 28.8 cm
	Bioelectrical impedance analysis
	  Fat percentage 19.5%
	  Fat free mass 34.2 kg
	  Muscle mass 32.4 kg
	  Fat mass 8.3 kg
	Grip strength dynamometry
	  Non-dominant arm 13.3 kg
	Physical activity – low score (incidental and planned activity questionnaire)
	Smoker for 40 years. Has reduced to 10/day from 20/day

Dietetic and Nutrition Case Studies, First Edition.
Edited by Judy Lawrence, Pauline Douglas, and Joan Gandy.

Companion Website: http://www.manualofdieteticpractice.com/

Assessment *(continued)*

Domain	
Biochemical and haematological	24 h urinary calcium 2.14 mmol/L Serum calcium 2.32 mmol/L Serum albumin 42 mmol/L ALP 90 mmol/L Phosphate 0.88 mmol/L Osteocalcin 21.7 mmol/L Parathyroid hormone 24.3 mmol/L C-terminal telopeptide of type 1 collagen (CTX) 0.273 mmol/L Procollagen type 1 N propeptide (P1NP) 37.6 mmol/L Serum 25 (OH)D 23 mmol/L WCC 7.0 mmol/L Hb 14.9 mmol/L Mean cell volume 95.9 f/L Platelets 283 mmol/L TG 1.1 mmol/L DXA results Total body BMD (0.868 g/cm^2) T-score 3.2 AP spine BMD (0.665 g/cm^2) T-score 4.3 Left femur BMD (0.663 g/cm^2) T-score 2.8
Clinical	Past medical history: Hypertension, hypercholesterolaemia, asthma, depression, osteoporosis – spinal fracture T10, T12, L2, L3 *Medication* Crestor, metoprolol, was on Fosamax for 4 years, but no improvement on recent DXA so switched to daily injection – parathyroid hormone Calcichew D3 Forte BD (non-compliant) Ventolin, becotide
Diet	24 h recall *Breakfast* Small bowl porridge (made with water and drop of low-fat milk (110 g)) Two slices white bread toasted (2× 27 g) with butter (20 g) and marmalade (2× 15 g) Cup of tea (190 mL)with teaspoon sugar (5 g) and drop of low-fat milk (15 mL) *Lunch* 1 slice white bread toasted (27 g) with butter (10 g) 1 sausage fried (40 g), scrambled egg (60 g) with low-fat milk (15 mL)

Assessment *(continued)*

Domain	
	Cup of tea (190 mL) with teaspoon sugar (5 g) and drop of low-fat milk (15 mL) *Dinner* 1 slice white bread (27 g) with tomato (17 g) and 1 slice ham (23 g) Cup of tea (190 mL) with 1 tsp sugar (5 g) and a drop of low-fat milk (15 mL) 2–3 glasses water during the day Note: Appetite has reduced significantly as a result of pain and she has experienced some nausea (possibly due to new medication) *Alcohol* <7 units/week underneath *Analysis of food diary* Estimated energy intake 1040 kcal Protein intake 39 g Total fat intake 55.6 g – 48% total energy Saturated fat intake 28.4 g – 25% total energy Monounsaturated fat intake 15.5 g 13% total energy Polyunsaturated fat intake 3.8 g 3% total energy Fibre 4.1 g Calcium from food 418 mg Sodium 3227 mg Iron 4.8 mg *Estimated requirements* Estimated energy requirements 1747 kcal (including weight gain factor) Estimated protein requirements 34–51 g protein/day

Questions

1. What is the nutrition and dietetic diagnosis? Write it as a PASS statement.
2. What are the main nutritional concerns for this lady?
3. Comment on the different methods used in this case to measure height to calculate BMI.
4. What are the aims and objectives of Mary's nutritional care plan?
5. What outcomes could you assess in order to monitor the success of your intervention?
6. What are the most important aspects of Mary's care that need to be documented?

7. Comment on the bioelectrical impedance analysis and hand grip results for this lady?
8. Discuss Mary's DXA results.
9. What other nutrients are important in patients with osteoporosis?
10. Would you advise Mary to see any other allied healthcare professionals? If so, who?
11. Describe the nutritional management when undergoing surgery for a broken head of femur.

References

Blackburn, B.R., Meini, B.S., Schianmm, H.T. *et al.* (1977) Nutritional and metabolic assessment of the hospitalised patient. *Journal of Parenteral and Enteral Nutrition*, **1**, 11–12.

Dawson-Hughes, B. (2003) Calcium and protein in bone health. *Proceedings of the Nutrition Society*, **62**, 505e9.

Delmi, M., Rapin, C.H., Bengoa, J.M. *et al.* (1990) Dietary supplementation in elderly patients with fractured neck of the femur. *Lancet*, **335**, 1013–1016.

Huang, Z., Himes, J.H. & McGovern, P.G. (1996) Nutrition and subsequent hip fracture risk among a national cohort of white women. *American Journal of Epidemiology*, **144**, 124–134.

Johnell, O., Gullberg, B., Kanis, J.A. *et al.* (1995) Risk factors for hip fracture in European women: the MEDOS study. Mediterranean Osteoporosis Study. *Journal of Bone and Mineral Research*, **10**, 1802–1815.

Kyle, U.G., Genton, L., Slosman, D.O. *et al.* (2001) Fat-free and fat mass percentiles in 5225 healthy subjects aged 15 to 98 years. *Nutrition*, **17**, 534–541.

Munger, R.G., Cerhan, J.R. & Chiu, B.C.H. (1999) Prospective study of dietary protein intake and risk of hip fracture in postmenopausal women. *American Journal of Clinical Nutrition*, **69**, 147–152.

Rizzoli, R., Ammann, P., Chevalley, T. *et al.* (2001) Protein intake and bone disorders in the elderly. *Joint, Bone, Spine*, **68**, 383–392.

Wardlaw, G.M. (1996) Putting body weight and osteoporosis into perspective. *American Journal of Clinical Nutrition*, **63** (**Suppl. 3**), 433S–436S.

Wolfe, R.R., Miller, S.L. & Miller, K.B. (2008) Optimal protein intake in the elderly. *Clinical Nutrition*, **27**, 675–684.

Resources

PEN: Practice Based Evidence in Nutrition. *Osteoporosis tool kit.* www.pennutrition.com/KnowledgePathway.aspx?kpid=553&tkid=21818.

Redmond, J. & Schoenmakers, I. (2014) Osteoporosis. In: J. Gandy (ed), *Manual of Dietetic Practice*, 5th edn. Wiley Blackwell, Oxford.

CASE STUDY 20

Eating disorder associated with obesity

Kate Williams

Maggie is seen in a primary care dietetics clinic at the health centre where her GP is based. She has had an NHS health check, which found an increased risk of heart disease and stroke, with raised LDL cholesterol and hypertension. She has been referred by her GP for help with her weight. The referral tells you that she is considering bariatric surgery. She has made many previous attempts to reduce her weight, but she has always regained weight rapidly. She also gained over 20 kg with her pregnancies.

Maggie is Caucasian, 42 years old, and lives with her husband and three children, who are at secondary school. She works part time as a classroom assistant, which she loves. Her mother lives alone nearby and is not in good health. Maggie has lived locally all her life, and her only sibling now lives abroad.

Maggie is not keen on having surgery as she has such a busy life, and it would be hard for her to take time away from her many responsibilities. She has never had surgery herself, but has a friend who had a bad reaction to an anaesthetic, and that makes her nervous. Maggie's height is 1.64 m and her weight on the referral (dated a month before) is 112 kg; her current weight is 115 kg. She is visibly upset and tearful that her weight has increased. She has used a variety of commercial weight loss plans and diets from books and magazines. She is concerned about the health risks that have been found, and her family is worried. She wants to try again to control her weight, to avoid surgery if she can, but is not confident that she can achieve any success.

Questions

1. What anthropometry would you assess? Would you measure Maggie's waist? Explain the reasons for your decision.
2. What information would you require from the blood tests?
3. What clinical information would you seek?
4. What information would you seek about Maggie's weight history? What information would you seek about her present eating and drinking?
5. What further information would you require about Maggie's life and the people in it?

Dietetic and Nutrition Case Studies, First Edition.
Edited by Judy Lawrence, Pauline Douglas, and Joan Gandy.

Companion Website: http://www.manualofdieteticpractice.com/

6. What would alert you to the possibility that Maggie may have binge eating disorder?
7. How would you investigate this possibility further?
8. What are the problems you need to work on with Maggie?
9. Which of these would form the basis of your primary nutrition and dietetic diagnosis?
10. Phrase the nutrition and dietetic diagnosis as a PASS statement.
11. How would you work with Maggie to develop a productive therapeutic relationship?
12. How would you respond to her obvious sensitivity about her weight and eating, to enable her to talk openly and honestly about it?
13. You confirm that Maggie binge eats at least once a week, sometimes more. How would this finding affect your approach to her care?
14. What outcome measures would you derive from these diagnoses to evaluate the success of your intervention?
15. Describe the dietetic intervention. What changes would you seek to make in Maggie's eating and drinking? How would you decide which to prioritise?

Further questions

16. How would you help her to develop her confidence in her ability to change?
17. How would you help Maggie to take forward healthy eating in the future without your support?
18. How might you work with a psychologist in primary care to support Maggie?
19. What sort of information would you need to share with the psychologist; do you need permission to do this?

References

Cotton, M.-A., Ball, C. & Robinson, P. (2003) Four simple questions can help screen for eating disorders. *Journal of General Internal Medicine*, **18** (**1**), 53–56.

Gable, J. (2007) *Counselling Skills for Dietitians*. Blackwell, Oxford.

Increasing Access to Psychological Therapies (IAPT) programme (2014) www.iapt.nhs.uk/about-iapt/ [last accessed on 7 August 2014].

Miller, W.R. & Rollnick, S. (2007) *Motivational Interviewing*. Guilford, New York.

Morgan, J.F., Reid, F. & Lacey, J.H. (1999) The SCOFF questionnaire: assessment of a new screening tool for eating disorders. *British Medical Journal*, **319**, 1467–1468.

Resources

Hunt, P. & Hillsdon, M. (1996) *Changing Eating and Exercise Behaviour: A Handbook for Professionals*. Blackwell, Oxford.

Miller, W.R., Rollnick, S. & Butler, C. (2008) *Motivational Interviewing in Healthcare: Helping Patients Change Behavior*. Guilford, New York.

Williams, K. (2014) Eating disorders. In: J. Gandy (ed), *Manual of Dietetic Practice*, 5th edn. Wiley Blackwell, Oxford.

CASE STUDY 21

Forensic mental health

Helen Bennewith & Eileen Murray

James is a 25-year-old, unmarried, Caucasian man. He has a dual diagnosis of treatment resistant paranoid schizophrenia with antisocial personality disorder. James has frontal lobe damage as a result of poly-substance misuse resulting in mild cognitive impairment.

James' personality disorder was brought to light at an early age after the death of a sibling, when he displayed signs of maladaptive behaviour. He ran away from home, fought with school peers and ill-treated the family pets. He was expelled from several schools and later he became involved with a rough crowd, abused alcohol and illegal substances that led to criminal behaviour and a short stay in an approved school.

As an adult he has served several brief prison sentences, and more recently he was referred for assessment to the local forensic mental health services from prison where he was remanded to custody on a charge of serious assault. (Patients may be remanded to hospital from court for assessment or/and treatment pending trial or sentence.) He has been referred to the dietitian due to his obesity.

Assessment

Domain	
Anthropometry, body composition and functional	Weight 120 kg Height 1.75 m Waist circumference 125 cm
Biochemistry and haematology on day 2 of admission	Total cholesterol 6.3 mmol/L HDL 0.8 mmol/L TG 3.0 mmol/L Glycosylated haemoglobin (hbA1c) 52 mmol/mol
Clinical	Chest infection reported prior to admission Dehydrated on admission Previous medical history Blood pressure 142/92 mmHg Hepatitis C virus positive Metabolic syndrome

Dietetic and Nutrition Case Studies, First Edition.
Edited by Judy Lawrence, Pauline Douglas, and Joan Gandy.

Companion Website: http://www.manualofdieteticpractice.com/

Assessment *(continued)*

Domain	
	Constipation *Physical appearance* Unkempt; poor personal cleanliness; poor dental health and oral hygiene *Medication* Clozapine 450 mg nocte Lactulose 20 mL bd Omeprazole 40 mg Simvastatin 40 mg nocte Metformin 500 mg with breakfast (SIGN 131, 2013); Amisulpride 400 mg bd Propranolol 80 mg bd Codeine phosphate 30 mg qds Loperamide 6 mg qds 1 L oral rehydration on admission
Diet	24 h recall *Breakfast (09:00)* (seldom taken) Corn flakes (30 g), semi-skimmed milk (200 mL), coffee with 2 tsp sugar *Lunch (12:15)* Lentil soup (300 g) Battered fish (225 g), chips (240 g), peas (100 g). White bread 2 × slices (72 g) buttered (20 g), 300 mL Coke *Evening (17:00)* Macaroni cheese (280 g), creamed potatoes (129 g), roasted tomatoes (170 g) White bread × 2 slices (72 g), butter × 2 (20 g); 300 mL Coke; Black Forest Gateaux (90 g) *Supper (20:00)* Egg mayonnaise sandwich (190 g); white coffee (260 g) with 2 tsp sugar (10 g) *Before bed (22:00)* Pot noodle (305 g, when made up); chocolate bar (58 g); 500 mL Coke Monthly take-away – replaces hospital meal. Patient choice is; large portion deep fried chicken (drumstick 131 g) with chips (165 g); or large meat feast extra cheese stuffed-crust pizza (1600 g); or chicken korma (200 g) with fried rice (180 g), garlic Nan (160 g), portion of mixed pakora (28 g each) Fluid (water, coffee, tea, sugar-free squash) and snacks (fruit and tea biscuits) are available throughout the day

Assessment (*continued*)

Domain	
	Restrictions are placed on patients' movements, to allow for equality in provision; a small shop is on-site. Limited shop storage space dictates the daily quantities of purchases to: 1 L soft drink 2 bars of chocolate 2 packets of crisps James buys the daily maximum, his choice being full sugar juice. In addition, to increase purchase opportunities, ward staff take the patients' shopping list to the local supermarket weekly. James' typical list: Family pack of crisps • 7 pot noodles (7 × 305 g). • 4 mini pork pies (4 × 75 g). • 6 tea cakes (6 × 60 g). • 5 bananas (5 × 100 g, without skin). Food gifts: Because of the stringent security arrangements, visitors are advised on the consumables they can bring for patients. James receives a large bar of chocolate (114 g) and 3 L Coke bi-weekly N.B. Patients have a right to make choices (European Convention on Human Rights (ECHR), 1998)
Environmental, behavioural and social	Walks 0.5–0.75 miles/day while smoking on the hospital grounds. He refuses to attend the hospital gym

James' energy requirements were calculated using the Mifflin-St Joer equation (Frankenfield *et al.*, 2005) and a personalised 600 kcal-deficit diet plan was explained to, and agreed by James; and added to his nutritional care plan. A food intake diary was given, and staff members were asked to support James with this as well as his choice of hospital or take-away meals or purchases (in house and from supermarkets).

This contact exhausted the patient's tolerance; therefore, further health improvement information was given over the following weeks. This comprised information on healthy snack exchanges, healthy take-away (carryout) meals and the consequences of obesity on physical wellbeing. James interacted appropriately, and the session concluded with James setting a goal to drink sugar-free fluids from the following day.

After 4 weeks, the diet review highlighted that James had not engaged with either completing his diary or with his diet plan. On examining his perceived barriers to change, James explained that he wanted to look 'big and strong' to keep him safe while in the hospital. (Psychotropic drug therapy requires time to effect change and influence behaviour; therefore, James' medical regimen was still under MDT review.)

After carrying out a risk assessment and in cognisance of his index offence, the dietitian acknowledged James' belief, and carefully suggested that he could lower his risks of ill-health if he reduced some sugar and fat from his diet. He was reassured that he would be supported in his attempt to do this in a slow manner so that he would not lose weight too fast. James agreed and he set a goal of replacing sugar with artificial sweetener and would start this at the end of the week.

After a further 2 weeks, his next review revealed no dietary changes. James admitted that it was not the right time for him to address his weight or his diet. He asked to be discharged from the dietetic service. The dietitian agreed, and requested the key ward staff to encourage James with his diet plan, and to re-refer when his mental health was stable. The dietitian closed the dietetic duty of care, but recommended that the psychologist explore his dietary ideation with cognitive behavioural therapy intervention.

Questions

1. What is James' BMI? What health risks are associated with this level of obesity?
2. What is the nutrition and dietetic diagnosis? Write this as a PASS statement.
3. Should his readiness to change have been assessed prior to dietetic intervention?
4. What are the barriers to change for James?
5. Was the dietitian right to discharge the patient?
6. Is it ethical for the dietitian to discharge the patient without treatment?
7. How should this be documented?
8. What were the objectives of the dietetic intervention?
9. What would a good outcome be?
10. How would you measure this?
11. What other members of the multidisciplinary team (MDT) do you think should be working with this patient?

Further questions

12. The Mifflin–St Jeor equations were used to calculate James' energy requirements; what other equation might be used? Why?
13. Why was James prescribed metformin?
14. What metabolic effects does Clozapine have on the patient?

References

BDA (2008) *Code of Professional Conduct*. BDA, Birmingham.

British Heart Foundation (2014) http://www.bhf.org.uk [accessed on May 2014].

European Convention on Human Rights (ECHR) (1998) http://www.echr.coe.int/Documents/Convention_ENG.pdf [accessed on 13 June 2015].

Foresight Trends and Drivers of obesity (2007) *A literature review for the foresight project on obesity*. https://www.gov.uk/government/publications/reducing-obesity-future-choices [accessed on 12 October 2015].

Frankenfield, D., Roth-Yousel, L. & Compher, C. (2005) Comparison of predictive equations for resting metabolic rate in healthy non-obese and obese adults: a systematic review. *Journal of the American Dietetic Association*, **105** (**5**), 775–789.

Philpot, U. (2014) Nutrition and mental health. In: J. Gandy (ed), *Manual of Dietetic Practice*, 5th edn. Wiley Blackwell, Oxford.

SIGN 131 (2013) *Management of schizophrenia. A national clinical guideline*. Edinburgh.

CASE STUDY 22
Food allergy

Isabel Skypala

Michael is a 46-year-old painter and decorator. He has had an egg allergy since infancy but has also recently started to experience symptoms of an itchy mouth when eating certain plant foods. He has also experienced several reactions in the past few months, which he attributes to egg, the most recent one being quite severe, prompting him to visit his GP surgery. His GP referred him to the dietitian with a request to assess his apparently worsening egg allergy and his symptoms in relation to multiple plant foods.

Assessment

Domain	
Anthropometry, body composition and functional	Not relevant to this consultation
Biochemical and haematological	Skin prick testing in clinic *Positive (≥3 mm)* House dust mite (4 mm), grass (6 mm), silver birch (6 mm), shrimp (3 mm), fresh apple (4 mm), fresh raw peanuts (5 mm) *Negative* Egg (1 mm), cod (0 mm), salmon (0 mm), peach (0 mm), fresh roasted peanuts (0 mm) Specific IgE blood tests *Positive (≥0.35 IU/mL)* Shrimp (0.45 IU/mL), peanut (0.61 IU/mL) *Negative* Egg white (<0.35 IU/mL), egg yolk (<0.35 IU/mL), salmon (0.1 IU/mL), apple (0.31 IU/mL)

Dietetic and Nutrition Case Studies, First Edition.
Edited by Judy Lawrence, Pauline Douglas, and Joan Gandy.

Companion Website: http://www.manualofdieteticpractice.com/

Assessment *(continued)*

Domain	
Clinical	*Medication* None prescribed Over the counter – antacid at least once a week for indigestion, especially when eating takeaways or fried foods No history of chronic disease including heart disease (FH of heart disease) Family history His mother had hay fever and asthma Sister 1 had hay fever, eczema as a child Sister 2 had hay fever Allergy history Eczema as a child but not as an adult Seasonal hay fever from early 20s (March to late July); uses OTC antihistamines and nasal spray when symptomatic
Diet	*History of recent reactions* Nausea and vomiting to eggs from infancy; avoids egg in all forms No allergic reactions until the past 12 months. Occasionally, itchy mouth and tickly, scratchy throat immediately after eating peanuts and other plant foods including apples and peaches. Symptoms go away quite quickly if he drinks some water The reactions of most concern to Michael are ones to foods, which are seemingly unconnected. He has experienced nausea immediately after eating a rice dessert he thought contained traces of raw egg. He has also had chest pain two hours after eating fried chicken, and flushing, difficulty breathing, croaky voice and itchy palms and feet 15 min after eating scampi. Michael feels both of these reactions are due to the egg in the breadcrumbs. The last reaction was severe and it was this that prompted the referral

Assessment *(continued)*

Domain	
	Assessment of current dietary intake – on questioning, Michael reports to be eating the following foods regularly: red meat, chicken, milk, cheese, white fish, Weetabix, bread, rice, pasta, pears, grapes, bananas, potatoes, broccoli, cauliflower, onions, peas, baked beans, lentils, cashew nuts, pistachio nuts, chocolate bars, sponge cake, Christmas cake, biscuits, desserts including fruit crumble and apple pie. He dislikes fish and shellfish and was not aware that scampi were a type of prawn until after he had eaten them
Environmental, behavioural and social	Patterns of consumption and any link to reactions – the itchy mouth has occurred to foods eaten both in and out of the home. The reactions to the rice dessert, chicken and scampi have all taken place when eating out Co-factors – there is no obvious link to any of the normal co-factors such as exercise, alcohol consumption or medication

The skin prick and blood tests suggest that Michael is no longer allergic to eggs despite the recent reactions that he attributed to egg. His dietary intake also suggested that he was eating some cooked egg without realising it. The symptoms to apples and peaches are likely to be linked to Michael's hay fever. His skin prick tests were positive to grass and trees, which fits with his hay fever pattern. Many people with springtime hay fever get an itchy mouth to raw fruits, known as pollen-food syndrome (PFS), also known as oral allergy syndrome (OAS). The reactions to peanuts could also be caused by pollen-food cross-reactions, but a peanut allergy cannot yet be ruled out. Shrimp was tested because one of the reactions involved scampi; however, Michael never normally eats fish or shellfish, and the other two reactions attributed to egg did not involve shellfish; therefore, the significance of the test is not clear and results for both SPT and specific IgE were borderline. It was proposed to undertake further tests with fresh foods and consider oral food challenges. In the meantime, Michael was advised to continue to avoid egg, peanuts, raw apples and peaches. Given his dislike for fish and shellfish, Michael is clearly not going to eat these but he was advised to also continue to avoid bread crumbed and battered foods until further testing could be carried out. He was also given some written information about PFS to take home.

Michael should be seen again to have further testing and an evaluation to ensure he has not had any further reactions.

Questions

1. What is the nutrition and dietetic diagnosis diagnosis? Write it as a PASS statement.
2. How prevalent is food allergy in adults and do most children with a food allergy grow out of it?
3. Is it likely that Michael still has an egg allergy? Give information on the natural history of egg allergy, an interpretation of the skin prick test results and his current dietary intake to support your answer.
4. What are the typical symptoms of a food allergy and were all the reactions Michael experienced of this type?
5. What food allergens would have been in the rice pudding, fried chicken or scampi and were any food allergens not tested for that should have been?
6. How do you interpret the peanut test results; does Michael have a peanut allergy or PFS?
7. Should Michael stop eating cashew and pistachio nuts and avoid foods with nut label warnings on them?
8. Why was the fresh apple skin prick test result positive but the blood test negative?
9. Should Michael avoid all raw fruits in case he starts getting reactions to other fruits?
10. What, if any, nutritional factors might be an issue for Michael if he is avoiding eggs, nuts and certain fruits?

Further questions

11. What further tests should be undertaken to determine his reactivity to eggs?
12. Is the shrimp test a good test for the reaction to scampi and should any further tests be done to find out if shellfish is a problem if he does not like or eat them?
13. Are people with PFS at a high risk of having a nutritionally poor diet?
14. Who has the primary responsibility for recording a patient's allergies, hypersensitivities, intolerances and adverse drug reactions.

Resources

Bock, S.A. (1987) Prospective appraisal of complaints of adverse reactions to foods in children during the first 3 years of life. *Pediatrics*, **79**, 683–688.

Ewan, P.W. (1996) Clinical study of peanut and nut allergy in 62 consecutive patients: new features and associations. *British Medical Journal*, **312**, 1074–1078.

Fleischer, D., Conover-Walker, M., Matsui, E. *et al.* (2005) The natural history of tree nut allergy. *Journal of Allergy and Clinical Immunology*, **116**, 1087–1093.

Mullins, R.J., Dear, K.B. & Tang, M.L. (2009) Characteristics of childhood peanut allergy in the Australian Capital Territory, 1995 to 2007. *Journal of Allergy and Clinical Immunology*, **123**, 689–693.

PEN: Practice Based Evidence in Nutrition. *Food allergies tools and resources*. www.pennutrition.com/KnowledgePathway.aspx?kpid=2446&trid=2425&trcatid=26.

Sicherer, S.H., Wood, R.A., Vickery, B.P. *et al.* (2014) The natural history of egg allergy in an observational cohort. *Journal of Allergy and Clinical Immunology*, **133**, 492–499.

Skolnick, H.S., Conover-Walker, M.K., Koerner, C.B. *et al.* (2001) The natural history of peanut allergy. *Journal of Allergy and Clinical Immunology*, **107**, 367–374.

Skypala, I. & Venter, C. (2009) *Food Hypersensitivity: Diagnosing and Managing Food Allergies and Intolerance*. Wiley Blackwell, Oxford.

Skypala, I., Venter, C. & Wright, T. (2014) Food hypersensitivity. In: J. Gandy (ed), *Manual of Dietetic Practice*, 5th edn. Wiley Blackwell, Oxford.

Venter, C., Pereira, B., Voigt, K. *et al.* (2007) Prevalence and cumulative incidence of food hypersensitivity in the first three years of life. *Allergy*, **63**, 354–359.

Wood, R.A., Sicherer, S.H., Vickery, B.P. *et al.* (2013) The natural history of milk allergy in an observational cohort. *Journal of Allergy and Clinical Immunology*, **131**, 805–812.

Zuberbier, T., Edenharter, G., Worm, M. *et al.* (2004) Prevalence of adverse reactions to food in Germany – a population study. *Allergy*, **59**, 338–345.

CASE STUDY 23
HIV/AIDS

Alastair Duncan & Clare Stradling

Andy is a 48-year-old Caucasian male living in an urban area in the United Kingdom. He has always been fit and healthy, although, for the past 6 months, gives a history of feeling tired all the time. Four weeks ago he was diagnosed with HIV by his GP. The next day he attended the HIV clinic at the hospital for counselling and phlebotomy, and saw the HIV consultant 2 weeks ago. During this appointment Andy was commenced on antiretrovirals. It is the standard clinical protocol that all patients newly diagnosed with HIV, and all patients commencing on antiretrovirals for the first time are referred for dietetic review. Andy was referred by the consultant, and attends the dietetic outpatient clinic today.

Assessment

Domain	
Anthropometry, body composition and functional	Weight 91.9 kg Height 1.78 m Weight has been stable at 86 kg past 10 years Left arm MUAC 41.5 cm Triceps skinfold 28 mm Waist 109 cm Hips 103 cm
Biochemical and haematological (Reference range)	CD4 90 cells/mL (300–1000) HIV viral load 880,050 particles/mL (<20) Sodium 139 mmol/L Potassium 4.1 mmol/L Creatinine 85 μmol/L eGFR 98 mL/min Hb 121 g/L

Dietetic and Nutrition Case Studies, First Edition.
Edited by Judy Lawrence, Pauline Douglas, and Joan Gandy.

Companion Website: http://www.manualofdieteticpractice.com/

Assessment *(continued)*

Domain	
	Liver function tests ALT 12 IU/L (<40) ALP 48 IU/L (40–129) GGT 60 IU/L (7–33) Total cholesterol 6.1 mmol/L Triglycerides 5.2 mmol/L Glucose 6.9 mmol/L Vitamin D 41 nmol/L (>59) NB: Results from a non-fasting phlebotomy 4/52 ago
Clinical	No previous medical history of note Physical examination – nothing of concern Andy continues to report feeling tired all the time BP 136/89 mmHg *Medication* Antiretrovirals D – darunavir, ritonavir, tenofovir and emtrcitabine (to be taken together at bedtime with a snack) Loperamide and cyclizine in case he experienced side effects because of the antiretrovirals but has not needed to use them No other medicines or supplements Appetite very good No oral or gastrointestinal problems
Diet	24-h recall *Breakfast 06:30* 4 slices white toast (4 × 27 g) with margarine (4 × 7 g) and marmalade (4 × 15 g) 250 mL orange juice (tetrapak carton) 2 mugs instant coffee with semi-skimmed milk (2 × 40 g) and 2 tsp sugar (2 × 10 g) *Mid-morning snack 09:30* 1 mug instant coffee with semi-skimmed milk (40 g) and 2 tsp sugar (10 g) 6 digestive biscuits (6 × 13 g) *Lunch 12:00* Ham sandwich made at home, 2 slices white bread (2 × 36 g), ham (46 g), mayonnaise (15 g), ½ tomato sliced (40 g) 1 banana (100 g) 500 mL blackcurrant squash (50 g concentrate)

Assessment *(continued)*

Domain	
	Mid-afternoon snack 15:00 1 mug tea with semi-skimmed milk (40 g) and 1 tsp sugar (4 g) 4 digestive biscuits (4 × 13 g) *Evening meal 17:30* Cottage pie (own-brand economy range ready meal single portion) (400 g) 1 Muller light yoghurt (175 g) *Supper 20:00* 500 mL red wine from a box pack Food frequencies Fruit – 1 portion per day plus 1 glass juice Vegetables – 1 portion per day Oily fish – 1 portion per week *Alcohol* 30–40 units/week, boxes of wine, and spirits, mostly during the weekend *Meal patterns* Always eats 3 meals per day when working, and takes food with him when on a night shift Often skips meals at weekend, usually when clubbing
Environmental, behavioural and social	Andy is single, lives alone in a council flat, works early, late and night shifts as a cleaner, and earns minimum wage. He seeks out bargains and buys from the economy range when food shopping. He has few friends and does not keep in touch with his family. He goes clubbing 3–4 times monthly and takes recreational drugs (usually crystal meth, mephedrone, or speed) at this time. He goes to the pub on Fridays, Saturdays and Sundays and admits to getting drunk sometimes. He says he is lonely but not depressed

Questions

1. What factors are important to bear in mind when working with a patient recently diagnosed with HIV?
2. Are there any specific record keeping issues that you should consider?
3. What are the implications of Andy's anthropometry measurements? Would you consider any other measurements or physical assessment at this stage?

4. How would you interpret the CD4 count and HIV viral load, and are these values of relevance to the dietitian?
5. Discuss the other blood test results.
6. Are there any clinical findings of note?
7. Andy describes feeling tired all the time, what may be causing this?
8. Are there any dietetic implications regarding the antiretrovirals Andy has been prescribed?
9. What is your impression of Andy's diet?
10. Do you have any observations regarding Andy's drug and alcohol use?
11. What is the nutrition and dietetic diagnosis? Write this as a PASS statement.
12. What advice would you give Andy at this appointment?
13. Would you request any other tests or investigations, or refer onwards to any other health professionals?
14. Would you consider any future dietetic plans at this stage?
15. How would you evaluate and monitor Andy's progress? What outcome measures would you use?

Further questions

16. Why is adherence to antiretroviral medicines important, and can the dietitian have a role in supporting this?
17. How would you calculate protein and energy requirements for an HIV patient?
18. What measures of anthropometry are routinely used in HIV care, and what is their utility?
19. Discuss the clinical pathway where all newly diagnosed patients and those initiating antiretrovirals are referred for dietetic assessment.
20. Are there any other situations where you think HIV patients should be referred for dietetic assessment?

References

Asboe, D., Aitken, C., Boffito, M. *et al.* (2012) British HIV Association guidelines for the routine investigation and monitoring of adult HIV-1-infected individuals. *HIV Medicine*, **13**, 1–44.

University of Liverpool (2015) *Food considerations for antiretrovirals*. www.hiv-druginteractions.org/data/NewsItem/100_ARV_Food_Final.pdf [accessed on 13 June 2015].

Resources

Dietitians in HIV/AIDS. *Competencies for dietitians working in HIV care*. http://dhiva.org.uk/wp-content/uploads/2013/01/DHIVA_Competencies_Jan_14.pdf.

Klassen, K. (2014) HIV and aids. In: J. Gandy (ed), *Manual of Dietetic Practice*, 5th edn. Wiley Blackwell, Oxford.

CASE STUDY 24

Type 1 diabetes mellitus

Paul McArdle

Harry is an 18-year-old male diagnosed with type 1 diabetes at 7 years of age. He lives with his parents and has recently begun an office-based apprenticeship. Harry has not attended specialist diabetes or dietetic services for several years, with his diabetes care being provided by his GP. The GP suggested a referral to the adult community diabetes service because of lack of engagement with specialist services and the high HbA1c recorded 6 months ago.

Assessment

Domain	
Anthropometry, body composition and functional	Weight Current 61.5 kg 6/12 ago 64.7 kg Height 1.7 m
Biochemical and haematological	HbA1c 115 mmol/mol 6/12 ago No self-blood glucose monitoring (SBGM) undertaken at the point of assessment
Clinical	Physical assessment: lypohypertrophy *Medication* Insulin detemir (background insulin) 47 units once daily at 10 pm Insulin lispro (quick-acting insulin) 16 units with breakfast, often missed at lunch, 18–20 units with evening meal. Not adjusted according to food eaten
Diet	Diet (typical work day) *Breakfast (06:30–07:15)* Cornflakes (30 g), full fat milk (100 mL) *Mid-morning snack (10:00)* Packet of crisps (40 g)

Dietetic and Nutrition Case Studies, First Edition.
Edited by Judy Lawrence, Pauline Douglas, and Joan Gandy.

Companion Website: http://www.manualofdieteticpractice.com/

Assessment *(continued)*

Domain	
	Lunch 12:30 Sandwich – cheese and pickle (185 g) or tuna and mayonnaise (165 g) May also eat packet crisps (40 g) and/or chocolate bar (54 g) *Dinner 17:00–18:00* For example, pizza with salad/spaghetti Bolognese 20:00 Occasionally: 2 slices of medium toast
Environmental, behavioural and social	Lives at home, parents shop and cook Socialises with friends 1–2 a week, likes to play football with younger brother occasionally. *Alcohol* 2–3 pints of standard lager once weekly (Sunday)

Harry is fearful of developing diabetes complications later in life and realises this is a significant risk for him, given his current HbA1c and that type 1 diabetes is life long. (NICE, 2004; Genuth, 2006). He is not intentionally losing weight. He has previous negative experiences of diabetes services and has a limited recall of previous education received regarding carbohydrate estimation. Harry lacks the knowledge, understanding and ongoing access to specialist health professional support to effectively self-manage his diabetes. This may partly be related to his earlier experience of services and poor or unstructured transition care being offered (or taken-up). The lack of quality transition care is well recognised, as is its importance in diabetes (NICE, 2004; Diabetes UK, 2008; Nakhla *et al.*, 2009; Bowen *et al.*, 2010; NHS Diabetes, 2012).

The focus in planning and implementing a dietetic intervention in this case is the development of a strong rapport and a positive therapeutic relationship with the patient in order to encourage attendance and engagement with the service. The embodiment of non-judgmental and person-centred approaches is therefore vital. This will allow an environment in which a comprehensive package of education can be delivered, either in a clinic setting or in a group setting depending on patient preference. However, it is also important to meet the patient's therapeutic expectations; that is, the patient is also expecting expert advice and guidance that will result in some discernible improvement in more immediate outcome measures, for example, blood glucose, sense of wellbeing.

The plan is to offer regular (monthly) appointments in the joint dietitian and diabetes nurse clinics for a period of 3–6 months initially. Harry will see the diabetes nurse for 30 min and the dietitian for 30 min at each visit. Support by telephone and email can be provided between appointments. The appointments will be a combination of education on all aspects of self-management for type 1 diabetes and motivational support to implement newly learnt self-management behaviours. Harry will be encouraged and supported to attend a recognised structured patient education programme for type 1 diabetes.

In the first appointment, Harry recognised the need to begin blood glucose monitoring and injecting insulin with all meals or relevant snacks. However, before implementing the education and support to achieve this, it was necessary to better understand Harry's current understanding of diabetes, his barriers to such changes, and potential requirements for insulin in order to provide some initial guidance, which is both safe and effective. These elements are jointly achieved by undertaking an informal (non-judgmental, non-threatening) and exploratory discussion with Harry regarding his current daily routines, how he currently makes decisions about his insulin doses, and what decisions or choices he might make given the new information available to him.

The diabetes nurse made a change to Harry's background insulin (detemir) to split the single dose of 47 units into two doses of 15 units each, morning and night.

The basic concepts of estimating carbohydrate and matching insulin doses to carbohydrates consumed were explained as part of the initial consultation. Based on Harry's diet and current insulin doses and his estimated carbohydrate intake, it was suggested he use a starting dose of 2 units of insulin lispro for every 10 g of carbohydrate consumed (referred to as the 'insulin to carbohydrate ratio'). Harry would be required then to monitor his blood glucose before each meal and before going to bed in order to assess the appropriateness of this and adjust accordingly.

Harry cancelled his next appointment and therefore was reviewed 2 months later. His weight had increased to 63.5 kg and Harry reported implementing changes as discussed and as a result he felt more alert. However, on turning 19 years he explained that he 'went off the rails', meaning he once again stopped routinely checking blood glucose and injecting insulin during the day. Barriers and reasons for this were explored, but Harry was unable to identify any, expressing feelings of guilt and remorse about not having continued the behaviour.

A revised plan was agreed for Harry to download the online app onto his smartphone, which would give him access to a carbohydrate portion list and to use the app as a blood glucose diary. Harry also committed to routinely check his blood glucose and to inject quick acting insulin with all meals. Harry was keen to attend the structured education course, so it was agreed that details would be sent in the post. Follow up was agreed for 1-month time.

Harry failed to attend his follow-up appointment and was discharged to be re-referred by his GP, as per the Trust's Access Policy.

Telephone calls with Harry since this time have resulted in him being re-booked into the diabetes clinic.

Questions

1. How would you assess Harry's current diabetes control? What additional information may be useful?
2. What is Harry's BMI and % weight loss between being referred by his GP and his first hospital clinic appointment?

3. What may be the relevance of this change in weight in relation to Harry's diabetes control?
4. How might Harry feel about his weight/body, etc. How could this be useful in motivating Harry?
5. What is lypohypertrophy? How could this affect his control? How is it treated?
6. Estimate the carbohydrate content of Harry's typical day. Give a range of carbohydrate portions, where 1 carbohydrate portion = 10 g of carbohydrate.
7. What is your assessment of Harry's current diet? What are your views of the effectiveness of advising Harry based on the eatwell plate at this stage?
8. Is it necessary for Harry to eat the toast before bed?
9. Why has Harry stopped engaging with the service? What action should be taken next to support him?
10. What is a structured education course? Give an example of a course used for type 1 diabetes with the rationale for its use.
11. What is the nutrition and dietetic diagnosis? Write this as a PASS statement.
12. What outcome measures would you use to assess Harry's progress?

Further questions

13. What are the important elements of good transition care in diabetes and what is the impact of this not being provided?
14. Suggest a rationale for splitting the background insulin at the initial appointment.
15. Is it necessary to document each phone contact with Harry? What about email contact?

References

Bowen, M.E., Henske, J.A. & Potter, A. (2010) Healthcare transition in adolescents and young adults with diabetes. *Clinical Diabetes*, **28** (**3**), 99–106.

DAFNE Study Group (2002) Training in flexible, intensive insulin management to enable dietary freedom in people with type 1 diabetes: dose adjustment for normal eating (DAFNE) randomised controlled trial. *British Medical Journal*, **325** (**7367**), 746.

Diabetes UK (2008) *Care Recommendation: Transition from Adult to Paediatric Services*. Diabetes UK, London, pp. 1–12.

Genuth, S. (2006) Insights from the diabetes control and complications trial/epidemiology of diabetes interventions and complications study on the use of intensive glycemic treatment to reduce the risk of complications of type 1 diabetes. *Endocrine Practice*, **12** (**Suppl 1**), 34–41.

Nakhla, M., Daneman, D., To, T. *et al.* (2009) Transition to adult care for youths with diabetes mellitus: findings from a Universal Health Care System. *Pediatrics*, **124** (**6**), e1134–e1141.

NHS Diabetes (2012) *Diabetes Transition. Assessment of Current Best Practice and Development of a Future Work Programme to Improve Transition Processes for Young People with Diabetes*. NHS Diabetes, Leicester.

NICE (2004) *CG15: Type 1 Diabetes: Diagnosis and Management of Type 1 Diabetes in Children, Young People and Adults*. National Institute for Clinical Excellence, London.

Resources

Carbohydrate counting. www.carbsandcals.com/about-us.

Carbs & Cals. *This is a series of books, apps and other resources for managing diabetes.* www.carbsandcals.com.

Diabetes UK. www.diabetes.org.uk.

Dose Adjustment for Normal Eating (DAFNE). www.dafne.uk.com.

Dyson, P. (2014) Diabetes mellitus. In: J. Gandy (ed), *Manual of Dietetic Practice*, 5th edn. Wiley Blackwell, Oxford.

UK Diabetes Education Network. www.diabetes-education.net.

X-PERT programme. www.xperthealth.org.uk.

CASE STUDY 25
Type 2 diabetes mellitus – Kosher diet

Ruth Kander

Rebekah is a 30-year-old housewife. She lives with her husband and 6 children (aged 6 months to 10 years). She was born in the United Kingdom but her parents and grandparents came from Europe to escape the Second World War. She speaks English and Yiddish at home. She is an ultra-orthodox Jew and follows strict kosher laws, observes the Shabbat and festivals along with all the other laws. She is obese with type 2 DM. Rebekah has been referred, as the GP is concerned with her continuing weight gain and high random sugar levels.

Assessment

Domain	
Anthropometry, body composition and functional	Weight 95 kg Height 1.60 m Waist circumference 90 cm
Biochemical and haematological	Random glucose 15 mmol/L Total cholesterol 6 mmol/L
Clinical	Obese Hypertension 150/90 mmHg *Medication* Metformin 1000 mg/bd Bendroflumethiazide 12.5 mg/d Ramipril 10 mg/d
Diet	24 hr recall mid-week *Breakfast* Nothing *Lunch* Crackers (15 g each), butter (6 g), sliced cheddar cheese (20 g), dried fruit bar (28 g) *Mid-afternoon* 3 digestive biscuits (3 × 13 g)

Dietetic and Nutrition Case Studies, First Edition.
Edited by Judy Lawrence, Pauline Douglas, and Joan Gandy.

Companion Website: http://www.manualofdieteticpractice.com/

Assessment *(continued)*

Domain	
	Supper Fried chicken breast (70 g), rice (180 g) and green peas (70 g) *Snacks* Cakes (25 g each), biscuits (11–20 g each) *Drinks* Fruit juice (180 mL), tea with sugar (10 g per cup)
Environmental behavioural and social	Housewife Shops weekly (supermarket for fruits/vegetables, bakery, kosher grocery shop, butcher) Works at home looking after her family and home Educated to GCSE level, married at 19 year Does not smoke or drink alcohol Does not do any formal exercise

Questions

1. What is Rebekah's BMI?
2. What is the ideal range for her waist circumference?
3. Comment on Rebekah's BMI and waist circumference (WC).
4. What is the nutrition and dietetic diagnosis? Write this as a PASS statement.
5. What are the objectives of the intervention?
6. What level of energy restriction would you recommend for achievable weight loss?
7. What is the recommended macronutrient content of a diet for someone of her age and size?
8. Would you calculate a meal plan based on requirements?
9. What are the dietary laws associated with being an ultra-orthodox Jew?
10. Describe the traditional foods that Rebekah would cook and eat and comment on their macronutrient content.
11. What are the co-morbidities associated with her degree of obesity?
12. What is the dietary intervention? How many sessions would you suggest over the next 6 months?
13. What advice can you give her to cope with festivals including Shavuot, which is associated with dairy foods?
14. What SMART goals would you propose to discuss with Rebekah that she might feel she can achieve?
15. What are the barriers to change?
16. How can you help her make the necessary changes?
17. What outcome measures would you use to monitor the objectives?

References

Foresight (2007) *Tackling obesities: future choices*. www.gov.uk/government/publications/reducing-obesity-future-choices [accessed on 4 November 2014].

International Diabetes Federation (2006) *The IDF consensus worldwide definition of the metabolic syndrome*. www.idf.org/webdata/docs/MetSyndrome_FINAL.pdf [accessed on 3 November 2014].

National Obesity Observatory (2009) *Body mass index as a measure of obesity*. www.noo.org.uk/uploads/doc789_40_noo_BMI.pdf [accessed on 3 November 2014].

SACN (2008) *The Nutritional Wellbeing of the British Population*. TSO, London.

Resources

Dyson, P. (2014) Diabetes mellitus. In: J. Gandy (ed), *Manual of Dietetic Practice*, 5th edn. Wiley Blackwell, Oxford.

Kander, R. (2013) Israel. In: A. Thaker & A. Barton (eds), *Multicultural Handbook of Food, Nutrition and Dietetics*. Wiley Blackwell, Oxford.

Thaker, A. (2014) Dietary pattern of Black and ethnic minority groups. In: J. Gandy (ed), *Manual of Dietetic Practice*, 5th edn. Wiley Blackwell, Oxford.

CASE STUDY 26

Type 2 diabetes mellitus – private patient

Barbara M. Arora & Juneeshree S. Sangani

Elizabeth is 50 years old and of African Caribbean descent; she was diagnosed with type 2 diabetes when she was 38 years old. She has hypertension and dyslipidaemia; in addition, she has recently been found to have peripheral neuropathy and diabetic retinopathy. Elizabeth is a divorcee and lives alone; she is an office administrator. She does not drive and therefore either takes the bus or walks. She would like to lose weight and consulted her GP. The GP expressed concern about her poor diabetes control and stressed that she had to pay more attention to her condition. When she was first diagnosed she saw an NHS dietitian. Previously she had attended a diabetes education group session and tried commercial slimming clubs. She did not gain a lot from the diabetes group. She disliked attending groups, as she did not like being told that she was overweight in front of the other group members. She said she was willing to pay for the necessary support and advice, and therefore her GP suggested a private referral to a dietitian for personal and detailed advice. Elizabeth was happy with this suggestion and made an appointment with a freelance dietitian.

Assessment

Anthropometry, body and composition	Weight 92 kg Height 1.55 BMI 38.2 kg/m^2
Biochemical and haematological	HbA1c 99 mmol/mol BP 157/123 mmHg Total cholesterol 4.40 mmol/L HDL 0.98 mmol/mol LDL 2.31 mmol/L TG 1.82 mmol/L

Dietetic and Nutrition Case Studies, First Edition.
Edited by Judy Lawrence, Pauline Douglas, and Joan Gandy.

Companion Website: http://www.manualofdieteticpractice.com/

Assessment *(continued)*

Clinical	Type 2 diabetes Dyslipidaemia Hypertension Medication – no information supplied
Diet	No information given
Environmental, behavioural, social	She has recently divorced her husband and has moved to a new area

Questions

1. Does the care pathway differ from an NHS pathway? If so, how?
2. What is the nutrition and dietetic diagnosis?
3. Is it appropriate to accept a self-referral for Elizabeth?
4. Assess the accuracy of the information provided. What additional information is required to complete the assessment?
5. Why is it important to gain Elizabeth's consent before you contact her GP?
6. Elizabeth has private medical insurance but is concerned that it will not cover these consultations. How would you advise her?
7. Detail how you would establish the client's expectations of the service. Give an explanation of the service you can offer and fee structure.
8. As with all dietitians those who are freelance are autonomous and therefore it is vital that they are familiar with, and adhere carefully to the Health and Care Professions Council's Standards of Proficiency. How can you ensure that you are adhering to these standards?
9. What should you do about record keeping?
10. What resources should you provide? What reliable resources are available?
11. Why should you establish Elizabeth's reasons for a private referral? How can you manage her expectations?
12. Are there advantages in consulting a dietitian privately?
13. Diabetes is a chronic problem. How can the private practice dietitian assist in the long-term care of this patient?
14. What components of the dietetic care process are common to both NHS and private dietetics?

Resources

BDA. *Code of Professional Conduct* https://www.bda.uk.com/publications/professional/codeofprofessionalpractice2015. NB Non members should contact BDA directly.

Diabetes UK (2011) *Evidence based nutrition guidelines for the prevention and management of diabetes.* www.diabetes.org.uk/nutrition-guidelines.

Dyson, P. (2014) Type 2 diabetes mellitus. In: J. Gandy (ed), *Manual of Dietetic Practice*, 5th edn. Wiley-Blackwell, Oxford.

Freelance Dietitians Group. www.freelancedietitians.org/. NB Non members should contact FDG directly.

Guidance for Dietitians for Records and Record Keeping (2008) Available to BDA members. https://www.bda.uk.com/publications/professional/practice_record_keeping. NB Non members should contact BDA directly.

HCPC *Standards of conduct performance and ethics*. www.hcpc-uk.org/assets/documents/10003B6EStandardsofconduct,performanceandethics.pdf.

HCPC *Standards of Proficiency – Dietitians*. www.hcpc-uk.org/assets/documents/1000050CStandards_of_Proficiency_Dietitians.pdf.

Information Commissioner's Office. https://ico.org.uk.

NICE (2009) *Type 2 diabetes: the management of type 2 diabetes*. http://www.nice.org.uk/guidance/CG87.

NICE (2011) *Obesity guidance on the prevention, identification, assessment and management of 8 overweight and obesity in adults and children*. www.nice.org.uk/guidance/CG43.

Nutrition & Diet Resources (NDR). www.ndr-uk.org/.

PEN: Practice Based Evidence in Nutrition. *Diabetes patient information leaflets*. www.pennutrition.com/SearchResult.aspx?portal=PEN&terms=ZGlhYmV0ZXMgaGFuZG91dHM=.

CASE STUDY 27
Gestational diabetes mellitus

Reena Shaunak

Badra is a 35-year-old Hindu Punjabi lady; she is married and lives with her husband and 8-year-old daughter. She works as a hospital pharmacist and her husband is an accountant. She was born in the United Kingdom but her parents were born and brought up in Kenya and therefore her diet has some influence of the Kenyan and Gujarati diet. She has a South-East Asian/Western diet and likes to eat out and has regular takeaways (Chinese, pizzas or Indian). Being a Hindu, Badra restricts beef in her diet. She is pregnant for the second time and her mother-in-law has moved in with her to help out. Her mother-in-law is insisting she should eat for two. She attended the antenatal clinic during her third trimester and presented with high blood glucose levels. She was referred by an antenatal consultant for dietary advice.

Assessment

Domain	
Anthropometry, body composition and functional	Weight Current 98 kg Pre-pregnancy 80 kg Height 1.61 m BMI 37.8 kg/m^2
Biochemical and haematological markers	Random glucose 7.8 mmol/L HbA1c 65 mmol/mol
Clinical	BP 150/95 mmHg Overweight since early childhood Pre-eclampsia in 1st pregnancy *Medication* Methyldopa 250 mg bd Folic acid 5 mg/day Ferrous sulphate 200 mg/day Metformin 500 mg bd Insulatard 4 U/day

Dietetic and Nutrition Case Studies, First Edition.
Edited by Judy Lawrence, Pauline Douglas, and Joan Gandy.

Companion Website: http://www.manualofdieteticpractice.com/

Assessment (*continued*)

Domain	
Diet	Diet history *Breakfast* Weekdays – often skips breakfast but sometimes has a latte (240 mL) and croissant (60 g) on her way to work Weekends – cheese (full fat cheddar) (60 g) on white toast (2 × 27 g), Indian milky spiced tea (190 g) (full fat milk (50 g), 2 tsp sugar (10 g)) or Take-away breakfast – sausage patty, hash brown (1), scrambled egg, toasted English muffin (160 g) *Mid-morning* Weekdays when missed breakfast – bacon (50 g) roll (50 g), coffee latte (240 g) (semi-skimmed milk, 2 tsp sugar (10 g)) or Muffin (120 g), latte coffee (240 g) (semi-skimmed milk, 2 tsp sugar (10 g)) *Lunch* Sandwich or 12-in baguette (chicken or ham, mayonnaise, salad (205 g)), crisps (30 g packet), regular fizzy drink (330 g) or Large jacket potato (220 g) with cheese (30 g), regular fizzy drink (330 mL) *Mid-afternoon* Tea (260 mL) (semi-skimmed milk (40 mL), 2 tsp sugar (10 g)), fruit (100 g) and/or crisps (30 g packet) Weekends may have samosa (2 × 70 g) (fried pastry filled with potatoes and peas) or handwa (60 g) (baked snack made with ground rice, lentils, vegetables and plain yoghurt) or dhokla (40 g) (steamed snack made with ground chickpea flour and plain yoghurt), Indian milky spiced tea (190 g) (full fat milk (30 g), 2 tsp sugar (10 g))

Assessment *(continued)*

Domain	
	Evening meal 2 medium chapattis (2 × 60 g) (roti) (made with wholemeal flour, 1/2 tsp spoon ghee), chicken/lamb curry (300 g), green salad, vanilla ice-cream (2 scoops × 60 g) NB: Her mother-in-law insists that she has ghee while she is pregnant, for easy delivery Takeaway Indian, Chinese or pizza 2× per week *other snacks in the day* Crisps (30 g), chevda (30 g) (Indian savoury snack; high in fat and salt) NB: Dislikes artificial sweeteners *Alcohol* 1 glass white wine 3–4 × per week (pre-pregnancy every day)
Environmental, behavioural and social	Non-smoker

Acknowledgement

Yvonne Jeannes for her contribution to this case study.

Questions

1. What is the nutrition and dietetic diagnosis? Write this as a PASS statement.
2. Describe the possible mechanism of gestational DM (GDM).
3. What are the risk factors for GDM? Why is Badra at risk of GDM?
4. What complications are associated with poorly managed GDM for the mother and foetus?
5. How is GDM diagnosed?
6. Estimate Badra's daily requirements for energy, macronutrients, iron, calcium, zinc, folate and vitamin C. Comment on her current diet.
7. What are the aims of the dietary intervention?
8. Describe the intervention.
9. Comment on the glycaemic index (GI) and glycaemic load (GL) of Badra's diet. What changes should she make to reduce both GI and GL?
10. What outcome measures would you use to monitor and evaluate the intervention?

11. What are the barriers to change? How can you help Badra overcome these barriers?
12. How will Badra's culture and ethnicity affect her dietary and lifestyle choices?
13. Badra is unaware of the problems of hypoglycaemia. How would you help her understand its effects and how to deal with it?
14. What would you include in your documentation of Badra's care?

Further questions

15. What advice would you give Badra about drinking alcohol and caffeine drinks? Explain your rationale.
16. Why is food safety important during pregnancy? What is the recommended advice to pregnant women?

References

Department of Health (DH) (1991) *Dietary reference values for food energy and nutrients for the United Kingdom*. Report of the Panel on Dietary reference values of the Committee on Medical Aspects of Food Policy. Report on Health and Social Subjects 41. London: HMSO.

Diabetes UK (2011) *Evidence-based nutrition guidelines for the prevention and management of diabetes*. http://www.diabetes.org.uk/nutrition-guidelines [accessed on 30 January 2015].

Henry, C.J.K. (2005) Basal metabolic rate studies in humans: measurement and development of new equations. *Public Health Nutrition*, **8**, 1133–1152.

NICE (2015) *Diabetes in pregnancy: management of diabetes and its complications from preconception to the postnatal period*. NICE guidelines [NG3] www.nice.org.uk/guidance/cg63/resources/guidance-diabetes-in-pregnancy-pdf [accessed on 7 October 2015].

SACN (2011) *Dietary Reference Values for Energy*. TSO, London.

WHO (2013) *Diagnostic criteria and classification of hyperglycaemia first detected in pregnancy*. http://apps.who.int/iris/bitstream/10665/85975/1/WHO_NMH_MND_13.2_eng.pdf [accessed on 18 November 2014].

WHO/IDF (2006) *Definition and Diagnosis of Diabetes Mellitus and Intermediate Hyperglycaemia*. http://whqlibdoc.who.int/publications/2006/9241594934_eng.pdf [accessed on 18 November 2014].

Resources

Rees, G. (2014) Preconception and pregnancy. In: J. Gandy (ed), *Manual of Dietetic Practice*, 5th edn. Wiley Blackwell, Oxford.

Royal College of Physicians of Ireland (2011) *Obesity and Pregnancy; Clinical Practice Guideline*. Version 1.0; Guideline No. 2; Revision date – June 2013.

Todorovic, V. & Micklewright, A. (2011) *A Pocket Guide to Clinical Nutrition*, 4th edn. Parenteral and Enteral Nutrition Group of the British Dietetic Association, BDA, Birmingham.

CASE STUDY 28

Polycystic ovary syndrome

Sema Jethwa

Nisha is a 31-year-old Asian woman who lives with her husband and parents; they are Hindu. She married 5 years ago and is eager to start a family but is unable to conceive so far. She has a family history of diabetes; her mother had gestational diabetes and developed type 2 diabetes later in life. She visited her GP to discuss her difficulties conceiving. Her GP noted a history of irregular menstruation, excess hair growth and acne.

Assessment

Domain	
Anthropometry, body composition and functional	Weight 95.4 kg Height 1.65 m BMI 35 kg/m^2 Waist circumference 80 cm
Biochemical and haematological	Random glucose 9.2 mmol/L HbA1c 45 mmol/mol Testosterone 4 nmol/L Prolactin 550 mU/L
Clinical	Acne and excess hair growth since adolescence Difficulty conceiving Multiple ovarian cysts confirmed by ultrasound Diagnosis – PCOS *Medication* Metformin 500 mg bd
Diet	Lacto-vegetarian Diet history *Breakfast* Monday–Friday none Weekends 2 slices toast (white, medium) (2 × 22 g), butter (2 × 10 g), jam (15 g)

Dietetic and Nutrition Case Studies, First Edition.
Edited by Judy Lawrence, Pauline Douglas, and Joan Gandy.

Companion Website: http://www.manualofdieteticpractice.com/

Assessment *(continued)*

Domain	
	or 5–6× 3 in. puri (5–6× 15 g) (deep fried white wheat flat bread or 2–3× 6 in. paratha (2–3× 140 g)(flaky flatbread made with white wheat flour cooked with butter/ghee), 1 tbsp (33 g) shop bought mango pickle or 2–3× 6 in. (2–3× 50 g) thepla (shallow fried spiced flatbreads made with white wheat flour, gram flour, fenugreek leaves and spices), 2 tbsp homemade full fat yoghurt Mug of tea (190 mL) – full fat milk (35 mL), 1 tsp (5 g) sugar *Mid-morning* Large milky coffee (latte) (480 mL) with 1 tsp (5 g) sugar Chocolate bar (54 g) *Lunch* Weekdays Cheese and tomato baguette (350 g) or Cheese and coleslaw sandwich (2 slices white bread) (200 g) or Jacket potato (180 g) with butter(2 × 10 g), cheese (25 g), baked beans (80 g) Medium sized bag crisps (40 g) Can fizzy drink (330 mL) Weekend May miss lunch if late breakfast or early lunch if missed breakfast 3–4 samosas (3–4× 40g) (deep fried triangle pastries filled with spiced vegetables) or 5–6 bhajiya (5–6× 28 g) (slices of potato or other chopped vegetables fried in a spiced gram flour batter) and Small cake (35 g) or 2–3 biscuits Mug of tea – as above

Assessment (*continued*)

Domain	
	Evening meal 2 × 6 in. chapatti (2 × 60 g) (roti) (made with white wheat flour, topped with butter) and 3 tbsp (3 × 40 g) white rice 1 serving spoon (30 g) vegetable (shaak) (e.g. cauliflower, spinach, potato and pea, aubergine) Small bowl of dahl (60 g) (split pigeon peas (tuvar dal)) or kadhi (200 g) (yoghurt based spiced 'soup')
Environmental, behavioural and social	University educated, works full time for an event management firm She has a moderately active social life and meets friends during the week but tends to spend time with her family at the weekend

Acknowledgement

Yvonne Jeannes for her reviewing and additional comments.

Questions

1. What is the nutrition and dietetic diagnosis? Write this as a PASS statement.
2. What are the clinical diagnostic criteria for PCOS?
3. What conditions are associated with PCOS?
4. Describe the dietetic intervention.
5. What are the short and long-term aims of the intervention?
6. How motivated is she to make dietary changes even though she states that she is motivated to get pregnant? How would you assess her motivation?
7. If you establish that Nisha is well motivated, how can you help her maintain this enthusiasm?
8. What dietary restrictions are associated with Hinduism?
9. How would you assess Nisha's physical activity level?
10. What can you do to encourage more physical activity? Select suitable SMART aims.
11. What are her possible barriers to change? How can these be overcome?

Further questions

12. Why has Nisha been prescribed metformin?
13. Describe the effects of insulin resistance in PCOS.
14. Nisha has been recommended dietary supplements by her friends. How would you counsel her about these?

References

ESHRE and ASRM Sponsored PCOS Consensus Workshop Group (2004) Revised 2003 consensus on diagnostic criteria and long-term health risks related to polycystic ovary syndrome. *Fertility and Sterility*, **81**, 19–25.

Jeanes, Y., Barr, S., Smith, K. *et al.* (2009) Dietary management of women with polycystic ovary syndrome in the United Kingdom: the role of dietitians. *Journal of Human Nutrition and Dietetics*, **22**, 551–558.

Public Health England (2009) *GP Physical Activity Questionnaire (GPPAQ)*. www.erpho.org.uk/viewResource.aspx?id=18813 [last accessed on 16 September 2014].

Tang, T., Lord, J.M., Norman, R.J. *et al.* (2010) Insulin-sensitising drugs (metformin, rosiglitazone, pioglitazone, D-chiro-inositol) for women with polycystic ovary syndrome, oligo amenorrhoea and subfertility. *Cochrane Database of Systematic Reviews*, **5** (**1**), CD003053.

Resources

Jeannes, Y. (2014) Polycystic ovary syndrome. In: J. Gandy (ed), *Manual of Dietetic Practice*, 5th edn. Wiley Blackwell, Oxford.

NICE (2013) *Clinical knowledge summaries: polycystic ovary syndrome*. http://cks.nice.org.uk/polycystic-ovary-syndrome [accessed on 24 November 2014].

CASE STUDY 29

Obesity – specialist management

A specialist community weight management service for severe and complex obesity (NHS tier 3)

Lucy Turnbull

Susan is a 41-year-old Black British woman. She is divorced and currently is not in a relationship. She lives with her son, and her daughter lives nearby with her 2-year-old twin daughters. Susan works in a nursery, so spends much of her day looking after young children and comes home at night very tired.

Susan reports she has always been bigger than others. As a child she remembers being bigger than other children and having to get clothes from a different shop as she was unable to buy from the normal school uniform shop. She puts her weight gain down to her mother giving her very large portions of food, and believing that she 'has to finish everything on her plate as there were starving children in Africa'. She says she was rarely allowed 'junk food' or takeaways, but reports that as she got older she started consuming more 'junk food', takeaways and large quantities of fizzy drinks especially in her teens and 20s and her weight really increased. She has tried losing weight in the past through increasing exercise, eating smaller portions and Weight Watchers and meal replacement shakes, but does not stick to it. Although she loses weight she regains when she finishes the diet.

Susan was referred for bariatric surgery (she wanted the gastric band as this was reversible), but after reading more about the operation and watching a documentary on TV she became afraid of what might happen and decided she wanted to lose weight 'the natural' way.

Susan was referred by her GP due to her high BMI and uncontrolled type 2 diabetes (diagnosed in 2005).

Dietetic and Nutrition Case Studies, First Edition.
Edited by Judy Lawrence, Pauline Douglas, and Joan Gandy.

Companion Website: http://www.manualofdieteticpractice.com/

Assessment

Domain	
Anthropometry, body composition and functional	Weight 150 kg Height 1.70 m Physical activity and functions of daily living Euroquol 5 dimensions (EQ5D) quality of life questionnaire indicated moderate difficulty in performing usual activities (e.g. functions of daily living including washing and dressing herself) and reported moderate pain in her left knee and lower back, especially when bending down to pick up the children at work She completed a 2 min sit to stand test in which she scored 32
Biochemistry and haematology	Total cholesterol 3.8 mmol/L HDL cholesterol 0.91 mmol/L LDL cholesterol 1.49 mmol/L TG 3.08 mmol/L HbA1c 67.2 mmol/mol (8.3%) BP 158/109 mmHg
Clinical	Type 2 diabetes *Medication* Gliclazide (160 mg, qd) Sitagliptin (100 mg, qd) Metformin (1 g bds) Hypertension *Medication* Ramapril (10 mg qd) Hypercholesterolaemia *Medication* Simvastatin (20 mg qd) Aspirin (75 mg qd)
Diet	*Breakfast* Nothing *Mid-morning* Fruit (110 g) *Lunch* Jacket potato (220 g) or spaghetti bolognaise (470 g) or chicken (161 g) and chips (165 g) from local shop *Mid-afternoon* A chicken wrap (175 g) from the local shop or sandwiches (145–205 g)

Assessment (*continued*)

Domain	
	Dinner – at home Usually chicken (250 g) and rice (300 g) or pasta (430 g) – very large portions. Take-aways such as Chinese, or pizza 2/7 Ice-cream (150 g) or cake (130 g) *Snacks throughout day* Crisps (will eat whole big bag in the day) (150 g) , sweets (120 g) *Drinks* 2 cups coffee with 1 sugar (5 g) and semi-skimmed milk (25 mL) and 5–6 cans (each 330 mL) fizzy drink per day *Alcohol* on special occasions she may have a glass of wine
Environmental, behavioural and social	Susan does all the shopping and cooking for the household, although she will get take-aways some evenings during the week when she is tired. She lives in a 2-bedroom flat on the first floor with no lift, so does have to climb stairs, with which she struggles especially with food shopping

Other validated measures

Susan completed the following other questionnaires as part of a multidisciplinary service:

Patient health questionnaire (PHQ) score = 12

Generalised anxiety disorder (GAD) score = 10

Epworth sleep score = 15

Psychological factors

The anxiety and depression score indicated moderate anxiety and depression. Susan also indicated during the consultation that she comfort ate when she is feeling sad or depressed. These foods are usually sweets foods such as cakes, biscuits, chocolate and ice-cream. She reports bingeing on these food approximately once per week. She did not report any purging measures such as vomiting or using laxatives to eliminate the food.

Intervention

Multidisciplinary Intervention

In her initial assessment, Susan was asked to keep a food and mood diary for a minimum of 3 days and bring to her next appointment in 2 weeks. It was also decided that an appointment would be booked with the team's clinical psychologist and physiotherapist (PT).

Dietetic intervention

Susan completed the food diary for a week and this revealed that she ate for negative emotions almost every day. Her comfort food choices tended to be sweet foods such as biscuits, cakes and chocolate. Therefore, her intervention started by working on how to deal with cravings, what she can do when craving foods or other tactics she could try when feeling sad.

The food diary also revealed that Susan would have take-away food more often than twice per week; she would usually have some form of takeaway every day.

It was also identified that Susan's portion sizes were much larger than normal; almost 3 times more. Susan reported that she often cooks far more than is needed for just her and her son (she says this is due to her culture), and she was always told not to waste food so she eats it all.

Susan identified that she never plans meals and just eats whatever she feels like at the time. The dietitian discussed with Susan tools about planning her meals and self-monitoring.

Throughout her intervention Susan was also provided with standard dietetic weight management advice.

Psychological intervention

Susan reported that her mood difficulties have been ongoing for a number of years, possibly as far back as aged 8 years. She explained that she has never had a strong relationship with either of her parents. Notably though, her relationship with her father has been more difficult. She described him as being very critical of her and a number of his negative comments have been about her weight. She stated that he would constantly criticise her about what she ate and the size of her portions. She spoke about him possibly doing this to either stop her or to motivate her but on the contrary it led her to comfort eat.

Also contributing to her mood is the break-up of her relationship 6 months ago. She reported that for the most part of the day she feels down and the behaviour of others towards her affects her mood. For example, when people made comments about her weight at work or in the street she will eat to make herself feel better. During her last emotional eating episode she ate chocolate, a big bag of crisps and an ice-cream cone. She admits that she sees food as a friend. During comfort eating episodes she can feel happy initially when eating but then upset when she looks at the wrappers and thinks 'Did I just sit and eat all of that?'

Susan admitted that when eating she does not have a 'stop button' and can just continue eating and eating. She also acknowledged over compensating as she over eats when she skips meals. In her head, the big portion sizes are normal and she does not see them as big portions.

Susan's reported symptoms of depression indicated in her PHQ9 score needs to be discussed and explored further. She may benefit from anti-depressants, which should be discussed with Susan and her GP.

In the psychological session the acceptance and commitment therapy (ACT) approach was used. In keeping with her values, Susan was able to identify a task that would be achieving her value of living, a healthier life as well as contributing to the lives of others. She acknowledged that if she continues living her life the way she has been doing then she will return to being depressed and retreat to her bed. Instead, she spoke about the fact that she would like her life to have purpose, where she can have something to look forward to.

Physiotherapist intervention

During the initial physiotherapist session, the following were addressed:

(a) The role of the physiotherapist within the specialist weight management service (SWMS).

(b) The benefits of exercise: endurance, fitness, general health and weight loss and how her current weight influences her knee and back pain.

(c) Susan's barriers to exercising.

(d) The NICE (2014) guidelines for obesity.

(e) The varieties of exercises she could try and which she prefers to do. Susan reported she enjoys walking. She does not like going to the gym as she feels very self-conscious.

The following plan was implemented for Susan:

- To incorporate a 20 min walk into her daily commute to work; and
- To attend the physiotherapist-led SWMS exercise class once per week.

Evaluation

After 3 months working with the SWMS dietitian, physiotherapist and psychologist, and attending the exercise classes, the same tests and forms were conducted as at the assessment.

Susan had lost 7 kg in weight bringing her weight to 143 kg and her BMI to 49.8 kg/m^2. She has been attending the weekly exercise classes, reports she has cut down her takeaways to 3× per week and reduced the portions of what she is eating. She says she feels much happier since losing weight and found the teams very supportive in helping her make difficult changes to her lifestyle and her psychological well-being.

BP 150/106 mmHg
PHQ score = 8
GAD7 score = 6
Epworth sleep score = 13
2 min sit to stand 35

Questions

1. What was Susan's initial BMI? What does this mean in terms of co-morbidities?
2. Why would the dietitian not measure Susan's waist circumference in the consultation?
3. Does this patient have normal blood lipid levels? What are normal blood lipid levels?

4. What other blood tests might you have wanted to ask the GP to organise?
5. Are there any other referrals or investigations that should be made for Susan?
6. What is the nutrition and dietetic diagnosis? Write this as a PASS statement.
7. How would you involve Susan in her dietetic goal setting?
8. What advice would you provide to a weight management patient?
9. What SMART goals might you hope to negotiate with Susan?
10. What could the dietitian do to help Susan reduce the number of takeaways she eats?
11. What tools can be used to help Susan identify normal portion sizes?
12. What self-monitoring tools could Susan use?
13. Can you think of any barriers to Susan changing her behaviour habits?
14. How would you document your care and ensure good communication with the MDT, particularly the physiotherapist and psychologist?
15. What outcome measurements would you collect to evaluate your care?

References

Chevette, C. & Balolia, Y. (2013) *Carbs and Cals*, 5th edn. Chello Publishing Ltd., London.

Foresight (2007) *Tackling obesities: future choices*. www.gov.uk/government/publications/reducing-obesity-future-choices [accessed on 4 November 2014].

NICE (2006) *Guideline CG43 Obesity: Guidance on the prevention, identification, assessment and management of overweight and obesity in adults and children*. www.nice.org.uk/guidance/cG43 [last accessed on 14 August 2014].

NICE (2008) *CVD risk assessment and management (CKS)*. http://cks.nice.org.uk/cvd-risk-assessment-and-management [last accessed on 7 October 2015].

NICE (2014) *Managing overweight and obesity in adults – lifestyle management services PH53*. http://www.nice.org.uk/guidance/ph53 [last accessed on 28 November 2014].

Resources

Hankey, C. (2014) Management of obesity and overweight in adults. In: J. Gandy (ed), *Manual of Dietetic Practice*, 5th edn. Wiley Blackwell, Oxford.

PEN: Practice Based Evidence in Nutrition. *Obesity: tools and resources*. www.pennutrition.com/KnowledgePathway.aspx?kpid=803&trid=22226&trcatid=27.

CASE STUDY 30
Obesity – Prader–Willi syndrome

Rachael Brandreth & Joanna Lamming

Prader–Willi syndrome (PWS) is a complex, genetic disorder associated with excessive appetite, low muscle tone, emotional instability, immature physical development and learning disabilities. Although infants with PWS may have feeding difficulties leading to growth faltering, children aged over 1 year often gain weight very rapidly due to hyperphagia. An estimated 3000 individuals in the United Kingdom have PWS.

Shelley is a 16-year-old girl with Prader–Willi Syndrome. Weight management has been a concern since birth. Initially, due to her poor suck and low tone, Shelley was naso-gastrically fed. As she transitioned to taking more milk orally the focus was on preventing faltering growth and she was given a high-energy density, age appropriate milk. Once solids were introduced there were also problems due to her low tone and the speech and language therapist gave guidance for the first couple of years to help Shelley move from puree and mashed foods to every day textures. Shelley is now able to manage all textures, but these early experiences affect her parents' current views on her diet.

Shelley was seen in the multidisciplinary clinic, which comprises the consultant paediatrician with a special interest in endocrinology, the community paediatrician and the children's dietitian.

Assessment

Domain	
Anthropometry, body composition and functional	Weight 77.3 kg Height 145.2 cm *Bioimpedance analysis* Fat 43.6% Total body water 41.3% *Growth history* 12 years 4 months 143 cm, 69 kg 13 years 6 months 144.1 cm, 73.3 kg 14 years 5 months 145 cm, 72 kg 15 years 4 months 145.2 cm, 71.7 kg

Dietetic and Nutrition Case Studies, First Edition.
Edited by Judy Lawrence, Pauline Douglas, and Joan Gandy.

Companion Website: http://www.manualofdieteticpractice.com/

Assessment (*continued*)

Domain	
Biochemical and haematological	Sodium 138 mmol/L Potassium 4.2 mmol/L Urea 3.2 mmol/L Creatinine 54 mmol/L Corrected calcium 2.38 mmol/L Phosphate 1.3 mmol/L ALT 19 U/L ALP 99 U/L Bilirubin 4 µmol/L Total protein 71 g/L Albumin 41 g/L Glucose 14.7 mmol/L Total cholesterol 5.3 mmol/L HDL cholesterol 0.96 mmol/L LDL cholesterol of 3.8 mmol/L HDL:LDL 5.5 TG 2.2 mmol/L *Glucose tolerance test* Fasting 7.1 mmol/L 120 min 15.4 mmol/L
Clinical	Blood pressure normal Growth hormone from 5 to 13 years Metformin 500 mg od started 1 week ago prescribed by the diabetologist Shelley uses a bilevel positive airway pressure (BiPAP) machine over night to help manage sleep apnoea
Diet	Notes: uses semi-skimmed milk, 50% white:50% wholemeal bread (50:50) *Breakfast* Branflakes (30 g) with milk (100 g) Slice of toast (50:50) (27 g) with scraping of marmalade (10 g) Tea (190) with milk (30 g) *Mid-morning* Low fat crisps (30 g) Banana (100 g) Water (500 mL bottle drunk throughout the school day)

Assessment (*continued*)

Domain	
	Lunch Chicken sandwich (2 slices of bread (2 × 36 g), salad cream and thin spread of butter (7 g)) Yoghurt drink (200 g) Oatmeal and hazelnut muesli bar (35 g) Blackcurrant squash (500 mL) *After school* Tea (190) with milk (30 g) 2 digestive biscuits (2 × 13 g) *Evening meal* Oven-baked battered fish (150 g) with chips (100 g) and peas (100 g) Sliced banana (25 g), strawberries (50 g) and raspberries (30 g) with ice-cream (1 scoop (60 g)) *Before bed* Glass of lemon and lime squash
Environmental, behavioural and social	Siblings Brother (18 years) diagnosed with Asperger syndrome Brother (14 years) who is very athletic

Shelley's mother works part time as a teaching assistant. She has recently been diagnosed with depression. Her father is a sales representative who travels regularly for work. Consequently, her mother usually does all of the household chores including the cooking and shopping.

Shelley attends an area resource base (for pupils with complex difficulties) attached to a secondary school and hopes to attend the local college from the beginning of the next school year. She is a well liked and sociable and loves to go out to cafes. This is encouraged by the school as part of developing independent living skills. Her favourite after school club is cookery and when her parents have time her favourite thing to do at home is to help with the cooking. Unfortunately, her mum finds cooking and mealtimes very stressful and so they often have ready meals or takeaways and therefore Shelley has little control over these meals. Shelley communicates using signing (Makaton) and her iPad. On the iPad she uses a specialist application (app), which allows a non-signer to see both the word and the sign. She can also write a little, but this is limited and slow. Shelley has a keen interest in food and nutrition and is keen to take more control over her own eating and drinking. To enable her to start doing this she keeps her own food diaries by taking photographs using her iPad. This allows better communication with the dietitian about her intake. Shelley is a very honest person, but sometimes she finds food so enticing that she forgets about her energy restriction.

Shelley attends a respite placement one night a fortnight; her carers view food as one of life's great pleasures. They view respite as a break from normal life and this includes a break from 'dieting'. Together they will often go out to do things such as watch a film at the cinema.

Questions

1. What charts should Shelley's growth be plotted on?
2. Plot Shelley's growth history on PWS growth charts available at http://www.pwsausa.org/publications/Growth%20Hormone%20booklet%20final.pdf. What centile is Shelley on for her height and weight? On comparing these centiles, what do you notice?
3. What patterns do you notice with Shelley's BMI and does this change your thought about her height and weight? Plot on the BMI centile chart avaialble at http://www.rcpch.ac.uk/system/files/protected/page/NEW%20Girls%202-18yrs(4TH%20JAN%202012).pdf. How does this change your conclusions about her BMI? What do the bioimpedance results indicate? Is this typical for somebody with PWS?
4. What do Shelley's blood results tell you?
5. What is the nutrition and dietetic diagnosis? Write this as a PASS statement.
6. What is the aim of the intervention? Include SMART goals and outcome measures.
7. What would Shelley's nutritional (macro and micronutrient) requirements be?
8. What is the potential impact of having an older brother with Asperger's and a very athletic younger brother on Shelley?
9. How would you involve Shelley in her dietetic goal setting, taking into consideration her social and family situation?
10. What are the possible barriers to change?
11. What aspects of Shelley's care would require collaborative working with other professionals. List the professionals and the care they manage.
12. What considerations need to be made, as Shelley gets older?
13. How does the recent diagnosis affect your dietetic intervention?

Further question

14. How would you take Shelley's diminished capacity for consent into account when documenting her care?

Acknowledgements

With special thanks to Chris Smith and Amanda Avery.

References

Borgie, K. (1994) *Nutrition Care for Children with Prader Willi Syndrome: A Nutrition Guide for Parents of Children with Prader Willi Syndrome ages 3–9 years*. PWSA, Sarasota, FL.

Butler, M.G., Hanchett, J.M. & Thompson, T. (2006) Clinical findings and natural history of PWS. In: L.R. Greenswag & R.C. Alexander (eds), *Management of Prader–Willi Syndrome*, 3rd edn. Springer-Verlag, New York, NY, pp. 23–24.

Butler, M.G. & Meaney, J.F. (1991) Standards for selected anthropometric measurements in Prader–Willi syndrome. *Pediatrics*, **88** (**4**), 853–860.

Hauffa, B.P., Schlippe, G., Roos, M. *et al.* (2000) Spontaneous growth in German children and adolescents with genetically confirmed Prader–Willi syndrome. *Acta Paediatr*, **89** (**11**), 1302–1311.

Miller, J.L. *et al.* (2013) A reduced-energy intake, well-balanced diet improves weight control in children with Prader–Willi syndrome. *Journal of Human Nutrition and Dietetics*, **26**, 2–9.

Nagai, T., Matsuo, N., Kayanuma, Y. *et al.* (2000) Standard growth curves for Japanese patients with Prader–Willi syndrome. *American Journal of Medical Genetics*, **95**, 130–134.

NICE (2010) *Human growth hormone (somatrophin) for the treatment of growth failure in children*. https://www.nice.org.uk/guidance/ta188/resources/guidance-human-growth-hormone-somatropin-for-the-treatment-of-growth-failure-in-children-pdf [accessed on 15 May 2015].

SACN (2011) *Dietary Reference Values for Energy*. TSO, London.

Resources

Prader Willi Syndrome Association (PWSA). UK http://pwsa.co.uk/.
Royal College of Psychiatrists. www.rcpsych.ac.uk.
The National Autistic Society. www.autism.org.uk.

CASE STUDY 31

Bariatric surgery

Gail Pinnock & Mary O'Kane

Abi is a 32-year-old teacher who presented in the outpatient clinic following a GP referral. She has been obese since she was aged 10 years. She arrives with details of bariatric surgery she had abroad 8 weeks ago. From the literature it appears that she has had Roux-en-Y gastric bypass. However, when discussing the procedure it becomes apparent that she is not entirely sure what was done or what, if any, follow-up will be arranged. The hospital has given her dietary advice that has to be followed after the surgery, but she finds it confusing because the English isn't clear. Her GP has referred her to the dietitian for dietary advice.

Assessment

Domain	
Anthropometry, body composition and functional	Height 1.75 m Weight 112 kg BMI 33.6 kg/m^2
Biochemical and haematological	Full blood count within normal range Urea and electrolytes within normal range Random glucose 12 mmol/L HbA1c 97 mmol/mol Self-reported random blood glucose 8.4–13.6 mmol/L
Clinical	*Past medical history* Abi has tried to lose weight many times and each time she has regained the weight lost, often gaining more weight than she lost. She has attended local commercial slimming groups and had consulted a dietitian 5 years ago. In the past, her GP prescribed a 3-month course of Orlistat (120 mg/day) but she stopped taking them as she found the gastric side effects too difficult to cope with. When she started Orlistat her BMI was 39 kg/m^2; it was 43 kg/m^2 at its highest

Dietetic and Nutrition Case Studies, First Edition.
Edited by Judy Lawrence, Pauline Douglas, and Joan Gandy.

Companion Website: http://www.manualofdieteticpractice.com/

Assessment (*continued*)

Domain	
	Abi was diagnosed with type 2 diabetes 3 years ago and initially prescribed metformin (500 mg tds); her dose is currently 850 mg tds due to poor control of diabetes. She does not keep a blood glucose diary but reports blood glucose levels in the range 7.0–14.1 mmol
Diet	Despite having a restricted diet, Abi is finding it difficult to know what to eat. She vomits a frothy, white liquid approximately three times a week. She describes feeling that foods such as bread get stuck. Over the past few weeks she has restricted her intake to foods that she finds easier to swallow and digest. These include soups, yoghurt and ice cream; she can also manage potatoes and mashed vegetables when they are mixed with gravy

Questions

1. Describe the NICE criteria for bariatric surgery? Was Abi eligible for surgical referral before she paid for private surgery abroad? Suggest possible reasons for her decision.
2. Describe the multidisciplinary team most suitable for managing bariatric surgery patients.
3. What other assessments would you make?
4. What other questions should you ask about her diet and eating habits?
5. What is the nutrition and dietetic diagnosis? Write this as a PASS.
6. What issues might patients who have bariatric surgery abroad encounter?
7. What is the dietetic intervention include SMART goal(s)?
8. Comment on her present diet. What advice would you give her to increase the variety of her diet and to continue to lose weight?
9. What rate of weight loss would you recommend? Justify your answer.
10. What are the key questions to ask her when she presents in the clinic?
11. Comment on her present diet. What advice would you give her to increase the variety of her diet and to continue to lose weight?
12. Describe the Roux-en-Y gastric bypass procedure. How does this affect the absorption of nutrients and medicines including the contraceptive pill?
13. What are the potential nutritional complications associated with this type of surgery?
14. What other procedures are used in bariatric surgery? Use diagrams to explain the procedures.

15. What is the likely effect of surgery and the appropriate dietary advice, on her blood glucose control? How would this affect her medication?
16. Abi's experience with dietitians in the past has not been successful. How can you make this experience different?
17. What are the possible barriers to change? How can you overcome them?
18. What follow-up or monitoring would you arrange? How should SMART goals be used to evaluate and monitor Abi's progress.
19. How can you involve Abi in goal setting?
20. Detail plans for her follow-up that include her GP and other healthcare professionals as appropriate.

Further questions

21. Abi is anxious to start a family, what advice would you give her about the timing of a pregnancy following surgery? Elaborate on the reasons for this advice.
22. What are the effects of rapid weight loss on a foetus?
23. Detail the dietary advice you would give her if she does become pregnant while losing weight rapidly?
24. How does obesity affect fertility?
25. Using the available literature assess the success of bariatric surgery in terms of weight loss and other affects to the client.
26. How cost-effective is bariatric surgery?

References

Abeezar, S.I. *et al.* (2012) Long-term follow-up after laparoscopic sleeve gastrectomy: 8–9 year results. *Surgery for Obesity Related Diseases*, **8** (**6**), 679–684.

Buchwald, H. *et al.* (2004) Bariatric surgery: a systematic review and meta-analysis. *JAMA*, **292** (**14**), 1724–1737.

CMACE/RCOG (2010) *Joint Guideline Management of women with obesity in pregnancy*. http://www.hqip.org.uk/assets/NCAPOP-Library/CMACE-Reports/15.-March-2010-Management-of-Women-with-Obesity-in-Pregnancy-Guidance.pdf [accessed on 24 November 2014].

Jeannes, Y. (2014) Polycystic ovary syndrome. In: J. Gandy (ed), *Manual of Dietetic Practice*, 5th edn. Wiley Blackwell, Oxford.

Kaska, L., Kobiela, J., Abacjew-Chmylko, A. *et al.* (2013) Nutrition and pregnancy after bariatric surgery. *ISRN Obesity*, **2013**, Article ID 492060. doi: 10.1155/2013/492060.

NHS England. (2013) *Clinical Commissioning Policy: Complex and Specialised. Obesity Surgery* NHS ENGLAND/A05/P/a http://www.england.nhs.uk/wp-content/uploads/2013/08/a05-p-a.pdf.

NICE (2006) *Obesity: a guidance on the prevention, identification, assessment and management of overweight and obesity in adults and children*. Costing Report.

NICE (2010) *Weight management before, during and after pregnancy PH27*. http://www.nice.org.uk/guidance/ph27 [accessed on 24 November 2014].

Nørgaard, L.N., Gjerris, A.C.R., Kirkegaard, I., Berlac, J.F., Tabor, A., Danish Fetal Medicine Research Group (2014) Foetal growth in pregnancies conceived after gastric bypass surgery in relation to surgery-to-conception interval: A Danish national cohort study. *PLoS ONE* **9**(3): e90317. doi: 10.1371/journal.pone.0090317

O'Brien, P.E. *et al.* (2013) Long-term outcomes after bariatric surgery: fifteen year follow-up of adjustable gastric band and a systematic review of the bariatric surgical literature. *Annals of Surgery*, **257** (**1**), 87–94.

Office of Health Economics (2010) *Shedding the pounds: obesity management, NICE guidance and bariatric surgery in England.*

Picot, J. *et al.* (2009) The clinical effectiveness and cost-effectiveness of bariatric (weight loss) surgery for obesity: a systematic review and economic evaluation. *Health Technology Assessment*, **13** (**41**), 1–190.

Siega-Riz, A.M1., Viswanathan, M., Moos, M.K. *et al.* (2009) A systematic review of outcomes of maternal weight gain according to the Institute of Medicine recommendations: birthweight, fetal growth, and postpartum weight retention. *American Journal of Obstetrics and Gynecology*, **201** (**4**), e1–14.

Sjostrom, L. *et al.* (2004) Lifestyle, diabetes and cardiovascular risk factors 10 years after bariatric surgery. *New England Journal of Medicine*, **351** (**26**), 2683–2693.

Sjostrom, L. *et al.* (2007) Effects of bariatric surgery on mortality in Swedish obese subjects. *New England Journal of Medicine*, **357**, 741–52.

Resources

PEN: Practice Based Evidence in Nutrition. *Practice question on impact of bariatric surgery on pregnancy outcomes.* www.pennutrition.com/KnowledgePathway.aspx?kpid=15324&pqcatid=146&pqid=17075 [accessed 24 November 2014].

Pinnock, G. & O'Kane, M. (2014) Bariatric surgery. In: J. Gandy (ed), *Manual of Dietetic Practice*, 5th edn. Wiley Blackwell, Oxford.

Rees, G. (2014) Preconception and pregnancy. In: J. Gandy (ed), *Manual of Dietetic Practice*, 5th edn. Wiley Blackwell, Oxford.

CASE STUDY 32
Stroke and dysphagia

Judy Lawrence & Pauline Douglas

Anne is a 74-year-old married, woman with six grandchildren; she worked as a teaching assistant before retiring 14 years ago. Anne has a wide circle of friends, volunteers in a charity shops 2 days a week and looks after two of her grandchildren 1 day a week. Anne smokes between 5 and 10 cigarettes a day, she has been 'giving up' for years but never quite manages to stop completely. Anne went to her GP a week ago following a dizzy spell, but no problems were diagnosed. She went on to have a stroke and has been admitted to the local stroke unit, where she had a speech therapy assessment for swallow and was referred to you for a thick puree dysphagia diet and thickened fluids.

The following information was available for Anne.

Domain	
Anthropometry, body composition and functional	Weight 74 kg Height 1.53 m Waist circumference 104 cm
Biochemical and haematological	TC 5.6 mmol/L LDL cholesterol 2.9 mmol/L HDL cholesterol 1.2 mmol/L
Clinical	Blood pressure 155/99 mmHg *Medication* Ramipril 1.25 mg od Simvastatin 20 mg od Speech and mobility are now impaired following CVA

Dietetic and Nutrition Case Studies, First Edition.
Edited by Judy Lawrence, Pauline Douglas, and Joan Gandy.

Companion Website: http://www.manualofdieteticpractice.com/

Domain	
Diet	Usual diet prior to admission *On waking* 1 mug of tea (260 g), including semi-skimmed milk (40 g) *Breakfast* Branflakes (30 g) or crunchy nut cornflakes (30 g) with semi-skimmed milk (100 g) or 2 × 50:50 bread (2 × 36 g) with marmalade (2 × 15 g) and butter (2 × 7 g) 1 mug of tea (260 g), including semi-skimmed milk (40 g) *Mid-morning* I mug of coffee (260 g), including milk (whole when volunteering (40 g)), 1 banana 100 g *Lunch* Homemade sandwich made with 50:50 bread (2 × 36 g) with either cheese (30 g) or cold meat (45 g), butter (20 g) and tomato (35 g) and lettuce (20 g), chocolate digestive (18 g) *Afternoon* Mug of tea (260 g), including semi-skimmed milk (40 g), chocolate digestive (18 g) or piece of cake (40 g) *Evening meal* Shepherds pie, made with meat (170 g), potatoes (mash 175 g) and vegetables boiled (cauliflower 60 g, or sweetcorn 85 g) or White fish (100 g), with potatoes boiled(120 g) and carrots (40 g) or kedgeree (300 g) or macaroni cheese (280), with peas (40 g) Fruit crumble (170 g) and custard (120 g) or fruit pie (bought, 54 g) and custard (120 g) or rice pudding (canned, 213 g) *Supper* Mug of tea (260 g), including semi-skimmed milk (40 g), 2 digestive biscuits (2 × 15 g) *Alcohol* Enjoys a glass of wine with family over Sunday lunch, might have a whisky before bed Adds salt to cooking, sometimes also at the table
Environmental, behavioural and social	Anne considers herself to be active, especially for her age. She does all the housework and walks into town to her charity shop job. She also has a dog that she walks around the block every morning

Questions

1. What are Anne's risk factors for stroke?
2. What is the nutrition and dietetic diagnosis? Write this as a PASS statement
3. What is the aim of your dietetic intervention plan?
4. Explain how you would implement the intervention.
5. What are the barriers Anne may have to making these changes?
6. What advice do you give to Anne to help her stay hydrated?
7. How would you document Anne's care?
8. What information would you need to collect to monitor and review Anne?
9. In terms of cardiovascular health, would you promote weight loss for Anne?
10. How would you ensure that you engage effectively with the MDT?
11. What are the challenges for Anne and her family when she goes home still on the modified diet.

Further questions

12. To reduce the risk of further stroke what risk factors would you advice Anne to moderate following a return to normal swallowing function?
13. Anne has been avoiding grapefruit juice because of her simvastatin prescription. Is this correct?

References

British National Formulary: BNF (2014) https://www.medicinescomplete.com/mc/bnf/current/bnf_int829-grapefruit-juice.htm [accessed on 18 September 2014].

Jenkins, F. (2014) Stroke. In: J. Gandy (ed), *Manual of Dietetic Practice*, 5th edn. Wiley Blackwell, Oxford.

Resources

He, F.J., Nowson, C.A. & MacGregor, G.A. (2006) Fruit and vegetable consumption and stroke: meta-analysis of cohort studies. *Lancet*, **367**, 323.

NICE (2014) *Stroke: diagnosis and initial management of acute stroke and transient ischaemic attack (TIA)* (CG68). www.nice.org.uk/guidance/cg68.

SIGN: Scottish Intercollegiate Guidelines Network (2010) *Guideline 118: Management of patients with stroke; rehabilitation, prevention and management of complications and discharge planning*. http://www.sign.ac.uk/guidelines/fulltext/118/.

Stroke Association. www.stroke.org.uk/.

CASE STUDY 33
Hypertension

Judy Lawrence, Pauline Douglas & Joan Gandy

John is 56 years old. He was diagnosed with type 2 diabetes 5 years ago and managed to lose 10 kg. His diabetes is controlled with metformin. He has had hypertension diagnosed at a routine diabetic clinic appointment. John had no symptoms and was surprised to be referred to the dietitian. John lives with his wife, and two of their three adult children. He travels abroad frequently on business and does not always have as much choice as he would like over his diet. He is aware that he drinks more than is probably good for him and worries about keeping his weight under control.

Assessment

Domain	
Anthropometry, body composition and functional	Weight 90 Kg Height 1.83 m
Biochemical and haematological	BP 160/95 mmHg HbA1c 59 mmol/mol TC 4.5 mmol/L LDL cholesterol 2.3 mmol/L HDL cholesterol 1.3 mmol/L
Clinical	Metformin 1000 mg bd
Diet	Diet history *Breakfast* Porridge – oats (40 g) full fat milk (200 mL) Sundays – grilled bacon (2 × 40 g), eggs (2 × 60 g), tomato (65 g) and mushrooms (44 g) *Lunch* Restaurant meal with clients, 2–3 times per week. Tries to stick to one course and choose fish (plaice 200 g) or chicken (190 g), with vegetables (potatoes, 3 × 40 g, or chips 165 g, leeks 75 g, courgettes 90 g, asparagus 125 g) or salad (250 g). Ham sandwich (180 g) at desk on other days, roast dinner on Sundays

Dietetic and Nutrition Case Studies, First Edition.
Edited by Judy Lawrence, Pauline Douglas, and Joan Gandy.

Companion Website: http://www.manualofdieteticpractice.com/

Assessment *(continued)*

Domain	
	Evening meal Another restaurant meal when travelling sticks to one course but usually chooses cheese (Danish blue 30 g, camembert 40 g) and crackers (5 × 25 g) if customers are having dessert, 2–3 glasses (175 mL each) of wine. At home food is usually cooked fresh but may include an Indian or Chinese take-away a couple of times a month *Snacks* Tries to avoid eating between meals but may have crisps (40 g), nuts (50 g) and bar snacks when waiting for clients or travelling *Drinks* Tea/coffee with milk (40 mL) no sugar, may have Scotch (2 measures, 46 g)
Environmental, behavioural and social	Enjoys cooking but tends to be confined to BBQ duty in the summer, as his wife usually has a meal ready in the evenings Finds travelling and work stressful but has no financial worries

Questions

1. What is the nutrition and dietetic diagnosis? Write this as a PASS statement.
2. What is John's BMI?
3. What are the diagnostic criteria for hypertension?
4. Why is hypertension a particular problem for people with diabetes?
5. What waist circumference would be considered to indicate increased morbidity?
6. What complications are associated with poorly managed high blood pressure?
7. What are the aims of the dietary intervention?
8. Describe the intervention.
9. Describe the lifestyle changes that help prevent and manage hypertension.
10. Comment on the main sources of salt in John's diet.
11. What outcome measures would you use to monitor and evaluate the intervention?
12. What are the barriers to change? How can you help John overcome these barriers?
13. John has been asked to be referred to a private dietitian who is able to offer him more easily accessible appointment times. What would you include in your referral letter?

Resources

Harnden, K. (2014) Hypertension. In: J. Gandy (ed), *Manual of Dietetic Practice*, 5th edn. Wiley Blackwell, Oxford.

National Institute for Health and Care Excellence (2011) *Hypertension the clinical management of primary hypertension in adults in primary care*, CG127. https://www.nice.org.uk/guidance/cg127.

PEN: Practice Based Evidence in Nutrition. *Cardiovascular disease – hypertension evidence summary*. www.pennutrition.com/KnowledgePathway.aspx?kpid=674&trid=1960&trcatid=42.

CASE STUDY 34

Coronary heart disease

Lisa Gaff

Jonathan is a 56-year-old married, Caucasian man with two adult children; he works as a builder. He is normally fit and well, but had a sudden onset of chest pain during the night followed by an episode of vomiting. He initially thought this was indigestion but his wife called an ambulance when symptoms did not resolve. He was taken to accident and emergency and admitted in the cardiology ward. He was given a diagnosis of a non-ST segment elevation myocardial infarction (NSTEMI).

Jonathan was invited to attend the hospital's cardiac rehabilitation service, which includes education on risk factor reduction. He was therefore booked into an initial appointment with a dietitian as part of this service. He will also receive on-going dietetic follow-up for 8 weeks during this service.

At the initial assessment, the following information was available for Jonathan.

Domain	
Anthropometry, body composition and functional	Weight 91 kg Height 1.83 m BMI 27.2 kg/m^2 Waist circumference 104 cm
Biochemical and haematological	*Troponin* Initial (ideally 2 h post initial onset of symptoms) 1481 ng/L (reference range: 0–56 ng/L) Second (12 h post-initial) 7210 ng/L (reference range: 0–56 ng/L) *Lipid profile* TC 4.9 mmol/L LDL cholesterol 2.8 mmol/L HDL cholesterol 1.3 mmol/L TG 1.5 mmol/L

Dietetic and Nutrition Case Studies, First Edition.
Edited by Judy Lawrence, Pauline Douglas, and Joan Gandy.

Companion Website: http://www.manualofdieteticpractice.com/

Domain	
Clinical	No past medical history Family history: Father died from heart attack at 66 years Smoker Blood pressure138/93 mm/Hg *Medication* Atorvastatin 80 mg Clopidogrel 75 mg Ramipril 1.25 mg o.d. Bisoprolol 1.25 mg o.d. Aspirin 75 mg o.d.
Diet	*Breakfast* Jonathan reports he has been trying to introduce breakfast as he has been advised by his medical team to have something to eat when he is taking his tablets. Prior to his heart attack he did not eat breakfast Cornflakes or rice crispies (30 g), milk (100 mL) Or 2 slices (2 × 35 g) 50:50 bread with jam (2 × 15 g), spread (2 × 10 g) 2 cups of tea with milk (2 × 15 mL) *Mid-morning* Coffee – milk (15 mL), 2 rich tea biscuits (2 × 7 g) or a piece of fruit *Lunch* Homemade sandwich made with 50:50 bread (2 slices–2 × 35 g) with either cheese/ham, spread 2 × 10 g) Crisps (40 g) Apple (112 g) Bottle of water *Afternoon* Tea – milk (15 mL) *Evening meal* Varies, for example, spaghetti Bolognese – spaghetti (230 g), Bolognese sauce (300 g) Meat (100 g) with potatoes (mashed 180 g or roast 200 g or boiled 200 g) and vegetables (boiled – 70 g), gravy (plenty - 150 g) Homemade chicken curry (300 g) and rice (290 g) Fish (salmon (150 g), mackerel (160 g), haddock (170 g)) 1/7 with potatoes (boiled 200 g) and peas (100 g) Fruit salad (120 g) with ice cream (90 g) in summer, crumble (200 g) and custard (110 g) in winter

Domain	
	Evening Cheese (cheddar 30 g), biscuits (2 × 7 g)2/7 *Alcohol intake* Wine with evening meal 7/7 He shares a bottle of wine (red or white) with his wife. Sometimes they drink the whole bottle over the course of the evening but they often split this over 2 days. On a Friday night, he has an additional gin and tonic Sometimes adds salt to food if he has chips or roast potatoes. Wife adds salt to vegetables, pasta and potatoes when cooking but does not use in other dishes, such as in Bolognese or curry
Environmental, behavioural and social	Jonathan plays 5-a-side football for an hour once a week with friends. He does not do any regular additional exercise during the week but feels that he is relatively active with his job as a builder. He drives to and from work. He has been a smoker since the age of 17 (15 per day) but since his heart attack he has stopped Jonathan's wife does the majority of cooking

Following taking of the diet history, you discuss with Jonathan about his diet and his weight and what the benefits of change would be. You discuss all aspects of a cardio-protective diet in relation to Jonathan's current intake. You ask Jonathan to consider his motivation to make changes. Jonathan chooses to focus on losing weight, reducing salt intake and reducing alcohol intake as he feels these are the most important to him.

Questions

1. What are Jonathan's risk factors for heart disease?
2. What are the main considerations of a cardio-protective diet and what information is missing from Jonathan's diet history that you would find beneficial when considering these areas?
3. What is troponin?
4. What additional information would you like to gather from Jonathans diet history?
5. What is the nutrition and dietetic? Write this as a PASS statement.
6. What are the aims of the intervention plan?
7. What barriers do you think Jonathan may have to making dietary changes?
8. In terms of cardiovascular health, would you promote weight loss for Jonathan? What would the benefits of weight loss be?

9. When discussing salt, what would you want to find out from Jonathan and his wife regarding meal preparation and what advice would you give on reducing salt intake?
10. Jonathan asks whether using rock/sea salt would be a better choice than table salt. What would you discuss with him regarding this?
11. What would you discuss with Jonathan regarding alcohol intake?
12. What drug–nutrient interactions may you need to discuss?
13. How would you ensure that Jonathan is engaged with the intervention?
14. What outcome measures would you suggest for monitoring Jonathan's goals?

Further question

15. Jonathan asks about dietary supplements such as folic acid, vitamin E and garlic and whether these are beneficial with heart disease. How would you advise him?

References

British National Formulary: BNF (2014) https://www.medicinescomplete.com/mc/bnf/current/bnf_int829-grapefruit-juice.html [accessed on 18 September 2014].

Hinchliffe, J. & Green, J. (2014) Coronary heart disease. In: J. Gandy (ed), *Manual of Dietetic Practice*, 5th edn. Wiley Blackwell, Oxford.

Kris-Etherton, P.M., Lichtenstein, A.H., Howard, B. *et al.* (2004) Antioxidant vitamin supplements and cardiovascular disease. *Circulation*, **110**, 637–641.

Rahman, K. & Lowe, G.M. (2006) Garlic and cardiovascular disease: a critical review. *The Journal of Nutrition*, **136**, 736S–740S.

Resources

British Heart Foundation. www.bhf.org.uk

CASH: Consensus action on Salt and Health (2014) http://www.actiononsalt.org.uk/less/faqs/index.html [accessed on 26 September 2014].

Drinkaware www.drinkaware.co.uk/check-the-facts/what-is-alcohol/daily-guidelines.

PEN: Practice Based Evidence in Nutrition. *Cardiovascular disease evidence summary*; www.pennutrition.com/KnowledgePathway.aspx?kpid=2671&trid=3489&trcatid=42.

SIGN (2010) *Guideline 115: Management of Obesity*. www.sign.ac.uk [accessed on 21 August 2014].

CASE STUDY 35

Haematological cancer

Nicola Scott, Natasha Jones, Seema Lodhia, Julie Beckerson,
Ellie Allen & Kassandra Montanheiro

A 35-year-old man, Terry, who is married with a 2-year-old daughter, has been admitted to the haematology ward following a diagnosis of acute myeloid leukaemia (AML). He was transferred from his local hospital following a visit to his GP where he reported fatigue, night sweats and weight loss. He commenced high-dose chemotherapy and is currently 2 weeks into his first cycle of treatment. Terry has been referred for dietetic input.

Assessment

Domain	
Anthropometry, body composition and functional	Weight Current 70 kg On admission 61 kg 68 kg 2/12 ago Height 1.75 m
Biochemical and haematological	Sodium 136 mmol/L Potassium 4.2 mmol/L Urea 5.0 mmol/L Creatinine 86 mmol/L Albumin 24 g/L CRP 160 mg/L Magnesium 0.5 mmol/L Phosphate 0.58 mmol/L Platelets 18×10^9/L Neutrophils 0.02×10^9/L Hb 85 g/L White cell count (WCC) 1.5×10^9/L

Dietetic and Nutrition Case Studies, First Edition.
Edited by Judy Lawrence, Pauline Douglas, and Joan Gandy.

Companion Website: http://www.manualofdieteticpractice.com/

Assessment *(continued)*

Domain	
Clinical	Temperature 38.4 °C (high) Complaining of taste changes and loss of appetite Current medications of relevance Loperamide Furosemide Meropenum Ciprofloxacin
Diet	*Breakfast* 1 slice of toast (30 g) with butter (10 g) and a probiotic yoghurt (125 g) *Lunch* 1/4 potatoes (40 g) and chicken (110 g), 1/2 crumble (70 g) and custard (120 g) with a glass of water (180 mL) *Evening Meal* 1/3 of a bacon, lettuce and tomato sandwich (60 g)
Environmental, behavioural and social	Daughter attends day nursery three times per week Works out at the gym 4 times a week Has a physically demanding job Terry is worried about something called neutropenia He is in isolation

Questions

1. Comment on Terry's weight history and calculate relevant anthropometry.
2. State and calculate the principle nutritional requirements for the patient.
3. What are the risks specific to this patient group?
4. What is the nutrition and dietetic diagnosis? Write it as a PASS statement.
5. What is the aim of your dietetic intervention plan?
6. Explain your dietetic intervention plan for this patient.
7. What are the important biochemical results and how did you interpret them?
8. Give a brief explanation of AML and the implications the treatment may have on clinical care.
9. What are the holistic needs of this patient?
10. What impact does neutropenia have on his diet and consider an appropriate approach to deliver this information in relation to his concern.

Further questions

11. Terry is planned for a stem cell transplant. You are asked to see him at pre-assessment to discuss artificial nutrition support routes. What further information would you need to consider when giving advice and preparing the patient for their transplant treatment?
12. If you were considering enteral tube feeding what additional points would you consider?
13. Discuss the reasons for low magnesium levels.

References

Beckerson, J. (2014) Haematological cancers and high dose therapy. In: J. Gandy (ed), *Manual of Dietetic Practice*, 5th edn. Wiley Blackwell, Oxford.

Henry, C.J.K. (2005) Basal metabolic rate studies in humans: measurement and development of new equations. *Public Health Nutrition*, **8**, 1133–1152.

Todorovic, V. & Micklewright, A. (2011) On behalf of the Parenteral and Enteral Nutrition Group of the British Dietetic Association (PENG). In: *A Pocket Guide to Clinical Nutrition*. British Dietetic Association, Birmingham.

Resources

BDA; *The Nutrition and Hydration Digest: Improving Outcomes through Food and Beverage Services*, (2012) page 87–90. BDA. www.bda.uk.com/publications/professional/NutritionHydration Digest.pdf [accessed on 27 January 2015].

Beckerson, J. (2014) Haematological cancers and high dose therapy. In: J. Gandy (ed), *Manual of Dietetic Practice*, 5th edn. Wiley Blackwell, Oxford.

Leukaemia and Lymphoma Association (2012) *Dietary advice for haematology patients with neutropenia* Leukaemia and Lymphoma Research. https://leukaemialymphomaresearch.org.uk.

Macmillan Cancer support. www.macmillan.org.uk.

CASE STUDY 36

Head and neck cancer

Sian Lewis & Rachael Donnelly

John is 61 years old and lives with his second wife; he has three children of his own and three stepchildren. He retired 6 years ago having worked as a supervisor in a factory. He presented with a 2-month history of swollen neck glands and a lump on the left side of his tongue. At presentation, he had discomfort in his mouth but no problems with eating, drinking or swallowing.

Previous medical history includes colour blindness, type 2 diabetes mellitus (diet controlled), asthma (controlled with inhalers) and he takes warfarin having had multiple pulmonary embolisms. He drinks 3 pints of beer a day, 7 days a week and in the past drank 17 pints a day for at least 10 years. He has never smoked.

He is diagnosed with T2 N2b M0 (Stage IVa) human papilloma virus positive squamous cell carcinoma left tongue base. His treatment plan is 2 cycles neoadjuvant chemotherapy (Carboplatin and 5-FU) given 3 weekly, followed by 6 weeks of intensity-modulated radiation therapy (IMRT) (65 Gy) with concurrent Carboplatin. A prophylactic gastrostomy was not placed.

As a result of fatigue, pain and poor nutritional intake, John is admitted to the cancer centre. At the time of assessment, John has completed 20 of 30 fractions radiotherapy and has had one cycle of concurrent chemotherapy to be considered for enteral feeding/intensive nutrition support

Assessment

Domain	
Anthropometry, body composition and functional	Weight Current 76.3 kg 4 months ago 82.4 kg 10 months ago 95.2 kg Height 1.74 m

Dietetic and Nutrition Case Studies, First Edition.
Edited by Judy Lawrence, Pauline Douglas, and Joan Gandy.

Companion Website: http://www.manualofdieteticpractice.com/

Assessment (*continued*)

Domain	
Biochemical & haematological	Albumin 32 g/L Protein 63 g/L Sodium 139 mmol/L Potassium 3.0 mmol/L Creatinine 62 mmol/L Urea 12.6 mmol/L Magnesium 0.57 mmol/L Hb 113 g/L
Clinical	*Common Terminology Criteria for Adverse Events (CTCAE) toxicity scoring* (Cancer Therapy Evaluation Program, 2010) Grade 3 mucositis Grade 2 dysphagia Grade 3 dehydration Grade 3 anorexia Grade 3 weight loss
Diet	*Breakfast* Ready Brek with extra milk, ate all (portion size not given) *Lunch* Soup, ate all *Evening meal* Minced beef and gravy (no potatoes, no vegetables, no pastry) reports eating 5 mouthfuls Pureed apple and custard, ate all Sips of water and 4 cups of coffee during day. *Alcohol* Stopped 1 week before admission Prescribed 4 × 200 mL oral nutrition supplements (ONS) (1.5 kcal/mL milk style) day, nil for last 5 days
Environmental, behavioural and social	Inpatient on ward

Questions

1. What other assessments will you require to plan and implement a dietetic intervention?
2. What biochemical results are the most important and are there any others you would advise?
3. Which predictive equation would you use to estimate energy and protein requirements? Give your reasons.
4. What may have contributed to John's loss of weight?

5. What medical interventions should John receive at this stage of his treatment?
6. What is the nutrition and dietetic diagnosis? Write this as a PASS statement.
7. What are the aims of the dietetic intervention?
8. How would you achieve these aims? Explain how you would implement the dietetic intervention?
9. Why is it important to document your implementation?
10. What aspects of John's care would require you to work collaboratively with other health care professionals (HCPs)? List the HCPs and the aspects of care they manage.
11. What exercises should John be doing regularly? When should they start?
12. What are the potential barriers to discharging John home with enteral feeding?
13. What outcome measures would you use to monitor the objectives?
14. How frequently would you recommend John be reviewed following completion of his radiotherapy treatment and discharge from the ward?

Further questions

15. What impact will Carboplatin and radiotherapy have on John's biochemistry results?
16. Which toxicity scoring system is the most relevant for grading treatment related problems and why?
17. When should enteral feeding be initiated?
18. What evidence is available to support nasogastric or gastrostomy feeding with this group of patients?
19. Describe the medical considerations that would need to be taken into account if John had been offered a prophylactic gastrostomy.
20. Describe how you would have managed this patient. If different to above, explain why.
21. As the number of reactive nasogastric tubes are increasing how could you implement more effective support within the community during and after discharge?
22. What supportive rehabilitation programmes would you suggest to reduce the risk of tube dependency? Which HCPs would you work collaboratively with at this stage?
23. What are the long-term side effects of treatment that John may require information about?
24. What initiatives may John benefit from once he has recovered from his chemoradiotherapy treatment and is disease free?
25. Compare prophylactic gastrostomy placement versus reactive nasogastric feeding in patients diagnosed with head and neck cancer and discuss the advantages and disadvantages of both.
26. What risk factors are associated with the decision making for gastrostomy placement?
27. There are different guidelines for refeeding syndrome; which would you adhere to and what is your justification?
28. How can you determine if a patient has refeeding syndrome or deranged electrolytes as a result of chemotherapy?

References

Cancer Therapy Evaluation Program (2010) *Common Terminology Criteria for Adverse Events (CTCAE).* http://evs.nci.nih.gov/ftp1/CTCAE/CTCAE_4.03_2010-06-14_QuickReference_5x7.pdf [accessed on 22 June 2014].

Findlay, M., Bauer, J., Bron, T. *et al.* (2011) *Evidence based practice guidelines for the nutritional management of adult patients with head and neck cancer.* http://wiki.cancer.org.au/australia/COSA [accessed on 13 June 2014].

Henry, C.J.K. (2005) Basal metabolic rate studies in humans: measurement and development of new equations. *Public Health Nutrition,* **8**, 1133–1152.

NICE (2006) *Nutrition support in adults: oral nutrition support, enteral tube feeding and parenteral nutrition.* www.nice.org.uk/nicemedia/live/10978/29979/29979.pdf [accessed on 13 June 2014].

Nugent, B., Lewis, S. and O'Sullivan, J. M. (2010) Enteral feeding methods for nutritional management in patients diagnosed with head and neck cancers being treated with radiotherapy and/or chemotherapy (Review). *Cochrane Database of Systematic Reviews,* **3**. http://onlinelibrary.wiley.com/doi/10.1002/14651858.CD007904.pub2/pdf/standard [accessed on 14 May 2014].

Radiation Therapy Oncology Group (2014) *Acute radiation morbidity scoring criteria.* www.rtog.org/researchassociates/adverseeventreporting/acuteradiationmorbidityscoringcriteria.aspx [accessed on 22 June 2014].

Talwar B (2011) Head and neck cancer. In: C. Shaw (ed). *Nutrition and Cancer.* Wiley Blackwell, Chichester.

Talwar, B. & Donnelly, R. (2011) Nutrition. In: N.J. Roland & V. Paleri (eds), *Head and Neck Cancer: Multidisciplinary Management Guidelines,* pp. 45–56. ENT UK, London.

Talwar, B. & Findlay, M. (2012) When is the optimal time for placing a gastrostomy in patients undergoing treatment for head and neck cancer? *Current Opinion in Supportive and Palliative Care,* **6** (**1**), 41–53.

Resources

PEN: Practice Based Evidence in Nutrition. *Improving outcomes in head and neck cancers: evidence update* (2012) www.pennutrition.com/KnowledgePathway.aspx?kpid=20918&trid=21699&trcatid=27.

Shaw, C. (2011) (ed) *Nutrition and Cancer.* Wiley Blackwell, Chichester.

Talwar, B. (2014) Head & neck cancer. In: J. Gandy (ed), *Manual of Dietetic Pratcice,* 5th edn. Wiley Blackwell, Oxford.

CASE STUDY 37
Critical care

Ella Segaran

Helen is a 34-year-old woman, previously fit and healthy. She is married with one son. She was admitted to intensive care following a fall down the stairs when out with friends.

Assessment

Domain	
Anthropometry, body composition and functional	Weight 65 kg Height 1.69 m Left arm MUAC 26.5 cm, Ulna 26.5 cm
Biochemical and haematological	Sodium 149 mmol/L Potassium 4 mmol/L Phosphate 0.73 mmol/L Corrected calcium 2.11 mmol/L Magnesium 0.8 mmol/L Albumin 25 g/L CRP 100 mg/dL
Clinical	CT scan – severe traumatic brain injury (TBI). Intubated and ventilated with mandatory ventilation Day 1 underwent decompressive craniectomy *Medication* Atracurium Propofol 250 mg/h Fentanyl Noradrenaline Insulin sliding scale Sodium docusate Lansoprazole Phenytoin IV
Diet	Enteral nutrition started per ICU out of hours feeding regimen
Environmental, behavioural and social	Lives with her husband and son in their own house. She normally does the cooking and housework

Dietetic and Nutrition Case Studies, First Edition.
Edited by Judy Lawrence, Pauline Douglas, and Joan Gandy.

Companion Website: http://www.manualofdieteticpractice.com/

She requires nutritional support and has a nasogastric tube in place. The dietitian is asked to manage her nutritional care.

Questions

1. Describe the metabolic response to critical illness.
2. What is the nutrition and dietetic diagnosis? Write this as a PASS statement.
3. What is the dietetic intervention? Give details of the feed type and rate.
4. How would you calculate energy and protein requirements accounting for stress and activity? Justify why you have selected these methods.
5. What clinical factors would influence energy expenditure in this case?
6. Why is the sodium high? Should you adjust your feeding regimen?
7. What factors need to be considered when interpreting anthropometric measures in the ICU setting?
8. What are the factors that could hinder enteral feed delivery on an ICU?
9. How would you monitor gastrointestinal tolerance to enteral nutrition in ICU patients?
10. If poor tolerance was identified, what steps could be taken to overcome this?
11. How would you evaluate and monitor her progress? What outcome measures would you use?

Further questions

12. Describe four different predictive equations that can be used to estimate energy requirements, stating the advantages and disadvantages of their use in the ICU setting.
13. Which predictive equation for energy would you now select and why?
    Insulin therapy has been commenced in this case.
14. The patient is not a known diabetic. What are the reasons for the poor glycaemic control?
15. Describe the rationale for using the medications listed above. Discuss any nutritional considerations.
16. This lady is sedated with 250 mg/h propofol. It has nutritional implications, so would you amend your feeding regimen accordingly?
17. What size of aspirate is now suggested as a definition of large and what evidence supports this?

References

Bessey, P.Q., Watters, J.M., Aoki, T.T. *et al.* (1984) Combined hormonal infusion simulates the metabolic response to injury. *Annals of Surgery*, **200** (**3**), 264–281.

Cerra, F.B., Benitez, M.R., Blackburn, G.L. *et al.* (1997) Applied nutrition in ITU patients. A consensus statement of the American College of Chest Physicians. *Chest*, **111**, 769–778.

Dhaliwal, R., Cahill, N., Lemieux, M. *et al.* (2014) The Canadian critical care nutrition guidelines in 2013: an update on current recommendations and implementation strategies. *Nutrition in Clinical Practice*, **29** (**1**), 29–43.

Frankenfield, D., Smith, J.S. & Cooney, R.N. (2004) Validation of 2 approaches to predicting resting metabolic rate in critically ill patients. *Journal of Parenteral and Enteral Nutrition*, **28** (**4**), 259–264.

Frankenfield, D., Hise, M., Malone, A. *et al.* (2007) Prediction of resting metabolic rate in critically ill adult patients: results of a systematic review of the evidence. *Journal of the American Dietetic Association*, **107** (**9**), 1552–1561.

Frankenfield, D.C., Coleman, A., Alam, S. *et al.* (2009) Analysis of estimation methods for resting metabolic rate in critically ill adults. *Journal of Parenteral and Enteral Nutrition*, **33** (**1**), 27–36.

Harris, J.A. & Benedict, F.G. (1919) *Biometric Studies of Basal Metabolism*. Carnegie Institute of Washington, Washington, DC.

Henry, C.J.K. (2005) Basal metabolic rate studies in humans: measurement and development of new equations. *Public Health Nutrition*, **8**, 1133–1152.

Ireton-Jones, C.S., Turner, W.W. Jr., Liepa, G.U. *et al.* (1992) Equations for the estimation of energy expenditures in patients with burns with special reference to ventilatory status. *Journal of Burn Care and Rehabilitation*, **13** (**3**), 330–333.

Kreymann, K.G., Berger, M.M., Deutz, N.E. *et al.* (2006) ESPEN guidelines on enteral nutrition: intensive care. *Clinical Nutrition*, **25** (**2**), 210–223.

McClave, S.A., Martindale, R.G., Vanek, V.W. *et al.* (2009) Guidelines for the provision and assessment of nutrition support therapy in the adult critically Ill patient: Society of Critical Care Medicine (SCCM) and American Society for Parenteral and Enteral Nutrition (A.S.P.E.N.). *Journal of Parenteral and Enteral Nutrition*, **33** (**3**), 277–316.

Montejo, J.C., Minambres, E., Bordeje, L. *et al.* (2010) Gastric residual volume during enteral nutrition in ICU patients: the REGANE study. *Intensive Care Medicine*, **36** (**8**), 1386–1393.

Singer, P., Berger, M.M., Van den Berghe, G. *et al.* (2009) ESPEN guidelines on parenteral nutrition: intensive care. *Clinical Nutrition*, **28** (**4**), 387–400.

Resource

Segaran, E. (2014) Critical care. In: J. Gandy (ed), *Manual of Dietetic Practice*, 5th edn. Wiley Blackwell, Oxford.

CASE STUDY 38

Traumatic brain injury

Kirsty-Anna McLaughlin

Steve is a 30-year-old man who was struck on the head with a blunt object on a night out. Paramedics recorded a Glasgow Coma Scale (GCS) of six. On hospital admission a repeat GCS was eight. A CT scan and X-ray were conducted, which showed he had sustained a skull fracture, epidural haematoma and diffuse axonal injury. A haematoma drain and craniotomy were performed and tracheostomy tube inserted. Steve went to ICU for monitoring where a urinary catheter and nasogastric (NG) tube were placed. Intracranial pressure was 23 mmHg. He was referred to the dietitian for a feeding regimen. At 14 days post injury Steve was in a minimally conscious state (MCS); tracheostomy secretions were thick.

Assessment

Domain				
Anthropometry	Weight (kg)	Admission	Day 14	
		72 kg	66.9 kg	
	Ulna length	26.6 cm		
Biochemistry		Day 1	Day 7	Day 14
	Sodium (mmol/L)	137	145	149
	Potassium (mmol/L)	5.0	—	—
	Urea (mmol/L)	—	7.7	8.0
	Glucose (mmol/L)	15	—	—
	CRP (mg/L)	180	75	84
	Albumin (g/L)	15	30	22
	Hb (g/dL)	15	—	13
	WCC $\times 10^9$ L	10	—	18
	ALT (U/L)	50	40	—
	ALP (U/L)	200	150	—

Dietetic and Nutrition Case Studies, First Edition.
Edited by Judy Lawrence, Pauline Douglas, and Joan Gandy.

Companion Website: http://www.manualofdieteticpractice.com/

Assessment *(continued)*

Domain				
Clinical	BP	90/60 mmHg		
	Temperature	38.0 C for 4 h		
	Gastric aspirate	4 h	8 h	12 h
		100 mL	120 mL	90 mL
	Stool chart	Day 1	Day 14	
	Whelan *et al.* (2001)			
		B2 × 1	D1 × 2, D2 × 1	
	Urine output (mL/d)	Day 1	Day 14	
		1500	1000	
		Clear	Cloudy	
	Perspiration	Day 1	Day 7	
		1 episode	5 episodes	
	Medication	Day 1	Day 14	
		IV Saline 0.9%	Ciprofloxacin	
		Phenytoin	Loperamide	
		Baclofen	Lansoprazole	
		Mannitol	Phenytoin	
Dietary	Alcohol drinker (intoxicated during assault)			
	NG tube *in situ*, placement confirmed			
Environmental, social	The patient lives with his parents in a flat He is a teacher			

Questions

1. What other initial assessments do you suggest? Why? Present your answers in the ABDCE format.
2. Interpret the biochemistry results on days 1, 7 and 14.
3. On initial assessment, what is the nutrition and dietetic diagnosis? Write this as a PASS statement.
4. What is the aim of the dietetic intervention? Include SMART goal(s) and outcome measures. Justify the outcome measures.
5. What needs to be considered when devising the enteral feeding regimen? Provide a feeding regimen based on the assessment.
6. What is the nutrition and dietetic diagnosis at day 14? Are there any changes to the initial assessment and plan?
7. What aspects would require you to work collaboratively with other health care professionals (HCPs)?
8. How would you obtain consent? Why is it important to document this?
9. How would you evaluate patient progress?

Further questions

10. What does the GCS Score mean for diagnosis and prognosis?
11. What long-term feeding would you suggest and why?
12. Discuss whether nutrition education can help to reduce TBI incidence.
13. Discuss the role of the dietitian in acute and rehabilitation stages of TBI.

References

BNF (2014) *Phenytoin: Additional Information, Interactions. British National Formulary* [online]. www.medicinescomplete.com/mc/bnf/current/PHP2958-phenytoin.htm [accessed on 4 June 2014].

Bombardier, C. & Turner, A. (2009) Alcohol and traumatic disability. In: R. Frank & T. Elliott (Eds.), *The Handbook of Rehabilitation Psychology*, 2nd edn. American Psychological Association Press, Washington, DC.

Department of Health (2005) *Mental Capacity Act 2005*. The Stationery Office Limited, London.

Haydel, M. Johnson, E. Ma, M. *et al.* (2013) Assessment of traumatic brain injury, acute. *British Medical Journal Best Practice* [online]. http://bestpractice.bmj.com/best-practice/monograph/515.html. [viewed on 1 June 2014].

HCPC (2008) *Standards of Conduct, Performance and Ethics*. Health and Care Professions Council, London [online]. http://www.hcpc-uk.org/publications/standards/index.asp?id=38 [accessed on 8 August 2013].

Henry, C.J.K. (2005) Basal metabolic rate studies in humans: measurement and development of new equations. *Public Health Nutrition*, **8**, 1133–1152.

London Health Sciences Centre (2012) *Neurological monitoring standards of nursing care in CCTC (SONC). Critical Care Trauma Centre* [online]. www.lhsc.on.ca/Health_Professionals/CCTC/standards/neuro.htm [accessed on 1 June 2014].

McLaughlin, K.-A. & Moore, G. (2014) Traumatic brain injury. In: J. Gandy (ed), *Manual of Dietetic Practice*, 5th edn. Wiley Blackwell, Oxford.

Morris, L., Whitmer, A. & McIntosh, E. (2013) Tracheostomy Care and Complications in the Intensive Care Unit. *Critical Care Nursing*, **33**, 18–30.

NICE (2006) *Nutrition support in adults: oral nutrition support, enteral tube feeding and parenteral nutrition*. National Institute for Health and Clinical Excellence Clinical Guideline 32 [online]. http://guidance.nice.org.uk/CG32/NICEGuidance/pdf/English [accessed on 1 June 2014].

NICE (2014) *Head injury: triage, assessment, investigation and early management of head injury in children, young people and adults*. National Institute for Health and Care Excellence Clinical Guideline 176 (Partial update of NICE CG56) Methods, evidence and recommendations [online]. http://guidance.nice.org.uk/CG176 [accessed on 1 June 2014].

Pinto, T., Rocha, R., Paula, C. *et al.* (2012) Tolerance to enteral nutrition therapy in traumatic brain injury patients. *Brain Injury*, **26**, 1113–1117.

Sanfilippo, F., Veenith, T., Santonocito, C. *et al.* (2014) Liver function test abnormalities after traumatic brain injury: is hepato-biliary ultrasound a sensitive tool? *British Journal of Anaesthesia*, **112**, 298–303.

SIGN (2009) *Early management of patients with a head injury: A national guideline 110*. Scottish Intercollegiate Guidelines Network. NHS Quality Improvement Scotland [online]. . www.sign.ac.uk/guidelines/fulltext/110/ [accessed 1 June 2014].

Smith, S., Fleming, C. & Taylor, S. (2011) Assessment of nutritional status. In: V. Todorovic & A. Micklewright (eds), *A Pocket Guide to Clinical Nutrition*, 4th edn. The Parenteral and Enteral Nutrition Group of the British Dietetic Association.

Stroud, M., Duncan, H. & Nightingale, J. (2003) Guidelines for enteral feeding in adult hospital patients. *Gut*, **52**, 1–12.

Ting, H., Chen, M., Hsieh, Y. *et al.* (2010) Good mortality prediction by Glasgow Coma Scale for neurosurgical patients. *Journal of the Chinese Medical Association*, **72**, 139–143.

Triebel, K. Martin, R. Novack, T. *et al.* (2012). Treatment consent capacity in patients with traumatic brain injury across a range of injury severity. *Neurology* **78**, 1472–1478.

Wang, X., Dong, Y., Han, X. *et al.* (2013) Nutritional support for patients sustaining traumatic brain injury: a systematic review and meta-analysis of prospective studies. *PLoS One*, **8**, 1–14.

Whelan, K. Taylor, M. & Judd, P. (2001). *The King's Stool Chart.* King's College London, London. www.kcl.ac.uk/medicine/research/divisions/dns/projects/stoolchart/index.aspx [accessed on 1 June 2014].

Resource

McLaughlin, K.-A. & Moore, G. (2014) Traumatic brain injury. In: J. Gandy (ed), *Manual of Dietetic Practice*, 5th edn. Wiley Blackwell, Oxford.

CASE STUDY 39

Spinal cord injury

Carolyn Taylor

Stan is a 30-year-old single man who fell from scaffolding. At the time of injury he was unable to move his legs and was taken to his local hospital where he was found to have a C3 complete spinal cord injury. The unstable spinal injury has undergone fixation. He is currently ventilated on an ICU unit. He is 6 weeks post injury and medically stable and is awaiting a bed at a specialist spinal injury centre for rehabilitation. The nearest specialist unit that will take ventilated patients is 105 miles away. He is unable to swallow and is being fed with an NG tube.

Assessment

Domain	
Anthropometry, body composition and functional	Pre-injury weight 97 kg Current weight, 6 weeks post injury, 88 kg Height 1.83 m
Biochemistry and haematology	Sodium 135 mmol/L Potassium 3.4 mmol/L Urea 8.7 mmol/L Creatinine 54 µmol/L Phosphate 1.2 mmol/L ALP 82 iu/L Total protein 57 g/L Albumin 32 g/L Bilirubin 9 µmol/L Adjusted calcium 2.47 mmol/L Hb 103 g/L WCC 6.9×10^9/L CRP 15 mg/L

Dietetic and Nutrition Case Studies, First Edition.
Edited by Judy Lawrence, Pauline Douglas, and Joan Gandy.

Companion Website: http://www.manualofdieteticpractice.com/

Assessment *(continued)*

Domain	
Clinical	Grade 3 sacral pressure ulcer Frequent type 6/7 stools (Bristol stool chart) Urinary catheter Ventilated with the aim to wean off. Previously managed a couple of hours but is now struggling with oral secretions and requiring regular suctions and twice daily chest physiotherapy Bed rest, but the doctors are keen for him to begin to sit out of bed
Diet	Nil by mouth Continuous 24 h NG feed Fluid requirements are being met with additional water flushes
Environmental, behavioural and social	Single, living alone but near parents. Car mechanic Proud of body image – developed upper body muscle mass (previously used protein shakes) and reported regular gym use before injury

You have been asked to develop a suitable feeding regimen for Stan as he begins to sit up in bed, taking into consideration the requirements for his bowel management and weight loss. A recent swallow assessment by the speech and language therapist indicates that the patient is likely to struggle to introduce food into his diet.

Questions

1. What other assessments do you suggest?
2. What is the nutrition and dietetic diagnosis? Write it as a PASS statement.
3. What is the aim of your dietetic intervention?
4. How would you involve Stan in the dietetic goal setting?
5. Explain how you would implement the dietetic intervention
6. How would you document Stan's care?
7. What aspects of Stan's care would require you to work collaboratively with other AHPs?
8. How would you assess the energy requirements for Stan considering that his spinal cord injury has resulted in loss of nerve supply to the body below the C3 level?
9. What could have contributed to weight loss?
10. What type of feed would you use?

11. Are there any specific nutritional recommendations to help pressure ulcer healing?
12. What information would you need to evaluate and monitor Stan's progress?
13. How would you recommend that the patient's weight be monitored?

Further questions

14. What long-term energy requirements would you recommend for Stan?
15. What type of bowel management would be most appropriate for Stan?

References

American Dietetic Association (2013) *Spinal cord injury (SCI) assessment of nutritional needs for pressure ulcers.* http://andevidencelibrary.com/template.cfm?key=2378&auth=1 [accessed on 10 July 2014].

Cameron, K.J., Nyulasi, I.B., Collier, G.R. *et al.* (1996) Assessment of the effect of increased dietary fibre intake on bowel function in patients with spinal cord injury. *Spinal Cord*, **34** (**5**), 277–283.

Cox, S.A.R., Weiss, S.M., Posuniak, E.A. *et al.* (1985) Energy expenditure after spinal cord injury: an evaluation of stable rehabilitating patients. *Journal of Trauma*, **25**, 419–423.

de Groot, S., Post, M.W., Postma, K. *et al.* (2010) Prospective analysis of body mass index during and up to 5 years after discharge from inpatient spinal cord injury rehabilitation. *Journal of Rehabilitation Medicine*, **42**, 922–928.

Henry, C.J.K. (2005) Basal metabolic rate studies in humans: measurement and development of new equations. *Public Health Nutrition*, **8**, 1133–1152.

Monroe, M.B., Tataranni, P.A., Pratley, R. *et al.* (1998) Lower daily energy expenditure as measured by a respiratory chamber in subjects with spinal cord injury compared with control subjects. *American Journal of Clinical Nutrition*, **68** (**6**), 1223–1227.

NICE (2014) *Pressure ulcer: prevention and management of pressure ulcers.* NICE clinical guideline 179. guidance.nice.org.uk/cg179 [accessed on 10 July 2014].

Resource

Twist, A. & Wong, S. (2014) Spinal cord injury. In: J. Gandy (ed), *Manual of Dietetic Practice*, 5th edn. Wiley Blackwell, Oxford.

CASE STUDY 40

Burns

Non-ventilated scald injury in an elderly patient

E. Mark Windle

Beryl is a 70-year-old lady admitted to the local burns unit following an accident in her home kitchen. She presented with a 17% total body surface area (TBSA) scald. She had partial thickness injuries affecting her lower abdomen, hands and forearms. Family members reported that Beryl had developed a chest infection a week prior to admission. Formal intravenous fluid resuscitation was required on admission. Following discussions on the multidisciplinary team (MDT) ward round, it was decided to manage her burns conservatively with dressings and full medical and nursing care. Because of her age, co-morbidity (chest infection) and the type of injury, the MDT agreed that it would not be appropriate to surgically intervene. Within 48 h of admission the unit made a referral to the dietetic department for assessment with a view to oral nutrition support, triggered by her Malnutrition Universal Screening Tool (MUST) score, which was 4.

Assessment

Domain	
Anthropometry, body composition and functional	Weight 69 kg (GP records also indicate weight at 77 kg, 4 months prior to admission) Height 1.62 m
Biochemical and haematological	Sodium 139 mmol/L Potassium 4.3 mmol/L Urea 15.1 mmol/L Creatinine 120 µmol/L Albumin 13 g/L CRP 129 mg/L WCC 14.6 × 109 L Hb 89 g/L Mean corpuscular volume 119 fl

Dietetic and Nutrition Case Studies, First Edition.
Edited by Judy Lawrence, Pauline Douglas, and Joan Gandy.

Companion Website: http://www.manualofdieteticpractice.com/

Assessment (*continued*)

Domain	
Clinical	Chest infection reported prior to admission Dehydrated on admission *Medication* Omeprazole 20 mg od Codeine phosphate 30 mg qds Loperamide 6 mg qds 1 L oral rehydration solution
Diet	As a consequence of her confused state, the patient offered very limited history Food record chart for the previous 24 h as recorded by nursing staff *Breakfast* Half cup of tea, with whole milk and 1 sugar Half a bowl of cereal with whole milk and sugar *Mid-morning* Half a cup of coffee with whole milk and 1 sugar *Lunch* Mashed potato, small portion Chicken with gravy, small portion, half left. Peas 1 tbs Apple pie, 2 spoonsful, custard – all eaten *Mid-afternoon* Half cup of tea, made with whole milk and 1 sugar *Dinner* Half an egg sandwich Cup of tea, with whole milk and 1 sugar *Evening* Half a cup of tea made with whole milk and 1 sugar
Environmental, behavioural and social	Elderly lady who lives alone. Beryl's son lives five miles away and assists with shopping. No regular alcohol consumption, non-smoker

Questions

1. What is the nutrition and dietetic diagnosis? Write this as a PASS statement.
2. Using the food record chart estimate Beryl's energy, protein and fluid intake for the past 24 h.
3. What is the aim/objective of your dietetic intervention plan?
4. What SMART goal(s) and outcome measures would you use to monitor the objectives?

5. What normal ranges would you use when assessing the blood results?
6. What are the important biochemical and haematological results and what is their dietetic relevance?
7. Calculate energy requirements using the Ireton-Jones *et al.* (1992) predictive equation for spontaneously breathing (i.e. non-mechanically ventilated) burned patients. Explain why this equation is used.
8. What metabolic and functional barriers would there be to optimising nutritional status?
9. What aspects of care would require you to work collaboratively with other health care professionals?
10. When would you document Beryl's dietetic care?
11. What arrangements would you need to make prior to discharge?

Reference

Ireton-Jones, C.S., Turner, W.W., Liepa, G.U. *et al.* (1992) Equations for estimation of energy expenditure in patients with burns with special reference to ventilatory status. *Journal of Burn Care and Rehabilitation*, **13**, 330–333.

Resources

Windle, E.M. (2004) Audit of successful weight maintenance in adult and paediatric survivors of thermal injury at a UK regional burn centre. *Journal of Human Nutrition and Dietetics*, **17**, 435–441.

Windle, E.M. (2014) Burn injury. In: J. Gandy (ed), *Manual of Dietetic Practice*, 5th edn. Wiley Blackwell, Oxford.

CASE STUDY 41
Telehealth and cystic fibrosis

Evelyn Volders

Justin is a 21-year-old man who has cystic fibrosis (CF). He has recently started his Master's degree in archaeology and will attend a dig in the desert for 3 months later this year. He currently lives in a shared house with friends. His university is in a small country town and is over 500 miles from his family home.

Justin was diagnosed with CF as an infant and attended the nearest tertiary paediatric hospital throughout his childhood. He was usually quite well and attended every 3 months for regular outpatient checks. He had some minor compliance issues with his pancreatic enzyme replacement therapy (PERT) through his teenage years and lost weight at that time. Consultation with the dietitian to explain the role of enzymes helped to increase his compliance and weight tracked along the 10th centile, while height was on the 50th centile.

At the age of 18 care was transferred to the adult tertiary hospital closest to his home where a dietitian works in the CF team. Nine months ago, during the summer holidays, he had his first admission to hospital in 5 years; he had a chest infection and a reported loss of 3 kg between his 3 monthly visits. He has not attended for review since.

This week you have received a call from a dietitian in the town of his university, to say that he has presented at her local hospital with influenza, has again lost weight and has been admitted. He is now 1.8 m tall and his BMI is 18 kg/m^2. He has been referred for dietetic input.

Questions

1. Arrange the assessment information in a table using the ABCDE format.
2. What do you suggest the dietitian could do for her initial consultation during this admission?
3. What important biochemical tests would you suggest?
4. How would you estimate energy requirements? What is the basis of the increased energy requirements in patients with cystic fibrosis?
5. What is nutrition and dietetic diagnosis? Write this as a PASS statement.
6. What is the aim of dietetic management?

Dietetic and Nutrition Case Studies, First Edition.
Edited by Judy Lawrence, Pauline Douglas, and Joan Gandy.

Companion Website: http://www.manualofdieteticpractice.com/

Justin is discharged 2 days later and has the district nurse coming to administer IV antibiotics each day. She calls you for further nutrition information and suggests you speak directly to Justin, who says Skype is easiest as he uses it regularly to talk to his family.

7. What precautions would you need to take to ensure confidentiality for Justin?
8. What might be difficult to manage during a telemedicine consultation compared with a face-to-face consultation?
9. You suspect that Justin has found it difficult to manage his CF as a young adult and that this has led to deterioration in his health and a susceptibility to infection. How will you broach this in your discussion with Justin?

   As a masters student and long time CF patient, Justin is likely to have some awareness of the relationship between poor CF management and susceptibility to infection; active listening and a supportive relationship should allow Justin to remind himself of the importance of self-care and self-developed goals to manage weight loss and compliance with enzyme usage and appropriate distribution.
10. You arrange a follow-up Skype call to support Justin to manage his condition. What is the new nutrition and dietetic diagnosis?
11. What is the aim of the follow-up Skype?
12. Justin is planning international travel shortly. What additional information can you provide to him?
13. The Cystic Fibrosis Trust recommends care by an extensive team for patients with CF. Who else is involved in the care of patients with CF?

Further question

14. One of the common complications of cystic fibrosis as patients get older is CF related diabetes. What is thought to be the aetiology of this and what is the recommended nutritional management?

References

Cystic Fibrosis Trust (2002) *Nutritional management of cystic fibrosis, a consensus report.* http://www.cysticfibrosis.org.uk/media/82052/nutritional-management-of-cystic-fibrosis-apr02.pdf [updated on 19 March 2013; viewed on 6 June 2014].

Cystic Fibrosis Trust (2011) *Standards for the Clinical Care of Adults and Children with Cystic Fibrosis in the UK*, 2nd edn. www.cysticfibrosis.org.uk/media/448939/cd-standards-of-care-dec-2011.pdf [viewed on 30 May 2014].

Cystic Fibrosis Trust (2013) *Cystic fibrosis related diabetes fact sheet.* http://www.cysticfibrosis.org.uk/media/127524/FS_Related_Diabetes_Mar_13.pdf.

Dietitians Association of Australia (2014) *Telehealth/technology based clinical consultations. Information Sheet.* http://daa.asn.au/wp-content/uploads/2014/04/Telehealth-Technology-based-Clinical-Consultations.pdf [viewed on 30 May 2014].

Dietitians of Canada (2011) *Cystic fibrosis. In: PEN: Practice-based Evidence in Nutrition®.* http://www.pennutrition.com [viewed 30 May 2014; access only by subscription].

Dietitians of Canada (2014) *Telehealth/teledietetics. In: PEN: Practice-based Evidence in Nutrition®.* 2011. http://www.pennutrition.com [viewed on 8 June 2014; access only by subscription].

Henry, C.J.K. (2005) Basal metabolic rate studies in humans: measurement and development of new equations. *Public Health Nutrition*, **8**, 1133–1152.

Moran, A., Burnzell, C., Cohen, R. *et al.* (2010) Clinical care guidelines for cystic fibrosis-related diabetes; a position statement of the American Diabetes Association and a clinical practice guideline of the Cystic Fibrosis Foundation, endorsed by the Pediatric Endocrine Society. *Diabetes Care*, **33** (**12**), 2697–2708.

Stapleton, D.R., Ash, C, *et al.* (2006) *Australasian Clinical Practice Guidelines for Nutrition in Cystic Fibrosis*. Sydney, Australia, Cystic Fibrosis Australia Publication. http://daa.asn.au/wp-content/uploads/2012/09/Guidelines_CF-Final.pdf [accessed on 29 November 2014].

Resources

BDA (2015) *Informatics*. https://www.bda.uk.com/professional/practice/informatics [viewed on 8 June 2014].

Morton, A. (2014) Cystic fibrosis. In: J. Gandy (ed), *Manual of Dietetic Practice*, 5th edn. Wiley-Blackwell, Oxford.

CASE STUDY 1

Veganism

Answers

1. A vegan diet excludes any food that comes from animals. This includes milk and dairy products, eggs and honey. Many vegans do not wear animal products, including leather, wool and silk. Vegans also strive to avoid using any products that contain animal ingredients, including medications.
2. You should explore her understanding of rheumatoid arthritis (RA) and what foods (if any) she considers are a problem. Specific food avoidance should not be recommended for RA. However, patient experiences should not be ignored and dietary assessment and advice should be given accordingly. Wendy avoids tomatoes, citrus fruits and potatoes as she believes these could worsen arthritic symptoms.
3. Incomplete knowledge of dietary regimen (problem) related to recent diagnosis of RA (aetiology) characterised by restricted eating pattern (signs and symptoms).
4. Studies have shown that vegan diets are appropriate for all ages (Craig & Mangels, 2009) but as with any diet where food groups are excluded care needs to be taken to meet all nutritional requirements. The following nutrients need to be considered:

   Protein: As a vegetarian Wendy was reliant on cheese as her main protein source, which she no longer eats. She does not vary her protein intake and tends to rely on grains and seeds. Kniskern & Johnston (2011) have suggested that the dietary reference intake (DRI) should be increased to 1 g/kg body weight (from 0.8 g/kg) when consuming <50% protein from animal sources. This is because plant proteins are not as easily digested as animal proteins. It was believed that food combining was necessary to meet all essential amino acid (EAA) requirements but it is now known that if energy intake is adequate and a mixture of plant proteins are eaten over the course of the day, the requirements for essential EAA will be met. Legumes are a particularly rich source of protein and include beans, peas, lentils, soya foods and peanuts. Other good sources of proteins are nuts but legumes are lower in fat. Choosing peanut butter, hummus or soya cheese in sandwiches as an alternative to sunflower seeds would improve protein intake. Quinoa is a high protein grain and could be suggested as an alternative to rice or other grain for the evening meal.

Dietetic and Nutrition Case Studies, First Edition.
Edited by Judy Lawrence, Pauline Douglas, and Joan Gandy.

Companion Website: http://www.manualofdieteticpractice.com/

Iron: Non-haem iron is absorbed at a lower rate than haem iron and vegans have been shown to have lower iron stores than the general population. There is no evidence of iron-deficiency anaemia being more common in vegans who tend to consume more iron than vegetarians or meat eaters (Mangels *et al.*, 2010). Vegan sources include beans, dried fruits and green leafy vegetables. Consuming vitamin C rich foods such as citrus fruits, green leafy vegetables and peppers with meals increases iron absorption.

Zinc: Absorption from plant foods is lower than from animal foods and studies have suggested vegans have lower intakes than meat eaters (Davis & Kris-Etherton, 2003) but no adverse health effects have been documented. Zinc rich foods include nuts, soya products and legumes. However, it has been suggested that vegans need to increase their intake by 50% above the RDA (Institute of Medicine, Food and Nutrition Board, 2001) as vegans typically eat high levels of legumes and whole grains, which contain phytates that bind zinc and inhibit its absorption. Soaking beans, grains, nuts and seeds in water before cooking, can increase zinc bioavailability.

Iodine and selenium: The amount of iodine and selenium consumed is dependent on the amount in the soil; studies suggest that levels may be low in vegans. However, iodine deficiency does not appear to be more common among vegans than in the general population and blood levels of selenium have been found to be adequate in vegetarians (De Bortoli & Cozzolino, 2009; Gibson, 1994). Iodine can be problematic because too much or too little can cause thyroid problems and there is a high potential for deficiency in vegan diets (Leung *et al.*, 2011), acceptable Iodine rich foods include iodised salt or sea vegetables or alternatively kelp fortified yeast extracts or an iodine supplement (75–150 μg, three times per week should be adequate but not excessive). Sources of selenium include nuts (especially Brazil nuts), seeds and cereals.

Calcium: Adequate calcium intake is necessary for healthy bones. Appleby *et al.* (2007) found that fracture risk in vegetarians was comparable to that in non-vegetarians with adequate calcium intake. It is possible to get adequate calcium from eating plant foods rich in calcium such as almonds, sesame seeds and dried figs but it can be difficult; even omnivores may not meet their calcium requirements. Therefore, fortified foods can be useful and vegan sources include calcium set tofu and fortified non-dairy milks. Encourage Wendy to consume calcium fortified milks and calcium set tofu.

Vitamin D: Vegans have been shown to have lower serum levels than meat eaters (Crowe *et al.*, 2011) and one study showed dietary intake to be insufficient to maintain normal ranges in winter months at northern latitudes (Outilia *et al.*, 2000). Vegans need to ensure adequate sun exposure or take a supplement that provides at least 10 μg/day. Calcium and vitamin D are important for bone health and weight bearing and high impact exercise, together with a healthy weight, can help prevent bone loss. Wendy takes regular weight bearing exercise; but having a history of anorexia is associated with bone loss.

Vitamin B_{12}: All vegans need to consume B_{12} fortified foods or take a supplement. Deficiency can result in nerve damage and may increase the risk for chronic conditions such as heart disease. A supplement of at least 10 μg/day or fortified foods is recommended. Fortified foods can include most non-dairy milks, nutritional yeast, yeast extract and soya 'meats'.

5. Her current BMI is 19 kg/m^2, which is within the normal range. It is important to be aware that it is not uncommon for those with an eating disorder to choose a vegan diet as a strategy to restrict further energy intake. However, she has been vegetarian since a teenager and the progression to a vegan diet has been a considered decision. However, her current dietary intake has the potential to be deficient in several nutrients including calcium, vitamin B_{12} and iodine.
6. Yes, you should follow the usual documentation guidelines when informing Wendy's GP.

Answers to further questions

7. Arachidonic acid (AA), docosahexaenoic acid (DHA) and eicosapentaenoic acid (EPA) found in oily fish are non-essential fatty acids and can be converted in the body from the short chain polyunsaturated fatty acids linoleic acid (LA) and alpha-linolenic acid (ALA) obtained from plants. The consumption of ALA, an $n-3$ fatty acid obtained from fish oil, is relatively low in vegan diets compared with $n-6$ PUFAs intakes, mainly LA from seed oils (Sanders, 2009; Kornsteiner *et al.*, 2008). This results in an unbalanced $n-6$ to $n-3$ ratio, which may inhibit endogenous production of EPA and DHA. Studies have shown that the tissue levels of long chain $n-3$ fatty acids are depressed in vegans (Kornsteiner *et al.*, 2008; Rosell *et al.*, 2005) but the actual effects of these lower levels are not clear. This is compounded by an inefficient conversion of ALA by the body to the more active longer chain metabolites EPA and DHA (Davis & Kris-Etherton, 2003). Total $n-3$ requirements may therefore be higher for vegans than for fish and meat eaters as they must rely on conversion of ALA to EPA and DHA. However, Welch *et al.* (2010) found that although non-fish eating meat eaters and vegetarians have much lower intakes of EPA and DHA than fish eaters, their $n-3$ status is higher than would be expected, which suggests a greater conversion of ALA to circulating long chain $n-3$ fatty acids in non-fish eating groups. As yet, there is no documented evidence of adverse effects on health from the lower DHA intake in vegans.

   Simpoulous (2009) demonstrated that western diets have become rich in $n-6$ PUFAs whilst $n-3$ PUFA consumption has reduced and the American Dietetic Association (Craig *et al.*, 2009) recommends that vegans 'should include good sources of ALA in their diets like flaxseed, walnuts, canola (rapeseed) oil and soya and this may be favourable with regard to the inflammatory process'. The significance of these oils (except olive oil, which is a MUFA) is that they contain greater quantities of ALA.
8. A vegan diet can easily meet the nutritional needs of pregnancy and breast feeding. A study of a vegan community (Carter *et al.*, 1987) found that vegan diets had no effect on the birth weights of infants and that the maternal weight gain during

pregnancy was adequate. Vegans generally have higher intakes of folic acid than omnivores, but not high enough to meet pregnancy needs, and as recommended for all women planning and up to 12 weeks of pregnancy, a folic acid supplement is recommended. In addition, a source of vitamin B_{12} is essential for all vegans and particularly important during pregnancy and for breast feeding. Cases of neurological damage in infants born of B_{12} deficient mothers have been cited (Erdeve *et al.*, 2009; Roed *et al.*, 2009; Mariani *et al.*, 2009; Mathey *et al.*, 2007; Weiss *et al.*, 2004; Smolka *et al.*, 2001).

9. Consider whether it is possible for your service to offer a service to all the clinical groups that would benefit from dietetic advice. Does your service offer general antenatal advice, and would Wendy be considered a special case? Are you able to offer a service to the rheumatology consultant; if not, is there a case for offering to develop a service?

CASE STUDY 2
Older person-ethical dilemma

Answers

1. Inadequate oral food intake (problem) related to depression (aetiology) as evidenced by estimated body weight less than 30 kg (sign/symptom).
2. At the end of life the nutrition and dietetic diagnosis would be inadequate oral food and fluid intake (problem) related to the end of life (aetiology), characterised by refusal of food and fluids (sign).
3. It is important to keep abreast of the latest guidance on all relevant topics. Local and national policy should be consulted. The current NICE recommendations for nutrition support in adults (NICE, 2006) give the following criteria for determining those at high risk of refeeding problems:
   - Patients with one or more of the following:
     - BMI < 16 kg/m^2;
     - Unintentional weight loss >15% within past 3–6 months;
     - Little or no nutritional intake >10 days; or
     - Low potassium, phosphate or magnesium levels prior to feeding
   - Or patients with two or more of the following:
     - BMI < 18.5 kg/m^2;
     - Unintentional weight loss >10% within the past 3–6 months;
     - Little or no nutritional intake >5 days; or
     - Receiving insulin, chemotherapy, antacids or diuretics or alcohol abuse

   High-risk patients should be cared for by health care professionals with appropriate skills and training who have expert knowledge of nutritional requirements and support. The nutrition prescription should:
   - Start nutrition support at a maximum of 10 kcal/kg/day, increasing slowly to meet or exceed full needs by 4–7 days.
   - Use only 5 kcal/kg/day in extreme cases (e.g. BMI < 14 kg/m^2 or negligible intake >15 days). Monitor cardiac rhythm continually in these people and any others who already have or develop any cardiac arrhythmias.
   - Restore circulatory volume and monitor fluid balance and overall clinical status closely.

Dietetic and Nutrition Case Studies, First Edition.
Edited by Judy Lawrence, Pauline Douglas, and Joan Gandy.

Companion Website: http://www.manualofdieteticpractice.com/

- Immediately before and during the first 10 days of feeding provide oral thiamine 200–300 mg daily, vitamin B compound strong 1 or 2 tablets, three times a day (or full dose daily intravenous vitamin B preparation, if necessary) and a balanced multivitamin/ trace element supplement once daily.
- Provide oral, enteral or intravenous supplements of potassium (likely requirement 2–4 mmol/kg/day), phosphate (likely requirement 0.3–0.6 mmol/kg/day) and magnesium (likely requirement 0.2 mmol/kg/day intravenous, 0.4 mmol/kg/day oral) unless prefeeding plasma levels are high.
- Prefeeding correction of low plasma levels is unnecessary.

4. You should consider that Rose is at the end of her life and may not benefit from the recommended treatment to prevent refeeding syndrome. You may also want to consider the ethical implications of not providing treatment to prevent refeeding syndrome.
5. Potassium requires correction. Liquid preparations such as Kay-Cee-L or Sando-K. should be considered. A dose of 20–40 mmol potassium 2–4 times per day should be sufficient to correct the problem (BNF, 2015). You could also consider IV infusions of potassium, to be given in normal saline infusion, if it is not possible to correct the deficit orally.

   The dosage of potassium given should also include consideration of the potassium content of an enteral feed.
6. There is no right or wrong answer, you could consider the following points:
   - What quality of life will she have after treatment?
   - How do we know she is depressed?
   - Are we prolonging life by artificial feeding and hydration?
   - What would Rose and her sister want?
   - Would feeding maintain her dignity?
   - If she is depressed and ECT works to improve this then she may have a better quality of life.
   - NG feeding is a short-term plan, what about long term if her appetite does not improve?
   - Would she survive a percutaneous endoscopic gastronomy (PEG) placement?
7. Gradual feeding regimen due to high risk of refeeding syndrome, increase in 10 mL/h from:

   Day 1 – 1 kcal/mL feed, for example, Jevity at 10 mL/h over 24 h and 8× 100 mL water flushes

   Final regimen – day 6 Jevity at 60 mL/h over 24 h and 2× 50 mL flushes

   Final regimen provides 1540 kcal, 57.6 g protein, 58.1 mmol sodium, 58 mmol potassium per day
8. Again there is no right or wrong answer, you could consider the following points:
   - Is Rose benefiting from the feed?
   - Are we promoting quality of life or prolonging it?
   - What would Rose and her sister want?
   - How do we maintain her dignity?

9. You could consider the following points:
   - How would staff know if an NG tube was in the correct position? (What is the national and/or local policy for this?)
   - How often should the position of an NG tube be checked?
   - What training would the staff require in order to care for a patient with an NG tube?
   - What would the advantages and disadvantages be of an NJ tube instead of an NG tube?
10. You could consider the following points:
    - Transferring between wards could increase her confusion (unfamiliar environment, unfamiliar staff)
    - At what stage did her mobility decrease? Rose was admitted with a fall and treated for an UTI – how did she end up bedbound and requiring hoisting?
    - What happened to the rehabilitation she was supposed to get in the community hospital?
    - Was she stimulated enough in the community hospital?
    - Were staff communicating effectively? There were differences in opinions, was there a case conference?
11. You could also consider the dilemma between knowing what Rose decided when she was well and what she would want in the future.

CASE STUDY 3
Older person

Answers

1. Unintentional weight loss (problem) related to reduced food intakes (aetiology) characterised by social isolation and poor cooking skills (signs and symptoms).
2.
   - Age-related height loss versus recalled height, especially in men;
   - Changes in proportions of body fat and lean body mass. Decrease in metabolically active lean mass caused by muscle mass loss (sarcopenia);
   - Re-distribution of adipose tissue with accumulation in the trunk and viscera;
   - The concept of frailty;
   - Decrease in grip strength;
   - Skeletal de-mineralisation;
   - Difficulty in taking anthropometric measurements;
     - Difficulty in measuring grip strength due to problems with grip, for example, arthritis or stroke;
     - Stooped posture making measuring height difficult thus needing alternative measurements: for example, demispan, knee height or ulna length;
     - Skin frailty making taking skinfold measurements more difficult without damaging skin;
     - Lack of validity of anthropometric standards in older people; and
     - Mobility, medical or moving and handling issues leading to difficulty obtaining a weight.
3.
   - Hospital – emotional and medical status may make recalling usual practices at home less accurate and comprehensive care planning difficult. Contact with other members of the multidisciplinary team may be easier. Focus can be on the inpatient stay rather than planning for home. The older person may be seen for an initial assessment and short-term plan put in place but may be discharged before a review and care planning for home can be carried out. There may then be a delay in commencement of community follow up. Patients may not want to discuss nutritional issues as they do not see them as relevant to their hospital admission or simply state that everything is ok. If a care plan involves a relative or carer it can be difficult to see them at a mutually convenient time. Patients may suffer from an overload of information from different medical,

Dietetic and Nutrition Case Studies, First Edition.
Edited by Judy Lawrence, Pauline Douglas, and Joan Gandy.

Companion Website: http://www.manualofdieteticpractice.com/

health and social care professionals and not remember advice given relating to nutrition. Written information may not be taken home or forgotten about. Medical records will give information care and interventions given whilst in hospital and an impression of the home situation.

- Outpatient clinic – onus can be on the patient to phone in to make an appointment, which can lead to appointments not being made. Transport may need to be arranged in order for the older person to attend the clinic. Key people involved in the care plan, for example, family member or carer may be able to attend or may need to be contacted after the appointment. Limited information may be given in the referral, which can make developing a holistic understanding of the older person difficult. Focus is on nutrition in the home situation. More natural setting than in hospital and information on a specific topic (nutrition) is being given, which is more likely to be remembered.
- Own home – easier to make an assessment regarding the home situation and food and drink provision. May prompt a fuller consultation and assessment as familiar cues for the older person. Assessment of mobility and ability to carry out food- and drink-related tasks can be more readily undertaken. Dietary recall can be easier in a familiar situation where food and drink are consumed.

4.
- What provision is there by the local authority, private sector and voluntary sector?
- What are the admission criteria for the varying schemes, costs, waiting times, travel to and from?
- How many times a week are meals provided and social events planned?
- Are there any additional services that the schemes offer, for example, laundry?
- If cooking skills are a problem are there any organisations that can offer help?
- Research the local area and check out what is available.
- Does the local authority have a database or webpage detailing what is available?
- What do the local social services, rapid discharge teams, intermediate care teams, rehabilitation teams, occupational therapists and so on know about and what can they offer older people?

5.
- Older people are set in their ways and are not willing to change their eating habits.
- Nutrition is not important in older life as it is 'too late'.
- Weight loss and decrease in appetite are a natural consequence of ageing.
- Malnutrition is not seen in this country.
- Coffee and tea are diuretics.
- Sandwiches are not a proper meal.
- Thirst is a good indicator of dehydration.
- Not drinking after mid afternoon leads to less trips to the toilet.
- All health care professionals are knowledgeable in nutrition.

6.
- Low body weight increases risk of falls and of harm from the fall.
- Reduced muscle mass and strength.
- Malnutrition leading to loss of function and mobility thus increasing risk of falls.

- Being overweight caused additional strain on muscles and joints.
- Being overweight can make it harder to correct a stumble.
- Inadequate calcium and vitamin D intake can slow the rate of bone demineralisation.
- Dehydration can lead to low blood pressure, increased risk of urinary tract infection, fatigue and confusion, which increase the risk of falls.
- Poorly controlled diabetes can increase the risk of falls.
- Excessive alcohol intake can increase the risk of falls.

7.
- Ensure all relevant information is used in the assessment and care planning process.
- Ensure that the older person's wishes and priorities are followed.
- Communication and explanation between the dietitian and the older person;
- Explain the risks and benefits of any proposed intervention act on the older person's feedback.
- Involve the older person and respect their decisions.
- Some older people may not feel comfortable being given a range of choices and expected to make a decision. They may be used to 'being done to' rather than a partnership between them and the health care professional.
- Think about the emotional needs of the patient and their impact on nutritional intake. Loneliness, depression and bereavement are common but do not affect everyone.
- Work with other members of the multidisciplinary team to address problems or concerns raised by the older person.
- Do not overwhelm the older person with multiple visits/assessments by different health care professionals and develop a team approach.
- Set goals and actions that meet the older person's priorities.
- Seek feedback on older people's experience of dietetic care in order to shape future service provision.

8. Care should be taken not to take other patient or client notes into people's homes. Notes should not be left unattended in a car.

CASE STUDY 4

Learning disabilities

Prader–Willi syndrome

Answers

1. PWS is a congenital disorder, resulting from an abnormality of chromosome 15. It is recognised as the most common genetic cause of life-threatening obesity. Hyperphagia, and in some cases polydipsia, are driven by a physiological abnormality that is highly resistant to motivational changes. Additional characteristics are mild learning disability (often masked by excellent language skills), emotional instability, small stature, skin picking and poor muscle tone (this includes the muscles around the heart). Food seeking behaviour can be extreme; stealing money or food from others, scavenging, eating unsafe or rotten foods are all behaviours, which may be associated with this disorder.
2. Quality of life is paramount. Other factors include:
   - Mastication;
   - Behaviour at meal times;
   - Weight history;
   - Choices;
   - Swallowing;
   - Macro- and micro-nutrient environment;
   - Pica;
   - Medication;
   - Diarrhoea;
   - Appetite;
   - Chronic constipation;
   - Physical anomalies;
   - Dentition;
   - Risk of aspiration;
   - Activity levels;
   - Blood test;
   - Reflux/regurgitation;
   - Budget;

Dietetic and Nutrition Case Studies, First Edition.
Edited by Judy Lawrence, Pauline Douglas, and Joan Gandy.

Companion Website: http://www.manualofdieteticpractice.com/

- Feeding ability;
- Therapeutic diet;
- Fluids; and
- Food aversion.

3. A central characteristic of the syndrome is an insatiable appetite for food, never feeling full even after a meal. This leads to severe overeating and a potential for marked obesity and associated health problems (heart disease, leg ulcers, diabetes) and premature death.
4. Normal predictive energy equations need to be employed with extreme caution in people with PWS while predicting the energy requirements from BMR equations, and the energy expenditure of physical activity should also be considered. The underdevelopment of muscle and any excess weight limits physical activity. The height/weight calculation of Hoffman *et al.* (1992) can be used; 10–14 kcal/cm height for weight maintenance and 7/8 kcal/cm for weight loss. Otherwise, the recommended energy intake for adults with PWS is around 800–1200 kcal/day, reducing to 800–1000 kcal/day for weight loss (International Prader–Willi Association, 2010; Prader–Willi Syndrome Association, 2010; Purtell *et al.*, 2015). A weight reduction diet should use low energy, nutrient-dense foods to ensure optimal vitamin and mineral intake (van Mil *et al.*, 2001; Lindmark *et al.*, 2010). As osteoporosis and low bone mineral density are common in PWS, calcium and vitamin D supplementation should be considered (van Mil *et al.*, 2001). Reduced gonadal hormones, and reduced inclination for exercise will further increase the risk of osteoporosis.
5. Unintentional weight gain (problem) due to the impact of a new environment on eating and drinking behaviours (aetiology) as evidenced by previous weight gain (signs/symptoms).
6. The aim of the intervention is to maintain John's weight within the normal range for an adult with PWS while maintaining his quality of life. The most significant outcome measure would be weight although it is also important to assess John's risk of heart disease and diabetes. This could be monitored by annual blood tests.
7. It is important to set goals that are short term and very gradual to allow acceptance and adjustment. The dietitian should give John clear messages and expectations leaving no room for misinterpretation, and a positive reinforcement to help establish new behaviours. Confrontation should be avoided. Eye contact and gentle encouragement will help when getting John involved in goal setting.
8. There should be regular training of carers and involvement in case conferences. Carers can also be involved in menu planning as they will have valuable insights into John's general and eating behaviours.
9. Other services and health care professionals include:
   - Social services;
   - Psychologist;
   - Physicians – GP and as appropriate to client, for example, orthopaedic specialist, gastroenterologist, respiratory physician, endocrinologist;

- Speech and language therapist;
- Occupational therapist;
- Physiotherapist; and
- Dentist.

Answer to further question

10. Both clients and carers should be involved when assessing capacity to consent. The assessment of ability to consent must be time- and decision-specific. All possible steps, for example, alternative forms of communication such as symbolised information or signing should be taken to help someone consent before reaching the decision that they lack capacity to consent. A decision made on behalf of someone who is deemed incapable to consent should be made in the person's best interest. Legislation provides a legal framework for decision making on behalf of adults who lack capacity to consent; this differs slightly between UK countries:

- Scotland: The Adults with Incapacity Act (Scottish Parliament, 2000);
- England and Wales: The Mental Capacity Act (MCA) (DH, 2005); and
- Northern Ireland: Seeking Consent (Department of Health, Social Services and Public Safety (DHSSPS), 2003).

CASE STUDY 5

Freelance practice

Pizza goes to school

Answers

1. The food-based standards were developed following an independent review in 2013 (School Food Plan) that found that the existing school food standards were difficult to understand and use. The new food-based standards were launched in January 2015. They form a framework, (underpinned by legislation) for schools and caterers, and being food based (not nutrient based) menus and recipes do not require nutrient analysis. The standards are based on the following food groups:
   - Starchy foods;
   - Fruit and vegetables;
   - Meat, fish, eggs, beans and other non-dairy sources of protein;
   - Milk and dairy;
   - Foods and drinks high in fat, sugar and salt; and
   - Healthier drinks.

   Variety is the key principle of the standards, which emphasises the importance of providing a variety of food across the week and thereby a good balance of nutrients. Standards are available for lunch and food other than lunch including breaks, breakfast clubs, vending machines, tuck shops and after school meals and snacks.
2. Many freelancers have earned fees analysing recipes and menus for the nutrient-based standards. This is no longer necessary, as the food-based standards have been piloted and found to be nutritionally sound; in fact, even better than the nutrient-based standards in some cases. However, there is still demand from schools, caterers and their suppliers for wider nutritional services.
3. It is important to keep your skills and knowledge abreast to the current market you are targeting, promote your practice by networking and other selling and marketing techniques, equip yourself appropriately, be ready to respond to demands in terms of business, pricing and branding and deliver the result to a high standard and on time.

Dietetic and Nutrition Case Studies, First Edition.
Edited by Judy Lawrence, Pauline Douglas, and Joan Gandy.

Companion Website: http://www.manualofdieteticpractice.com/

4. It is important to build a good rapport with the client and discuss their requirements before accepting the commission. In this case, the nutritional attributes of the product range and existing recipes were compared with the standards. This exercise highlighted where the products and recipes could be improved nutritionally, and also built a comprehensive database of their products and generated detailed specifications for them.
5. - Coaching and advisory services to staff on nutrition and standards and the resultant needs of their school clients.
   - A nutritional strategy, tightly integrated with their positioning, budget and marketing aims.
   - Sales and marketing support materials.
   - Analysis, creation and development of dozens of recipes for pizzas.
   - Reformulation of several products to make them more nutritious.
6. Freelance dietitians mostly work on their own success or failure depending on their personal knowledge, experience, flair, resources, drive and inter-personal skills. Getting and keeping corporate clients demands these elements in large measure. Professional networks, for example, Linkedin BDA's Freelance DIetitian's Group are invaluable for support and networking.
7. Freelancers must continue to improvise on their portfolio throughout their careers and must maintain continuous professional development in order to remain competent enough to practice and stay HCPC registered. CPD activities may be available through professional networks. Resources such as diet sheets may be expensive to develop and reproduce and therefore it is important to keep abreast of available resources that may be cheaper, for example, Nutrition and Dietetic Resources (NDR) (www.ndr-uk.org).
8. The freelancer pays for it. Clients do not expect to pay for anything over and above the fee and they expect freelancers to be over-equipped to deliver the results they want quickly, and to assimilate their needs at once. There is no training, induction or supervision and the client does not pay to get up to speed.
9. Occasionally, clients have a very clear idea of what exactly they want, with a timeframe and budget. The freelancer must then decide whether the project is feasible. More often, clients need to talk through their situation and get the freelancer's suggested actions at the proposal stage. They can feel overwhelmed by too much scientific and legal information and too many ideas, resulting in the project being delayed or abandoned altogether. Managing the initial contact is therefore an important skill that the freelancers have to master.
10. Many simply use online search engines such as www.freelancedietitians.org, the website of the BDA's specialist group. Many will go to their networks and ask around, relying on word-of-mouth. Clients will generally select two or three freelance dietitians and telephone or email them to explore their suitability. Thanks to social media, managers' networks are far wider today than ever before and include many people with whom they have only indirect or tenuous relationships. Potential clients are thus able to assess a freelancer within moments without the freelancer's knowledge. From the freelancer's perspective, getting work by word-of-mouth and online promotion is cost-effective, but not

without risk. A freelancer must always excel in order to build and protect his or her reputation.

11. Setting up a freelance practice is a big investment, not only of your time, but also of significant amounts of money. When you launch your freelance career, you must be confidant that you know what services you can offer, how much to charge for them, where your prospect base is to be found and what is different about you. If you cannot express this simply and briefly, you will lose out to established freelancers. You will also need a clear grasp of your tax, insurance, accountancy, and resource requirements. Many corporate clients are seeking a long-term relationship with their freelance providers. If they feel you are only in it for the short run, they will often look elsewhere. Include developing a business plan, setting up and equipping an office, keeping accounts, paying taxes and so on.

12. It is inadvisable because a new graduate has no experience and so cannot practise. You need to build up a range of experiences in order to decide where your strengths lie and to have a wide enough array of services to offer.

13. Your fee is part of your marketing strategy. If you pitch it too low, your prospective clients may assume you are not as good as others who charge more. In addition, at low fees you will not have enough money to invest in your practice. Remember from your fee you must pay personal income tax, national insurance, pension provision and all the costs involved in your work such as transport, insurance, subscriptions, training, stationery, office equipment, phone bills, clothes and all other resources.

14. You need to provide a written quotation for the work you propose to do, specifying when you will invoice and when it will be paid. You also need terms of business, which set out other elements of the contract such as your liabilities, your legal relationship with the client, that the contract is for services (not employment) and how the client can use your outputs.

CASE STUDY 6

Public health – weight management

A multi-faceted approach

Answers

1.
   - National prevalence rates for overweight and obesity alongside the local community health profile and local primary health care plans and targets were used.
   - An asset based community consultation. Individual face-to-face interviews were carried out door to door, in public areas, for example, outside supermarkets, and at established groups running in the community, for example, a mother and toddler group. Local residents were asked:
     - Where do you source your food?
     - How do you keep active?
     - How could either of these factors be improved for you?
   - A food access survey was carried out using the healthy eating indicator shopping basket instrument (Food Standards Agency Scotland, 2008). All retail outlets selling food in the four communities were identified and the availability and price of defined healthy food items were recorded.
2. Nutrition and dietetic diagnosis can be used to help shape a community intervention. Restricted diet pattern (problem) potentially exacerbated by poor uptake of available healthy food (aetiology) evidenced by community consultation and profile.
3. Some residents may live a significant geographical distance from services such as leisure facilities and healthy food but this should not be assumed of everyone living in rural areas.

   Another point to note is that irregular demographic spread is often a feature of rural areas, so postcodes are not necessarily a useful indicator to identify areas that are most deprived of services.
4. A number of commercial programmes are now available such as Counterweight, Slimming World and Weight Watchers. There may also be locally designed and developed evidence-based weight management programmes.

Dietetic and Nutrition Case Studies, First Edition.
Edited by Judy Lawrence, Pauline Douglas, and Joan Gandy.

Companion Website: http://www.manualofdieteticpractice.com/

5. Tourism is a major source of local employment and, thereby, income. Increased income is related to improved health status. However, tourism places extra demands on local resources including food supply and medical services.
6. Numbers of people in different age groups, health statistics, employment, transport. Demographics can shift and change over time; therefore, it is important to ensure that the most up-to-date information is used.
7. Specific factors will include:
   - Number of food retail outlets;
   - Type and brand of food retail outlet (stimulates competition in value, quality and price of products);
   - Type, variety and price of food on sale;
   - Local food networks;
   - Home-grown produce;
   - Hunted or gathered foods (e.g. fish, shellfish, venison, rabbits, berries);
   - Geographic distance and terrain to travel to shops;
   - Transport to shops;
   - Internet shopping options; and
   - Home delivery services.
8. Every area has a unique combination of groups and activities from national initiatives, for example, 'Paths for All' or local groups, funded by local or national grants or awards such as the Big Lottery Fund.
9. The voluntary sector, for example, charitable organisations and support groups, which often play a significant role in public health; consider both local and national bodies such as Age UK, Step It Up Highland, housing associations.
10. The company could talk to:
    - Participants who engaged in the activities;
    - Community members who did not engage;
    - Members of staff from the organisations and groups collaborating in the whole project;
    - Project leaders;
    - Managers; and
    - Funders.
11. That participants:
    - Enjoyed taking part;
    - Were empowered to make changes to improve their health and continue to be involved;
    - Felt improvement in their health and well-being; and
    - That the project activities were sustainable.
12. Across the NHS Highland Health Board, public health strategy reduction in levels and rates of obesity in the long term across the population would be assessed as an outcome.

    In the individual Counterweight programme delivered through the medical practice, weight would be measured and monitored as an outcome.

In the community activities, weight would not be recorded and other aspects of improving health and well-being, rather than weight targets, were measured as outcomes.

All local residents were eligible to participate in the community activities. Overweight or obese residents had the additional option of referral to the Counterweight service on an individual basis, alongside any community activities they chose to participate in.

13. How could you document any comments regarding how people felt about taking part?

Participants were asked for feedback after each session. This could be done in a variety of ways such as short surveys, questionnaires, comments recorded on "post it" notes and flip charts or audio/video recordings, and collated.

14. Other methods could include:

- Paper or electronic survey forms distributed to each household;
- Use of local media to advertise the campaign;
- Posters at doctors surgeries', community centres, post offices, schools, library and service points, shops and leisure facilities;
- Online networks – see what exists locally through the council or the third sector; and
- Virtual social networks, for example, Facebook pages.

Answers to further questions

15. The following actions are included in the case study to illustrate the principles:

- Identifying and working with stakeholders to identify needs, priorities and actions (human dignity);
- Collaborative decision making with stakeholders (ownership);
- Gradually transferring decision making power from the project team to the community (adaptiveness);
- Recruiting and training local community members (empowerment);
- A focus on sustainability (relevance);
- Education elements included where appropriate, for example, cookery classes emphasised how the recipes were in line with healthy eating recommendations (learning); and
- Involving the local community in defining indicators for success, ongoing progress reviews and evaluation of the project (participation).

16. The *performance story technique* provides a framework for reporting on the contribution of a programme to long-term targets or outcomes using mixed methods and a participatory process. It results in a report that is easy for stakeholders to understand and provides a depth of information to enable the impact of a programme to be assessed.

In this case study, *performance story technique* was appropriate because:

- There were numerous learning and reflection opportunities throughout the programme to involve stakeholders, a key aspect in the participatory process;
- It was also possible through the framework to include other gathered data information; and
- It provides a common language for comparison with other programmes, which would be required for future planning strategies.

It does not however examine the cost effectiveness of the programme and this technique can be criticised for bias. As a result, this technique should complement other reporting processes rather than replace them totally.

CASE STUDY 7
Public health – learning disabilities

Answers

1. People with learning disabilities have a shorter life expectancy and increased risk of early death when compared to the general population (Emerson *et al.*, 2011). They have higher rates of obesity, coronary heart disease, respiratory disease, some types of cancers, osteoporosis, sensory impairment, dementia and epilepsy and may also have physical disabilities associated with certain conditions (DHSSPS, 2012). It is estimated that people with learning disability are 58 times more likely to die prematurely (DHSSPS, 2012).

   Unemployment, poverty and social exclusion are higher among the learning disabled and contribute to the significant health inequalities compared with the general population (Emerson & Hatton, 2008).
2. Difficulty preparing food for eating, (problem) related to communication problems (aetiology) characterised by inappropriate written material and lack of cooking experience (sign).
3. The *Cook it!* programme was developed for those with an 'average' reading ability; it includes printed recipes, quizzes and other written activities.

   Research estimates that between 50% and 90% people with a learning disability have significant communication problems making it difficult to read and understand written material, thereby creating barriers to accessing health information (DHSSPS, 2012).

   All written information would require modification to make it more accessible, including the recipes and quiz sheets. The use of fewer words and more photographs, pictures or symbols is more helpful in printed information (Mencap, 2002).

   It would be preferable to use fewer written materials and more interactive activity and discussion.
4. Other factors include:
   - Participants' physical disabilities and/or inexperience, which may present challenges when handling kitchen equipment including knives, peelers and so on;

Dietetic and Nutrition Case Studies, First Edition.
Edited by Judy Lawrence, Pauline Douglas, and Joan Gandy.

Companion Website: http://www.manualofdieteticpractice.com/

- The safety hazards presented by, for example, saucepans of boiling food, hot ovens, grills;
- Clients will require more time to complete tasks; and
- Making the recipes appealing to participants to encourage full participation in the programme.

  These factors highlight the need to consider the complexity of the recipes used, the time allocated to the sessions and the number of sessions required for the essential topics whilst remaining true to the ethos of the Cook it! programme to prepare nutritious, low cost dishes that use readily available equipment.

5. Evaluation is essential to guide the development and implementation of a pilot programme and to assess the outcome from the intervention. The methods used to evaluate the pilot were:
   - The Talking Mats® tool at the beginning of the first session and the end of the final session to assess if the learning disabled participants' knowledge of healthy eating and/or food hygiene and safety increased as well as to canvas their views of the pilot programme.
   - Semi-structured interviews with the facilitators at the end of the pilot to seek feedback on the materials and practical issues relating to the delivery of the pilot sessions.
6. Key issues could include the following:
   - A lack of support from carers

     Carers of learning disabled individuals are a valuable stakeholder group. Lack of support from carers could include practical issues such as insufficient time to check if someone in independent living is awake and preparing to attend the programme; or transport not being available at the correct time to bring a participant. It is important that carers see the value of the programme as they are then more likely to support attendance.
   - Timekeeping

     This can be difficult for many people with learning disabilities, and so using strategies such as calendars and planners can be helpful. Use of text messaging to issue a reminder immediately before a session can be a useful option.
   - Fitting *Cook it!* sessions in with other appointments

     People with learning disabilities may have many other appointments with, for example, health care professionals and social services. These appointments are often rigid with no option for flexibility, and can therefore make it difficult for learning disabled individuals to attend all sessions in an extended programme such as Cook it!
   - Lack of clarity or understanding about the programme

     The details concerning the programme, as well as its importance and value, may not be fully understood by learning disabled participants. Ensuring clear communication and engagement with the participants in the early stages is essential to the programme's success. One-to-one discussions, although time consuming, may be required to help a person with learning difficulties connect with those running the programme and ensure engagement.

7. BME groups would each require individual adaptations, dependent on their ethnicity, to take into account issues such as:
   - Foods, eating patterns and culture specific to each group;
   - Health and lifestyle issues prevalent within the groups; and
   - Language.

   Many people from BME groups have well developed skills in using spoken English; however, for others it may be necessary to use translators during the delivery of *Cook it!* sessions. This can change the dynamics of sessions and add significantly to the time required to deliver the sessions; factors which will need to be considered by facilitators.

   Consideration should also be given to the need to translate printed materials as many adults from BME groups, even those with good skills in using spoken English, may lack confidence and/or competence in reading materials published in English.

   It would be essential to engage with BME group(s) in the adaptation of the programme, including the development of the programme, recipes and other materials, the delivery of pilot sessions and the evaluation. Useful contacts within the BME voluntary organisations should be identified as stakeholders. Examples of potential organisations include the National Council for Voluntary Organisations and Voice4Change in England and in Northern Ireland, the Northern Ireland Council for Minority Minorities.

   The Public Health Agency (Northern Ireland), in partnership with community dietitians from local health and social care trusts, is currently engaged in adapting the *Cook it!* programme for use with the main minority ethnic groups in Northern Ireland, including Chinese, Polish, Lithuanian, Bulgarian, Muslim, Indian/South Asian and East Timorese groups as well as Irish.

Answers to further questions

8. A range of stakeholders, including:
   - service users with a learning disability;
   - families of the learning disabled;
   - support workers for the learning disabled;
   - community/voluntary organisations who work to support people with learning disabilities, for example, Mencap NI, Disability Network;
   - speech and language therapists;
   - health improvement specialists; and
   - dietitians.
9. Piloting new interventions with the target audience is good practice. It provides an opportunity to check if they are suitable for use and that they will achieve the intended outcome as well as to identify any refinements that are required prior to final publication.

   Identifying a long list of recommendations provides clear direction on how the intervention can be strengthened for maximum benefit.

10. The recommendations directly related to the programme and the supporting materials were prioritised initially and have been tested with learning disabled clients. At present, they are being finalised for printing and use across Northern Ireland.

    The published resources will include a folder for each learning disabled participant to build over the eight sessions. This will include a 'certificate of achievement' for each session, outlining the key messages and skills developed during the session, and a pictorial copy of the recipe(s) prepared. It is hoped that this will help to build engagement and support from family members/carers to continue skills development at home.

    The development of a facilitators' forum is under discussion and Talking Mats® will be considered as an evaluation tool as the programme is disseminated.

CASE STUDY 8

Public health – calorie labelling on menus

Putting calories on menus to create a healthier food environment

Answers

1. Two stakeholder groups – food service businesses (FSBs) and health professionals were identified. While representative bodies for health professionals were easily identified, this proved difficult for FSBs. Only a small proportion of FSBs are chain outlets, the majority (~90%) are small-to-medium size outlets. However, even within these two groups there is much disparity and no single body represents either group of FSBs.
2. The Food Safety Authority Ireland (FSAI) held an on-line national public consultation to find out what consumers and FSBs wanted regarding calorie menu labelling. The consultation provided information on what calorie menu labelling would look like and whether it would be mandatory or voluntary. The Minister for Health launched the national consultation. There was intense media interest throughout the 4-week consultation period, which helped ensure a good response. Over 3200 submissions, mostly from consumers, were received. This response was five-fold larger than any previous national consultation held by the FSAI.
3. To increase the limited feedback received from FSBs in the national consultation, the FSAI undertook an additional survey of FSBs attending a large Hospitality Expo using an interview-assisted questionnaire. This facilitated assessment of FSB views on calorie menu labelling by gender and age.
4. An obesogenic environment (problem) that is fuelled by increasing consumption of take-away foods and eating outside of the home (aetiology) as evidenced by increasing levels of obesity and associated health problems (signs/symptoms, for example, type 2 diabetes, cardiovascular disease, cancer).
5. A comprehensive evaluation of FSBs voluntary uptake of calorie menu labelling across the country was required. This needed to include assessment of the benefits, drawbacks and barriers involved. A telephone survey was developed to

Dietetic and Nutrition Case Studies, First Edition.
Edited by Judy Lawrence, Pauline Douglas, and Joan Gandy.

Companion Website: http://www.manualofdieteticpractice.com/

evaluate uptake of calorie menu labelling among FSBs. The sample was selected to ensure that geographic location and outlet type (e.g. coffee shop, fast food outlet) were represented. In addition, this evaluation included a quality assessment of calorie menu labelling in terms of best practice principles that enable consumers to use the information, which was conducted in outlets reporting to display the calories on their menus in the main city area. This included taking food samples to assess the accuracy of calorie information displayed (food samples were disaggregated, ingredients weighed and assessed for energy content using appropriate food–nutrient composition software).

6. The team should have experts in nutrition and dietetics, software engineering and development; food business training. Most importantly, the end-users (chefs, cooks, food business managers and catering students) were recruited to develop the calculator.
7. An on-line interactive training programme was developed to guide food service personnel through the entire process of 'getting recipe information in order' to 'displaying calorie information for consumers'. This provided essential guidance in a cost-effective manner.
8. On-going engagement of both the public and FSBs has been critical to the success of this voluntary obesity-prevention scheme. This has involved using every opportunity to communicate comprehensively through the media and stakeholder bodies on all aspects of this initiative. Releasing the findings of the evaluation and the launch by the Minister for Health represented two opportunities for such engagement. All feedback received during these communication sessions was valuable for identifying barriers and formulating workable solutions to guide the process successfully. Throughout all stages of implementation and evaluation of calorie menu labelling, learning about the needs of stakeholders and consumers has been prioritised. Problem solving with the involvement of these groups has enabled the project to develop to meet the specific needs of these key stakeholders. For example, a key learning identified the importance of on-going acclaim and praise of FSBs who are implementing calorie menu labelling towards honouring their commitment to this initiative, which requires arduous effort from them.

There is no single solution that can halt the increasing levels of overweight and obesity. A large number of strategies at all levels of society are needed if the rise in obesity is to be reversed or even just halted. Therefore, calorie menu labelling needs to be continually evaluated on its own terms. This involves on-going evaluation of the numbers and types of food outlets implementing calorie menu labelling. It also involves assessing the quality of such labelling in terms of best practice to enable consumers use the information. The findings of such on-going evaluation will inform the development of this obesity-prevention initiative. By evolving to help FSBs meet the changing nature of food fashions and consumer demands is the only way calorie menu labelling can remain relevant and effective.

CASE STUDY 9

Genetics and hyperlipidaemia

Answers

1. BMI = 24.7 kg/m^2.
   For populations of Asian descent, a BMI > 23 kg/m^2 is classified as overweight and at an increased risk of cardiovascular diseases (NICE, 2013). The rationale for a separate BMI classification for Asian populations is based on epidemiological studies recognising higher levels of metabolic conditions (e.g. cardiovascular disease) amongst Asian when compared with European populations at the same BMI level (WHO, 2004). Importantly, given the limitations of BMI, it should be used in the context of other risk factors when considering risk of disease.
2. Measurement of her waist circumference is recommended to assess abdominal adiposity. Hannah's waist circumference places her above recommended thresholds for a Chinese women (<80 cm) (NICE, 2013). In combination with her BMI, Hannah's anthropometry suggests she may be at increased risk of cardio-metabolic conditions.
3. Hannah presents with several risk factors for CVD (i.e. family history, anthropometric and clinical), which may have prompted her GP to measure her biochemistry. Since blood cholesterol and glucose are sensitive to dietary change, fasting glucose and lipids are therefore more accurate in predicting impaired glucose tolerance and CVD (British Cardiac Society, British Hypertension Society *et al.*, 2005; IDF, 2005).
4. Risk factors

Modifiable	Non-modifiable
Diet Anthropometry – increased risk BMI, waist circumference Hyperlipidaemia – total cholesterol, LDL cholesterol, triglycerides (TG)	Family history – mother had a premature CVD event Asian descent

Dietetic and Nutrition Case Studies, First Edition.
Edited by Judy Lawrence, Pauline Douglas, and Joan Gandy.

Companion Website: http://www.manualofdieteticpractice.com/

5. Further assessments

Domain	
Anthropometry, body composition and functional	No further assessment needed
Biochemistry and haematology	No further assessment needed
Clinical	Smoking status Alcohol intake Family history of CVD Secondary causes of dyslipidaemia, for example hypothyroidism, hepatic, renal disease Previous attempts of weight loss
Diet	Meal procurement and preparation arrangements. Who is involved? Clarification of the size of bowls Consumption of other foods high in saturated fat, sugars and sodium (e.g. soy sauce, soy bean paste, oil use for cooking, meat preparation) Clarification of the ingredients of Chinese foods, for example Chinese, Kaya, Chinese soymilk, deep fried Chinese donuts Types of dishes chosen at Yum Cha
Environmental, behavioural and social	Hannah appears to be the sole income provider for 4 people. Given her current working status, this may place additional financial strain on accessing healthy food choices. It may be worthwhile sensitively probing her need or interest for financial assistance Does Hannah think she is overweight?

6. Combined hyperlipidaemia is characterised by a combined elevation of cholesterol and triglycerides (TG) with individuals having an increased risk of premature coronary artery disease (Brouwers *et al.*, 2012). There are two broad forms:

a. Familial combined hyperlipidaemia (FCH) is a genetic form of dyslipidaemia, with recent research indicating a polygenic (multiple genes) mode of inheritance (Brouwers *et al.*, 2012). The pattern of inheritance is more complex compared with monogenic (single gene) conditions. Genes affecting metabolism and clearance of plasma lipoprotein particles have been implicated in its aetiology. Inheritance is more evident and often manifests earlier in life. As a result of the intra-individual and intra-family variability of its phenotype, clinically it is often difficult to distinguish from the metabolic syndrome (Gaddi *et al.*, 2007). Diagnostic criteria includes elevated fasted apolipoprotein B100 and TG concentrations plus the presence of elevated levels of these in at least two first degree relatives, on at least three repeated measures, with potential to use genetic markers in the future (Gaddi *et al.*, 2007).

b. Acquired combined hyperlipidaemia is multifactorial and explained by an interaction between genes (of lower penetrance than those implicated in FCH) and environmental factors such as body weight, diet and exercise. It is often associated with the metabolic syndrome. Endocrine disorders such as hypothyroidism, liver or renal disease may also induce dyslipidaemia. Development is often sporadic although it may cluster in families.

7. Impaired nutrient utilisation (problem) related to acquired combined hyperlipidaemia (aetiology) characterised by abdominal adiposity, and slightly elevated blood pressure (signs).

8. Diet appears low in fibre because of low intake of wholemeal and wholegrain products. Folate, vitamins C and A intake may be limited because of low intake of vegetables. In view of her acquired combined hyperlipidaemia and increased CVD risk, excessive energy intake appears to be because of high intakes of saturated (and potentially trans) fat-rich foods such as cakes, biscuits, pastries and deep fried foods as well as refined carbohydrates from sugar sweetened beverages. Her diet also appears to be high in sodium, which is evident in her choice of condiments. Currently, there is no regular intake of oily fish.

9.
- Encourage a reduction in abdominal adiposity (waist circumference) and associated weight loss.
- Reduce the risk of metabolic conditions, especially CVD, via normalisation of blood lipids and blood pressure.
- Optimise nutritional adequacy to improve nutritional status.

10.
- Advice on dietary changes to reduce total energy intake, to replace saturated and trans-fats with unsaturated fats, increase long chain omega-3 fatty acid intake and fibre and reduce sodium intake. Specific advice may include:
  - Replace discretionary high fat and sugar foods (such as biscuits, pastries and cakes) with a variety of fruit and, nuts and/or Chinese rice cakes. Limit intake of sugar sweetened beverages;
  - To save money, preparing home-made wholegrain sandwiches with fillings such as salad vegetables and oily fish varieties including salmon, sardines or pilchards, would be a better option over purchasing meat pie, pasties and so on;
  - Limit intake of deep fried foods and choose lean meats for cooking. Choosing steamed options at Yum Cha. Include fish at least twice a week, at least one of which should be an oily variety; and
  - Limit pickled vegetable intake. Gradually replace soy sauce, soy bean paste and oyster sauce with Chinese herbs and spices.
- Advice to increase physical activity, perhaps by walking to work.
- Encourage diversity in nutrient intake.

- Advice should be given in line with appropriate national and/or international guidelines (Lichtenstein *et al.*, 2006) in the context of general healthy eating guidelines such as those given by NHS choices in the United Kingdom. www.nhs.uk/livewell/healthy-eating/Pages/Healthyeating.aspx.

11. Outcome measures
- A healthy waist circumference for a Chinese woman <80 cm. Weight loss and BMI may be monitored but should be used to supplement, rather than be the focus of, the outcome of Hannah's main goal.
- Normalisation of blood lipid levels and blood pressure.
- Assess changes in dietary intake; use a 4-day food diary including at least one weekend day.
- Increased physical activity levels, which could be assessed by a physical activity questionnaire.

12. Consideration of Hannah's self-efficacy and barriers to change may aid in improving adoption of behaviour change. It is important to find culturally acceptable changes that will also be acceptable to the family. Careful consideration of her culture and traditional ways of cooking and eating should enable Hannah to make the necessary changes. Nutritional advice will need to be financially appropriate; may consider referral to a social worker for financial assistance, if required.

Answers to further questions

13. As shown in Table 9.1

Table 9.1 **Dietary interventions for lipid abnormalities.**

Lipid abnormality	Suggested dietary interventions (Reiner *et al.*, 2011)
Elevated total cholesterol and/or LDL-C	Reduce saturated (<10% total energy) and trans-fats (<2% total energy) and replace with unsaturated fatty acids ($n-6$ PUFA or MUFA) Increase dietary fibre (>18 g/day) Increase exercise Use of foods enriched with phytosterols or stanols Maintenance of a normal waist circumference and body weight
Elevated TG	Maintenance of a normal waist circumference and body weight Reduce alcohol intake Reduce intake of simple carbohydrates (<10% total energy) Increase exercise Increase intake of foods rich in long chain $n-3$ polyunsaturated fatty acids (mainly from oily fish). Aim to consume at least 2 portions of fish weekly, one of which is oily (providing ≥0.45 g/day long chain $n-3$ PUFA)
Low HDL-C	Reduce trans-fats and increase unsaturated fatty acids (PUFA or MUFA) Increase exercise Maintenance of a normal body weight

14. • Assessing Hannah's understanding of how genes may affect her risk of CVD may help elicit any misconceptions and/or cultural beliefs to better direct your communication.

• Explain that for common CVD, especially for her form of hyperlipidaemia (multifactorial), both genes and lifestyle factors, including diet, may be involved.

• Acknowledge that emerging research shows apolipoprotein (APOE) is involved in lipid metabolism and genetic variations in the *APOE* gene may affect blood lipid response to dietary fat (Lovegrove & Gitau, 2008). However, there is currently insufficient scientific evidence to enable personalised dietary recommendations according to genetics (Camp &Trujillo, 2014).

• It is important to be aware that patients can be referred for genetic testing by their GP, if necessary.

• Carriage of the genetic ε4 variant means that Hannah may have a greater chance of developing CVD if she consumes high quantities of saturated fat and excessive dietary cholesterol as a result of its effect on plasma LDL-cholesterol concentrations. Individuals who are *apoE4* carriers (particularly if homozygote) respond well to reduction in dietary saturated fats and therefore general healthy eating advice is reinforced and appropriate. Hannah's understanding about the role of genetics in her condition may be used to empower her. You may wish to channel this and her interest in preventing CVD to emphasis her need to be more vigilant with the diet and lifestyle advice you have given her, than someone without the genetic variant.

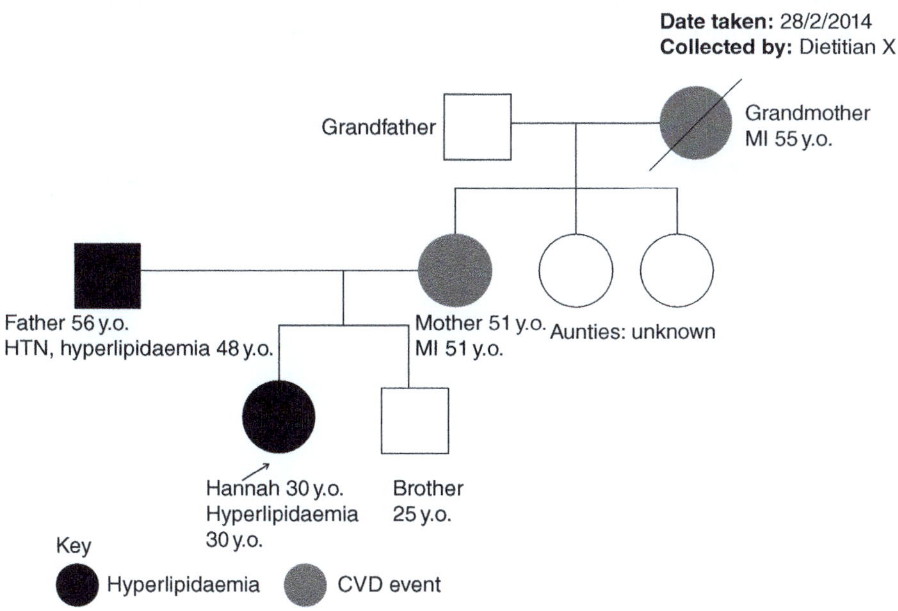

Figure 9.1 Three generation family pedigree for hyperlipidaemia and CVD

- In respect to the supplements supplied, it would be prudent to determine what these contained and explain that if a balanced diet is followed then dietary supplements are not generally required.

15. Dietitians will not be expected to perform a detailed genetic assessment or genetic counselling, but should be able to identify whether a patient is at risk of a rare genetic condition as well as to explain to a patient their risk.

16. The large number of affected relatives, all closely related to Hannah and their early onset of disease, suggests an increased role of genetics in the development of her hyperlipidaemia. You should alert her GP who can better assess Hannah for genetic causes of hyperlipidaemia. The GP may then determine the need for referral to specialist lipid clinics.

17. Currently, there are no dietary guidelines targeting individuals with FCH. Given the larger role that genetics may play in contributing to Hannah's hyperlipidaemia you may need to set realistic expectations about her lipid levels following therapy. The aim should be to use the knowledge of her condition's aetiology to empower her to make a more conscientious dietary change. Greater emphasis should be on preventing the development of other risk factors associated with CVD (e.g. type 2 diabetes) and more frequent monitoring may be beneficial. Therefore, dietary management should be more intensive. If Hannah is prescribed drug therapy, nutrient–drug interactions should be considered (Gandy, 2014).

18. Diagnosis of FCH has implications for her children, who may or may not demonstrate any overt symptoms in the near future. They will have a higher chance of developing FCH. Screening her children via referral to her GP or a specialist lipid clinic should be recommended and acknowledging the benefit of lifestyle advice for her whole family should be encouraged (HeartUK, 2014).

CASE STUDY 10

Intestinal failure

Answers

1. Unintentional weight loss (problem) related to malabsorption, infection and inadequate intake (aetiology) as evidenced by 17.5% weight loss in 3 months, and dehydration (signs and symptoms).
2.
   - Restrict oral fluids to 1 L of an oral rehydration solution plus 1 L of all other fluids.
   - The diet needs to be high in energy, protein, fat, and salt but low in fibre. He will need to eat 30–60 kcal/kg and 0.2–0.25 g/kg of nitrogen per day to compensate for the malabsorption caused by short bowel.
   - He may need to fortify foods if his appetite is poor and he may require oral nutritional supplements (1.5 kcal/mL polymeric recommended), which will need to be included in his fluid restriction.
   - The codeine phosphate and loperamide will need to be taken 30–60 min before his main meals and before sleeping.
   - He may benefit from not eating and drinking at the same time.
3.
   - Prevent dehydration by aiming for urine sodium >20 mmol/L by encouraging adherence to fluid restriction and consumption of an oral rehydration solution over the next 2 weeks.
   - Improve nutritional status by showing an increase in lean body mass; as evidenced by an increase in mid-arm muscle circumference and handgrip strength over the next 4 weeks.
4.
   - Goal 1 – urine sodium >20 mmol/L, consistently over next 2 weeks.
   - Goal 2 – Increase mid-arm muscle circumference by 1 cm in 4 weeks.
5.
   - Provide written information on the intestinal failure regimen and explain how the regimen will help him achieve his goals of increasing his strength by preventing dehydration.
   - Encourage him to take responsibility for recording his own fluid balance.
6. Provide written information to Jack and inform nursing staff of the monitoring requirements, that is, daily weight, strict fluid balance, twice weekly urine sodium, biochemistry as requested.

Dietetic and Nutrition Case Studies, First Edition.
Edited by Judy Lawrence, Pauline Douglas, and Joan Gandy.

Companion Website: http://www.manualofdieteticpractice.com/

7.
   - Medical and dietetic notes/electronic records.
   - Jack's care should be recorded accurately, signed, dated, clearly written and easy to read.
   - Records should say what has been done and why, so that any decision made can be justified, should this prove necessary at a later date (BDA, 2008). Informed consent required for any aspect of Jack's care be obtained and documented.
8.
   - Consultant gastroenterologist/surgeon – overall clinical care of the patient.
   - Stoma care nurse – teach patient how to manage stoma.
   - Nutrition nurse specialist – teach the patient how to infuse fluid and electrolytes safely using an aseptic technique.
   - Pharmacist – check for drug–drug or drug–nutrient interactions and monitor for side effects of medications.
   - Physiotherapist – provide exercises to improve functional capacity.
   - Psychologist/psychiatrists – help the patient come to terms with the change in his health situation.
9. Weight, BMI, MAC, TST, Handgrip, biochemistry, urine sodium, fluid balance, blood pressure, temperature, thirst, medication changes and food intake.
10. Patient questionnaire and evaluation of written information provided.

Answers to further questions

11.
    - Urinary sodium – this is a useful test as it often falls earlier than plasma sodium.
    - Malnourished patients may have normal or low plasma urea and creatinine and therefore dehydration may be difficult to identify using these parameters alone.
12.
    - Thirst may result in excessive amounts of unsuitable (low sodium) fluids being consumed, which will increase the stoma losses and lead to dehydration.
    - Jack may become depressed, which could affect appetite and behaviour and therefore he may not be able to adhere to the intestinal failure regimen or consume a suitable diet.
    - It may be difficult for his boyfriend to understand the changes required and as he does most of the cooking it would be important to include him in the discussions.
13.
    - Recommend the use of ice chips to ease thirst.
    - Discuss ways of making the fluid allowance appear to last longer, for example by using a smaller cup, drinking between rather than with meals.
    - Check room temperatures are not exacerbating thirst by being overly hot.
    - Refer to MDT for help dealing with depression or use cognitive behaviour therapy (CBT) if appropriate.
    - Make an appointment at a suitable time to include Jack's boyfriend, it should be possible to speak on the telephone if a face-to-face appointment is not possible.

CASE STUDY 11
Irritable bowel syndrome

Answers

1. Coeliac disease – symptoms may be similar. Coeliac screening should be done while the individual has been including gluten in their diet in more than one meal every day for at least 6 weeks before testing (Ludvigsson *et al.*, 2014; NICE, 2009).
2. Impaired nutrient utilisation (problem) possibly caused by lactose intolerance (aetiology) as evidenced by relationship between ingestion of milk and occurrence of bloating and flatulence (symptoms).
3. First line: check for healthy eating. Second line – restriction of short-chain fermentable carbohydrates (a low fermentable oligosaccharides, disaccharides, monosaccharides and polyols (FODMAP) diet).
4. To take time over meals, sit down to eat and chew food thoroughly, encourage good food variety and ensure nutritional adequacy in line with general healthy eating guidelines, including calcium intake adequacy.
5. Provide acknowledgement and focus on symptom improvement through appropriate, evidence-based dietary change. Diarrhoea and bloating with distension may limit physical activity and therefore the ability to reduce weight. Symptom improvement, which may also be associated with lethargy reduction, enables individuals to become more physically active, supporting a negative energy balance and intentional weight reduction.
6. Jackie's estimated fibre intake (g):

Breakfast: porridge + fruit	7
Lunch	5
Evening meal	8
Snacks: fruit	4
Low calorie wafer	0.3
Total	24

Dietetic and Nutrition Case Studies, First Edition.
Edited by Judy Lawrence, Pauline Douglas, and Joan Gandy.

Companion Website: http://www.manualofdieteticpractice.com/

7. Whole grains, for example, whole grain rice, wild rice, quinoa grains, pasta, buckwheat flour, pasta, noodles, 100% sourdough spelt bread, also rice noodles, polenta.

   She might be reluctant to have a starchy food at lunch/evening meal because she might think they will make her gain weight.
8. Her estimated calcium intake mg/day:

Skimmed milk	366
Cottage cheese, 2/7	20
WW yoghurt, 3/7	128
Petit Filous, 2/7	42
Hard water	200
Total	*756*

   The RNI for women of this age (non-lactating) is 700 mg/day and therefore, her intake is not compromised. If she were on a low lactose diet she could use low lactose skimmed milk and yoghurt.
9. You could discuss her reasons for not taking the analgesic. Sometimes individuals do not take it because they hear that it is an antidepressant and do not appreciate that at a low dose it is used for pain relief, for example, starting at 10–30 mg, taken at night. Many individuals are keen to try dietary intervention before medication, which they may not want to take long-term. Medication may improve some, but not all, symptoms.

   It is preferable to keep dietary and medication changes separate in order to appreciate which therapy is most satisfactory to the individual.
10. This is usually a patient-driven question. The effect of a specific probiotic may be difficult to interpret if other dietary changes are being made simultaneously. Systematic review and meta-analysis show them to be effective, although which individual species and strains are the most beneficial remains unclear (Ford, 2014).

    In line with NICE (2015) recommendations, individuals could trial one product at a time for 4 weeks at the dose recommended by the manufacturer, and continue to take it if it provides symptom benefit.
11. Assess the following:
    - Gut symptoms – belching/burping, borborygmi (stomach rumbling), incomplete evacuation, nausea, heartburn, acid regurgitation, mucous.
    - Non-gut symptoms – lethargy, backache and bladder symptoms, headaches.
    - Other dietetic outcomes – reduction in number of IBS medications taken, that their diet is not IBS symptom causative.
12. Impaired nutrient utilisation (problem) possibly caused by fructose malabsorption (aetiology) evidenced by gut symptoms not fully relieved by low lactose diet (sign/symptom).

Answers to further questions

13. FODMAPs are short-chain fermentable carbohydrates – fermentable oligosaccharides, disaccharides, monosaccharides and polyols.

14. Examples of foods high in FODMAPs include wheat and rye based staples (e.g. bread, pasta, pizza), onion, garlic, pulses, apple, pear, stone fruits, sugar-free chewing gum, mammalian milks and yoghurts.

15. FODMAPs:

- Are rapidly fermented by ileal and colonic bacteria, which may result in an increase in gaseous production and luminal distension and lead to abdominal discomfort or pain, bloating and flatulence.
- Are osmotically active: fructose draws fluid into the small bowel and has a laxative effect.

These physiological effects induce symptoms in people susceptible to functional gut symptoms. Aside from IBS, functional symptoms are also common in about a third of those who have had a gastrointestinal infection, for example, helicobacter pylori, food poisoning, and those with coeliac disease, Crohn's disease or ulcerative colitis.

16. Within 1–3 weeks (Halmos *et al.*, 2014; Staudacher *et al.*, 2012).

17. At least 4 weeks and for up to 8. Thereafter, if the intervention provides satisfactory symptom improvement the individual should undertake planned, systematic re-introduction of foods high in short-chain carbohydrates (Halmos *et al.*, 2014; Staudacher *et al.*, 2012).

18. It is very important as the low FODMAP diet modifies the colonic bacterial profile (Halmos *et al.*, 2014; Staudacher *et al.*, 2012) but it is not known what the long-term effects are of avoiding short-chain carbohydrates. It is also important to identify which FODMAPs she is most sensitive to as not everyone reacts to all FODMAPs. Additionally, identifying how much of a high FODMAP food can be consumed before it triggers symptoms, supports long-term self-care and making the diet more varied and healthy.

19. To return to her usual, healthy diet. Weight reduction is important for the prevention of colorectal cancer and other disorders and diseases associated with excess adiposity. With persisting diarrhoea, refer back to the referrer for further investigation/treatment, for example, consideration of bile acid-induced diarrhoea.

CASE STUDY 12
Liver disease

Answers

1. Inadequate oral food intake (problem) due to increased nutritional requirements caused by decompensated ARLD (aetiology) characterised by poor appetite, potentially steathorrea, weight loss, decline in functional ability and early satiety secondary to ascites (signs/symptoms).
2. Assessment

Domain	
Anthropometry, body composition and functional	Estimated dry weight 70–6 for moderate ascites = 64 kg Height 1.80 m BMI dry weight = 19.8 kg/m^2 12 months ago 86 kg 22 kg weight loss = 25.6% dry weight loss Request dry weight after paracentesis or adjust weight to his dry weight Handgrip strength 26 kg = 65% – indicative of protein energy malnutrition MAMC 18.3 cm ≤ 5th centile
Biochemistry and haematology	Request: Albumin, bilirubin as high bilirubin can be associated with steathorrea Sodium, potassium, urea, creatinine and haemoglobin Fat soluble vitamins – replace if necessary
Clinical	Drug history – thiamine 300 mg and vitamin B Compound Strong 2 tablets tds due to ARLD and not abstinent Calcium 1 g and 800 iu/d Vitamin D as per British Society of Gastroenterology guidelines (Collier *et al.*, 2002)

Dietetic and Nutrition Case Studies, First Edition.
Edited by Judy Lawrence, Pauline Douglas, and Joan Gandy.

Companion Website: http://www.manualofdieteticpractice.com/

Assessment (*continued*)

Domain	
Diet	Dietary intake from 24 h recall does not meet his calculated nutritional requirements Full dietary history obtained and consideration of variation in intake according to the timing of last paracentesis drain Establish food preferences, meal pattern and portion size Not received previous dietary advice
Environmental, behavioural and social	Lives at home with fully supportive wife who prepares meals. She leaves him a sandwich for lunch but often comes home and finds he has not eaten. Some financial difficulties due to the loss of his salary; currently receiving sick pay

3. Energy and protein requirements

   In clinical practice, either the ESPEN (Plauth et al., 2006) guidelines of 35–40 kcal/kg dry body weight per day or calculation of basal metabolic rate (BMR) (using dry weight) using Henry (2005) equations with added stress and activity factors according to PENG handbook (Todorovic & Micklewright, 2011) guidelines.

   Use PENG handbook guidelines to determine protein requirements.

   Equations that estimate energy and protein are estimates and the key to evaluating if energy and protein requirements are being met is through close monitoring and review.

4. Estimated Energy and protein requirements

   Maintenance

   Energy

   Using his dry weight, determine BMR using either Henry equations or ESPEN guidelines (35–40 kcal/kg/day)

   Using Henry equations

   Male 48 years $(14.2 \times 64) + 593 = 1502\,\text{kcal/day}$

   Adjust for stress using liver disease specific stress factor, that is, decompensated liver disease +30–40%

   +40% stress factor = 600 kcal

   Adjust using +25% activity factor = 376 kcal

   Total energy requirement for maintenance = 1502 + 600 + 376 = 2478 kcal/day

Protein (Todorovic & Micklewright, 2011)
In decompensated liver disease

Protein requirements = 1.2–1.5 g/kg dry body weight per day
Nitrogen 0.2–0.25 g/kg dry body weight per day

Using a dry weight of 64 kg

Protein requirements = (1.2×64) 76.8 to $(1.5 \times 64) = 96.0$ g/day
Nitrogen requirements = (0.2×64) 12.8 to $(0.25 \times 64) = 16$ g/day

However you should aim for repletion due to Richard's clinically significant weight loss and muscle depletion.

For repletion/weight gain
Energy
Using Henry equations
Total energy requirement for maintenance = 1502 + 600 + 376 = 2478 kcal
Add 400–1000 kcal for repletion
For repletion
Maintenance = 2478 kcal
Repletion = +400 to 1000 kcal = 2878–3478 kcal/day

Protein
1.5–2 g/kg dry weight
1.5 to $2 \times 64 = 96$–128 g protein/day

Nitrogen
0.25–0.3 g/kg dry weight
0.25–0.3 $\times 64 = 16$–19.2 g nitrogen/day

5. Salt
Large volume paracentesis (LVP) every 3 weeks = Refractory ascites Grade 2
EASL guidelines (2010) 90 mmol/d sodium restricted diet = 5.2 g salt (90 mmol sodium) per day
6. Dietetic intervention plan
24 h recall = 1490 kcal; 52 g protein; 4.1 g salt
Estimated nutritional requirements 2878–3478 kcal and 96–128 g protein per day
Therefore, dietetic advice needs to aim to add 1388–1988 kcal and 44–76 g protein to the diet
Aims
a. To improve and prevent further decline in nutritional status
   - Aim to initially stabilise weight with appropriate nutritional support via food first oral nutritional supplements (ONSs) to meet calculated requirements for kcal and protein.
   - Aim to provide advice to achieve a minimum of 1200 kcal and 42 g protein to calculated requirements for repletion including the following measures:
     - Advise a small frequent meal pattern and supplementary dietary advice.
     - Educate and advise a late evening 50 g CHO snack.

        - Provide ONS as required. Often, low-volume 2 kcal/ml sip feeds required to meet requirements and low volume protein and fat supplements are helpful when there is early satiety.
    - Back up with written information and contact details.
    - Recommend ascorbic acid and vitamin A, D, E and K supplementation.

  b. Potentially provide symptomatic relief from accumulating ascites by restricting sodium intake:
    - Salt intake is not excessive from dietary recall.
    - Provide education on higher salt foods and advise not to exceed 5.2 g per day.
    - Assessment of daily fluid intake may be appropriate. Formal fluid restrictions are only advised if serum sodium is below 125 mmol/L (EASL, 2010)
    - However due to early satiety and frequency of drains an assessment of fluid intake and pattern is appropriate to ensure is not excessive or hindering food intake.

  c. Exclude steathorrea and maximise absorption with appropriate dietary fat adaptation:
    - Patients with ARLD can often have chronic pancreatitis, which can be investigated with a faecal elastase test to assess pancreatic exocrine activity and pancreatic enzyme repletion introduced
    - If there is no pancreatic insufficiency, dietary fat may require adaptation. Fat may be reduced to tolerance and energy replaced from carbohydrate and protein sources. The use of medium-chain triglyceride products for energy replacement can be considered.

7. Appropriate meal pattern

A grazing pattern of 4–6 small meals per day can reduce fasting gluconeogenesis, nocturnal amino acid breakdown and improve nitrogen balance and reduces muscle catabolism. This pattern may also help patients with early satiety caused by reduced abdominal volume as ascites increases (Tsien *et al.*, 2011).

A late evening snack of 50 g carbohydrate can improve nitrogen balance as it reduces fasting periods overnight and an improvement in nutritional status has been demonstrated as a result (Plank *et al.*, 2008).

8. Nutritional monitoring

Domain	
Anthropometry, body composition and functional	Weight, BMI % weight loss Handgrip, MAMC Functional ability
Biochemical and haematological	Potassium and sodium levels as on diuretics Reassess ascorbic acid, vitamins A, D, E, K levels post replacement Assess compliance with B vitamins, thiamine and calcium

Domain	
Clinical	Bowel opening – frequency and form Frequency of LVP Any other symptoms relevant, for example, hepatic encephalopathy (HE), reflux
Dietary	Nutrient intake from food and oral nutritional support products including any changes in condition that are affecting food intake To ensure that patient is receiving nutrients to meet requirements, and that the dietary advice given is the most appropriate for clinical condition To assess tolerance to ONS and allow alteration of intake/ONS as indicated To reassess nutrient intake and meal pattern
Environmental, behavioural and social	Ability for daily activities of living Any social concerns that impact on intake

9. Outcome measures that may be used include:
   a. Direct nutrition outcomes
      - Knowledge gained;
      - Change in eating pattern;
      - Food and nutrient intake changes; and
      - Improved nutritional status.
   b. Clinical outcomes
      - Increase in weight BMI, handgrip and MAMC;
      - Improvement in bowel opening; and
      - Reduced frequency of paracentesis.
   c. Patient-centred outcomes
      - Able to walk his dog;
      - Improved quality of life scores; and
      - Reduced fatigue enabling increased activities of daily living.
   d. Health Care Related Outcomes
      - Medication changes to improve absorption and bowel opening; and
      - Increased number of days between LVP if fluid intake was excessive. This will result in fewer days as a hospital inpatient.
10. Documentation should be as per dietetic care process and to BDA's standards for record keeping.

Answers to further questions

11. Nutritional requirements should be calculated as per energy and protein requirements with the aim to achieve a positive nitrogen balance. However, he is at risk of developing hepatic encephalopathy (HE); therefore, while nutritional support is important, the guidance is not to exceed the upper limit of calculated requirements for protein and ensure adequate energy is made available. A small frequent meal pattern of 4–6 small meals and snacks should be recommended with oral intake every 2–3 h to meet nutritional requirements. Late evening 50 g carbohydrate snacks are crucial as this reduces protein catabolism during overnight fast and promotes a positive nitrogen balance (Tsuchiya *et al.*, 2005; Yamanaka-Okumura *et al.*, 2006).

12. Periods of fasting should be minimised as endogenous waste from protein catabolism can precipitate HE. A small frequent meal pattern of 4–6 small meals and snacks should be recommended with oral intake every 2–3 h to meet nutritional requirements. It is important to ensure Richards's bowels are opening 2–3× per day as constipation can precipitate encephalopathy (Amiodo *et al.*, 2013).

13. Vitamin B deficiency is common in ARLD, in particular thiamine, folate, pyridoxine and riboflavin. Thiamine is an essential cofactor in the metabolism of carbohydrate and alcohol. Non-abstinent people with ARLD are at high risk of developing clinical vitamin B group deficiencies and Wernicke's encephalopathy (NICE, 2010).

14. It is inappropriate to consider long-term outcomes unless he becomes abstinent for 6 months, when liver transplantation may be considered (Guevara *et al.*, 2005; Moreau *et al.*, 2004). The development of ascites in cirrhosis indicates a poor prognosis with the mortality approximately 40% at 1 year and 50% at 2 years. Once refractory ascites has developed, the median survival of patients is approximately 6 months (Guevara *et al.*, 2005).

15. Diuretics are prescribed when patients present with the first episode of grade 2 (moderate) ascites; Richard is within this category.

- Aldosterone antagonists such as spironolactone are potassium sparing and weak natrietics. If patients develop hyperkalaemia >6 mmol/L in the absence of renal failure it should resolve with the discontinuation of the drug and long-term potassium restriction is unlikely to be necessary.
- Loop diuretics such as furosemide, which may be used in combination with aldosterone antagonists. These are powerful natrietics and are potassium loosing. If patients develop severe hypokalaemia <3 mmol/L loop diuretics need to be discontinued (Angeli *et al.*, 2010).
- Hyponatraemia may occur with both diuretics.

CASE STUDY 13
Renal disease

Answers

1. Assessment

Anthropometry, body composition and functional	Body mass index, weight history, % weight change
Biochemical	CRP, urinary protein loss and fluid status should be considered if monitoring serum albumin
Clinical	Physical appearance, presence/absence of oedema, blood pressure
Diet	Food frequency questionnaire or 3 day food diary
Environmental, behavioural and social	Motivation and readiness to change. Shopping habits, housing, cooking facilities, language and literacy

2. • Excessive dietary intake of potassium (problem) related to consumption of foods highin potassium and reduced renal function (aetiology) as evidenced by diet history and recent biochemistry (potassium 6 mmol/L) (signs/symptoms).
   • Unintentional weight loss (problem) related to inadequate dietary intake and reduced kidney function (aetiology) as evidenced by poor appetite, looser cloths and reduction in eGFR (signs/symptoms).

   Note: The diagnoses should be prioritised according to their severity and taking into account the patient's perspective. From the dietitian's perspective, reducing the potassium level is the most important, due to the increased mortality rates in these patients. However, weight loss is also significant (8%) and should be treated.

Dietetic and Nutrition Case Studies, First Edition.
Edited by Judy Lawrence, Pauline Douglas, and Joan Gandy.

Companion Website: http://www.manualofdieteticpractice.com/

3. Aim

   To achieve serum potassium levels within an acceptable range whilst ensuring a nutritionally balanced diet.

   Goals
   - Understand benefits of dietary advice;
   - Motivated to make dietary changes;
   - Be able to make appropriate dietary changes;
   - Achieve nutritional adequacy;
   - Achieve serum potassium levels within target range;
   - Improve nutritional status/gain weight; and
   - Patient achieves what is important to him.

   Outcome measures
   - Patient reported level of understanding;
   - Patient reported knowledge of foods that were high/low in potassium;
   - Patient reported level of motivation (using scales for confidence and importance);
   - Patient reported diet history;
   - Serum potassium level;
   - Weight; and
   - Patient reported experience.
4. Agree goals with Martin is he motivated to make dietary changes?
   What is important to Martin?
   Agree suitable timescales to achieve goals with patient.
5. - Assess Martin's knowledge and understanding of the dietary changes required and his level of motivation to make these changes.
   - Reassess dietary intake to evaluate if dietary changes have taken place and if they were having a nutritionally adequate diet.
   - Objective measures such as serum potassium level and weight should provide further evidence of this.
6. A patient experience questionnaire can be provided at the end of the episode of care such as the CARE measure (Nursing Midwifery and Allied Health Professions Research Unit).
7. - Potassium and eGFR are the most important results.
   - Urea and creatinine are also helpful – uraemia can adversely affect appetite.
   - Low serum albumin levels can reflect poor nutrition but are more likely to reflect inflammation, co-morbidity and fluid overload (Jones, 2001).
8. For kidney patients, the complexity of a diet has been one of the most frequently identified barriers to patient compliance (Caggiula & Milas, 1993). Dietary priorities may often change over time, which can be confusing.
   - For Martin, there are two different dietary priorities, which could be confusing.
   - Other barriers can be lack of understanding and the provision of conflicting information from other sources such as from the Internet.
   - Lack of motivation can be a barrier, but appears to be unlikely in this case.
9. Agree priorities and educate patient using appropriate methods and at an appropriate level.

Plan:

- Assess initial motivation and understanding regarding potassium.
- Educate patient as to the benefits and risks of reducing dietary potassium.

Rationale: Angiotensin converting enzyme inhibitors (ACEI) lower blood pressure and reduce proteinuria in those with CKD, but can cause hyperkalaemia. If serum potassium level rises to ≥6 mmol/L, ACEI should be stopped and causes of raised potassium levels, including diet, should be investigated (NICE, 2008).

Benefits: Once potassium levels have reduced to 5 mmol/L, ACEI can be restarted (NICE, 2008).

Risks: Some patients with a low potassium intake have been found to have low serum vitamin levels (Pollock *et al.*, 2005). As a result, though most patients should be encouraged to consume five 80 g portions of fruit and vegetables daily, they should also be educated regarding those that are particularly high in potassium. A low potassium diet should be individualised according to dietary intake and blood levels and should not be too restrictive (Perry & Hartley, 2014).

Explain how to make appropriate dietary changes

Limit the 'non essential' nutrient poor high potassium foods first. Care should be taken not to restrict nutrient rich foods more than necessary (Perry & Hartley, 2005).

- The 24 h dietary recall provided is high in potassium (approx. 100 mmol). Removing the supplement drinks would reduce the potassium by 25%. Changing the roast potatoes to boiled potatoes, limiting the soup and coffee would also help to reduce the potassium intake still further. Sprouts are one of the vegetables that are higher in potassium, but such a small quantity makes very little difference to overall potassium intake. A large glass of pure fruit juice contains a significant amount of potassium; swapping this for a small glass would still ensure that he has sufficient vitamin C.
- Establish which foods he currently enjoys and jointly agree to replace higher potassium foods with foods lower in potassium.
- If Complan was removed, this would reduce the protein intake to less than that recommended. Hence, additional sources of protein need to be considered. Energy intake is also inadequate.

Assess initial motivation and understanding regarding ensuring adequate nutritional intake

Educate patient as to the benefits and risks of increasing nutritional intake

Rationale: Malnutrition becomes more prevalent as GFR falls, particularly from stage 4 CKD onwards and is associated with increased morbidity, greater health care requirements, and reduced functional ability.

Benefits: Early identification and dietetic treatment of any reduction in nutritional status is important in order to prevent established malnutrition.

Risks: Dietary protein intake should not be less than 0.8 g/kg in stage 3 CKD, but as renal disease progresses it is prudent not to have more than 1.0 g/kg IBW (SIGN, 2005; Renal Association, 2011). As a result of the prevalence of hyperphosphataemia, high protein intakes are not recommended in stage 4 CKD and may also increase metabolic acidosis.

Though energy requirements are not increased by the presence of CKD, it is important to ensure an adequate energy intake to prevent negative nitrogen balance and weight loss (Perry & Hartley, 2014).

Explain how to make appropriate dietary changes

First line dietetic advice should be to fortify the existing diet with additional nutrient-dense foods. The use of sugary foods and sweet drinks should be encouraged and fats are a useful source of energy. This is a greater priority than a strict cardio-protective diet at this time. Encourage an adequate protein intake; provide suggested quantities (either as weights or handy measures).

10. Monitoring

- Dietary intake and serum potassium levels should be regularly monitored (NICE, 2008)
- Nutritional status should be monitored by means of weight, diet history and appetite. Other methods including measuring handgrip strength or MUAMC.

NB: When the target serum potassium has been achieved, the low potassium diet may need to be relaxed or stopped. Inform the GP as the patient may be able to restart ACEI.

If the patient's dietary intake continues to be inadequate, oral nutritional supplements (ONSs) may be required. If potassium levels remain high, ONS that are low in electrolytes should be considered (Cano *et al.*, 2006). This is because they enable the consumption of adequate protein and energy without the provision of additional potassium, facilitating a less restrictive diet (Perry & Hartley, 2014).

Answers to further questions

11. Educate using appropriate methods and at an appropriate level

Rationale: The main aims of dietetic treatment are to reduce the progression both of CKD and cardiovascular disease (CVD).

- Initially, the main focus should be on ensuring a healthy weight and limiting salt intake to less than 6g per day (Jones-Burton *et al.*, 2006).
- The 'DASH' diet may not be appropriate due to the potential for increased potassium and phosphate levels (SIGN, 2008).
- A cardio-protective diet also helps those at high risk of CVD.
- By CKD stage 4, other factors become more important including:
  - Regular monitoring of nutritional status; and
  - Regular monitoring and dietetic advice as required for potassium and phosphate (Perry & Hartley, 2014).

12.
- The use of a variety of nutritional markers is recommended including appetite and dietary intake.
- Subjective Global assessment has been validated for use with patients with kidney failure.

- Skinfold calipers can be used to assess mid upper arm circumference, triceps skinfold thickness and mid upper arm muscle circumference; they have been found to correlate well with other measures such as weight and BMI.
- Handgrip strength has been found to correlate well with lean body mass (Perry & Hartley, 2014)

13. Yes, as the incidence of malnutrition increases from stage 4 CKD onwards. By this stage, complications such as fluid and electrolyte imbalance, metabolic acidosis, anaemia and the accumulation of metabolic waste products (such as urea) are more common, which have an adverse effect on nutritional status. Martin has several of these complications already.

14.
- Low serum bicarbonate levels may require treatment with sodium bicarbonate.
- Martin's eGFR had reduced significantly over 3 months, but this could be an acute problem caused by the UTI. Monitoring eGFR changes over a longer timescale will determine the rate of progression of CKD.
- Most patients with CKD stage 4–5 (or with CKD stage 3 and rapidly declining eGFR) should be referred for assessment by nephrology (Perry & Hartley, 2014).

CASE STUDY 14
Renal – black and ethnic minority

Answers

1. Excessive dietary intake of potassium and phosphate (problem) related to over-consumption of foods high in potassium (aetiology) characterised by potassium 6 mmol/L, and phosphate 1.99 mmol/L (sign Symptom).
2. Low phosphate and low potassium diet.
3. • To restrict dietary potassium and phosphate intake whilst maintaining a well-balanced diet.
   • Reduced intake of sodium by suggesting to add less salt in cooking and not to add anymore whilst at the table.
4. • Diet history reveals some foods high in potassium included on a regular basis.
   • Dietary phosphate intake does not appear to be unduly high so raised phosphate level more likely influenced by elevated PTH.
   • As dried fruit and nuts are high in potassium, discuss alternative snacks she can have instead.
   • Limit high potassium fruits such as bananas and exotic fruits, aim for 2 portions of fruit per day; include lower potassium options such as apples, Clementine's and pears and 2 portions of vegetables per day.
   • Suggest low potassium cereals such as weetabix or porridge rather than bran flakes, which is high in potassium and phosphate.
   • Reduce dietary intake of phosphate rich foods that she includes whilst ensuring she has an adequate protein intake. Although pulses (dals) are high in phosphate and potassium, they are a good source of protein in her diet.
   • Discuss use of rice milk or soya milk, which are lower in phosphate.
   • Limit intake of kheer and mithai, as Asian desserts are high in milk, fat and sugar. They would be an additional source of phosphate and potassium. Dried fruit and nuts are often added to these dishes.
   • Suggest using rice milk when making Asian desserts or buttermilk (lassi).
   • Discuss with patient to avoid having dal and meat curry at one meal, encourage one of these dishes at one meal time.

Dietetic and Nutrition Case Studies, First Edition.
Edited by Judy Lawrence, Pauline Douglas, and Joan Gandy.

Companion Website: http://www.manualofdieteticpractice.com/

- Discourage the use of adding butter to rice or chapatti (roti) as this will increase the phosphate intake, and encourage her to have plain roti over the oiled bread (parata).
- Make sure the patient understands the correct way of taking phosphate binders, the dose and distribution.
- Discuss the role of Calcichew as a phosphate binder, the importance of timing and distribution with meals.
- Consider any changes that have been made to the diet or lifestyle since diagnosis in order to be realistic about future expectations.
- Suggest reducing intake of salt both in cooking and from processed foods and Indian snacks.
- Evening meal which patient has is high in potassium therefore suggest alternatives, keep in mind the patient's cultural background and if she prefers a light option for dinner.

5. Reduce potassium intake.
   - Discuss cooking methods.
     - Potatoes can be parboiled before frying; however, she may prefer to cook her vegetables the South Asian way, which is usually sautéed in oil/ghee with spices and steamed.
   - Limit intake fruit.
   - Limit milk intake or change to soya or rice milk.
   - Consider alternative phosphate binders that may be easier to take with snacks.
6. As with any patient, make sure they are in agreement with what advice you give and explain the rational, which is always important. Consider saying to Amina what goals does she think she can achieve till your next appointment. Explain to her why potassium and phosphate can affect her if too high, and that the symptoms she may be having may reduce when she makes those changes.
7. - To optimise nutritional status, maintaining potassium and phosphate within target levels is very important.
   - Aim for a healthier weight, which will include moderate weight loss.
8. - Ensure Amina has a healthy balanced diet encompassing all the food groups from the eatwell plate.
   - She would benefit from a modest weight loss. Discuss what changes she can make to her diet and how she can modify her cooking methods to reduce the fat content.
   - Increasing her physical activity level, considering barriers for certain exercises due to her culture and dress.
9. Guidelines are to use ideal body weight (IBW) as BMI = 25 kg/m^2 in this case (Renal Association, 2009).

Estimated dietary intake	Estimated dietary requirements
Energy – 1750–1990 kcal/day	1860 kcal/day (30 kcal/kg IBW)
Protein – 64–75 g/day	60/72 g/day (0.8–1/ kg IBW) (1–1.2 g/kg IBW for dialysis.)

Also consider the following:

- Reduce potassium level to acceptable range for pre-dialysis 3.5–5.5 mmol/L Highlight high potassium foods, and advice on low alternatives.
- Aim to keep phosphate level to 0.9–1.5 mmol/L. This can be achieved with diet and phosphate binders.
- Consider the nutritional status of the patient – ensure adequate energy, protein, minerals and vitamins are provided to achieve a balanced diet.
- Ensure that the patient's cultural practices are considered and taken into account in order to personalise dietary advice to her needs.
- Consider appropriate literature to give to patient.
- Consider the raised PTH levels influencing the phosphate levels and consider management with the medical team.

10.
- Cultural barrier – take into account patient's cultural dietary habits and the foods the patient can or cannot eat because of religious or personal choices.
- Language barrier – ensure communication and written material is provided in the language that is native to her and that she is literate. If necessary, use a translator.

11.
- Diet history.
- Serum potassium.
- Serum phosphate.
- Weight.

12. Under Islamic rulings, it is not obligatory for a person to fast if they have poor health or if fasting can cause adverse effects on health. It is important to discuss with the medical team before discussing with the patient, as each patient will be at an individual stage of disease and treatment. If the medical team suggests that Amina should not fast, then explain the adverse effects and suggest to Amina to discuss with her local imam and give to charity instead. If the medical team agrees that Amina can fast then consider what dietary changes will affect her dialysis. For example, she will be drinking less fluid and therefore less will be needed to be removed by dialysis. You may find her potassium and phosphate levels drop too much in which case you may have to encourage her to have higher potassium and phosphate foods when she breaks her fast. It will be a challenge to maintain them protein and energy intakes at this time so encourage Amina to make the right food choices.

CASE STUDY 15

Motor neurone disease/amyotrophic lateral sclerosis

Answers

1. 12% unintentional weight loss, body mass index 21.6 kg/m^2
   Dysphagia assessment – bedside swallowing assessment, other assessments may be available, for example, videofluoroscopy.
2. Inadequate oral food intake (problem) secondary to dysphagia including difficulty swallowing food and liquids (aetiology) as evidenced by unintended weight loss of 12% usual body weight (sign/symptom).
3. The aim of the dietetic intervention are as follows.
   - To improve quality of intake to meet nutrition and energy requirements.
   - To reduce risk of aspiration.
4. - Weight gain/prevention of further weight loss.
   - Nutritionally adequate diet in terms of quality and quantity.
   - Changes in swallowing, choking episodes and report of increasing difficulty with particular foods and fluids.
   - Screen for occurrence of fever or chest infection.
5. - Discussion with Peter and his wife regarding their priorities and wishes around Peter's food goals.
   - Education regarding realistic goals through the course of the disease
     - Weight maintenance/prevention of further weight loss;
     - Appetite changes due to early satiety/changes in intake due to fatigue, constipation, dysphagia; and
     - Being proactive in modifying foods and fluids to reduce the risk of aspiration.
   - Peter to keep food records to review adequacy and to record problem foods (BDA, 2008).
6. Discussion with patient and wife concerning current status.
   - Written instructions regarding recommended food choices considering texture modification/liquid consistency, food preparation methods, available resources
   - Nutritional intake – increase dairy intake, increase energy density of intake, for example, increase fat intake, nutritional supplements (homemade or commercial), and small more frequent meals/snacks

Dietetic and Nutrition Case Studies, First Edition.
Edited by Judy Lawrence, Pauline Douglas, and Joan Gandy.

Companion Website: http://www.manualofdieteticpractice.com/

- Dysphagia – appropriate food texture/liquid consistency, avoid high risk foods and problem foods
- Education – resources, for example, recipes

7. In accordance with BDA/HCPC guidelines all entries would be signed and dated and written as soon as possible after seeing Peter.
8.
   - Speech and language therapist (SLT) – swallowing assessment to determine most appropriate food texture and liquid consistency.
   - Occupational therapist – adapted utensils to aid in self-feeding.
   - Nurse – bowel management.
   - Respirologist – pulmonary function tests to assess disease progression, risk associated with PEG/RIG procedure.
   - Pharmacist – medications in liquid/crushable form versus pills/tablets.
   - Social work – funding, emotional support.
   - Community/home support.
9.
   - Record weight (%change), appetite, changes in intake and reasons, problem foods/beverages (new/changes).
   - Interventions recommended, implementation – what has been implemented/note challenges, barriers.

   Goals may be adjusted through the course of the disease, for example, goal of weight gain may become prevention of further weight loss. Focus on intake may be to optimise nutrition and hydration and eating for quality of life and eating for pleasure (with or without nutrition via PEG).
10. By asking directly and/or by using an evaluation questionnaire.
11. The ALS specific equation to estimate energy requirements (Kasarskis *et al.*, 2014) should be used. This is a web based calculator that is based on total daily energy expenditure measurements measured for 10 days over a 40 week period in MND/ALS patients. It also includes a surrogate for physical activity. The surrogate is based on six elements of the amyotrophic lateral sclerosis functional rating scale (ALSFRS), which is a disease specific rating scale that estimates a patient's degree of impairment in performing common tasks (ALS CNTF Treatment Study (ACTS) Phase I-II Study Group, 1996). The elements are speech, handwriting, dressing and hygiene, turning in bed/adjusting bedclothes, walking and dysphagia. The ALSFRS is routinely measured on clinical visits enabling recalculation of energy requirements as the disease progresses.
12.
   - Face-to-face – SLT would be involved for assistive and augmentative communication (AAC), handwritten notes while hand/arm is functional and latterly a speech-generating device (Lightwriter, iPad, etc.);
   - Distance – it is common to communicate by e-mail although this requires agreement with patient and his consent regarding privacy concerns; and
   - Through family/friends with patient's consent.
13. Peter may have difficulty accepting the diagnosis, making decisions (this could be a previous part of his personality or may be new as a result of the diagnosis). He may also have some difficulty anticipating risk and therefore be resistant to making the changes recommended.

Answers to further questions

14. • Nutritional intake – increase dairy intake, increase energy density of intake, for example, increase fat intake, nutritional supplements (homemade or commercial), and small more frequent meals/snacks.
    • Dysphagia – appropriate food texture/liquid consistency, avoid high risk foods and problem foods.
    • Education – resources, for example, recipes.
    • Discussion on PEG/RIG – indicators (declining respiratory function, dysphagia, weight loss), pros and cons, risks and benefits, decision-making.
15. Discussion with Peter regarding challenges meeting energy requirements which are resulting in further undesirable weight loss
    • High energy output – distance running, increased effort for ADLS and hypermetabolic aspect of MND/ALS;
    • Decrease in intake related to self-feeding difficulty in addition to dysphagia; and
    • Recommendations regarding increased energy density of intake, energy conservation, exploring alternate methods of stress management.

    NB Recommendations may vary at each visit depending on patient's status and needs.
16. Indicators for PEG/Rig feeding include declining FVC (safety of procedure), dysphagia (risk of aspiration pneumonia and decreased intake), weight loss (inadequate intake). It is important to assess patient readiness for discussion and may include the following points; acceptance of diagnosis, recognition that there is a problem, attitude to enteral feeding, for example, importance of oral eating.

    Peter has had
    • A significant weight loss – >5–10% unintended weight loss is considered a 'red flag' for initiation of this discussion; and
    • Decreased pulmonary function
        ◦ Decline in FVC which is approaching the 50% of predicted that is considered the cut-off point for safety of the procedure and.
        ◦ Peak cough flow (PCF) is now 250 L/min and he would be considered to have an 'ineffectual' cough for airway clearance.

    The discussion regarding PEG/RIG should be initiated now if it has not already been done.
17. • Indicators are declining respiratory function, dysphagia, weight loss.
    • Provision of information (verbal and written) to aid in patient's decision making.
    • Pros/cons, risks and benefits and potential complications of procedure.
    • Strategies for use of feeding tube (complete nutrition, supplementation of oral intake, hydration, administration of medications).
    • Enteral feeding administration (syringe, gravity, pump).
    • Where to obtain enteral feeding supplies and financial considerations.

CASE STUDY 16

Chronic fatigue syndrome/myalgic encephalopathy

Answers

1. Assessment

Domain	
Anthropometry	Current weight 52 kg Weight 1 year ago 56 kg Height 1.69 m BMI 18.2 kg/m^2
Biochemical and haematological	Low ferritin levels 2 years ago
Clinical	CFS/ME, 1 year duration Headaches, eye pain, muscle and joint pain, poor sleep and concentration, sensitivity to light, palpitations and dizzy spells and nausea Prescribed amitriptyline (10 mg ods)
Diet	Coffee, 1 average mug, 260 g Milk in coffee 40 g occasional energy drinks, 250 g Evening meal Chicken stew or casseroles, 260 g roast chicken, breast 130 g fish, 100 g with vegetables, 60–70 g/portion and potatoes, boiled 175, or roast 85 g Avoids lactose and gluten Magnesium and coenzyme Q10 supplements
Environmental, behavioural and social	Recently resigned from work Lives with partner in parents' home

Dietetic and Nutrition Case Studies, First Edition.
Edited by Judy Lawrence, Pauline Douglas, and Joan Gandy.

Companion Website: http://www.manualofdieteticpractice.com/

2. Inadequate energy intake (problem) caused by the exclusion of gluten and lactose and continuing nausea (aetiology) characterised by 4 kg weight loss (sign/symptom).
3. A number of diets claim to promote recovery and relieve CFS/ME symptoms such as the anti-candida diet but are often based on unreliable evidence. Many of these diets can be very restrictive and create more work for the patient whether in food preparation, or in visiting various shops to buy food ingredients or products (Luscombe, 2012). NICE (2007), Baumer (2005), and Morris and Stare (1993) recommend dietary advice in line with a balanced diet as in the Eatwell plate. In addition working with the patient to overcome any barriers secondary to symptoms, be this is a practical barrier (such as ability to cook or shop) or physical such as nausea, sore throat and intolerances (McIntosh, 2014; NICE, 2007).
4. • To maintain energy levels throughout the day.
   • To prevent further weight loss.

   For Melissa and many other people with CFS/ME, eating little and often is beneficial. Eating every 3–4 h and choosing low GI foods for both meals and snacks aids in maintaining blood sugar levels which can help to improve energy levels throughout the day (Maclintosh, 2014; NICE, 2007).
5. • Weight.
   • Verbal feedback.
   • Patient satisfaction survey, which includes:
   • 5 point rating scale from excellent to very poor.
   • Questions regarding what has been good about the service received and how this could be improved.
6. Energy drinks have a high GI and would not be recommended as they cause large fluctuations in blood sugar. Patients should be encouraged to eat regular balanced meals and to include low GI foods rather than high GI items (McKenzie, 2014). Energy drinks also contain caffeine along with drinks such as cola, tea and coffee. Caffeine can impact on energy levels and bowel symptoms. Good sleep hygiene routines should be advised for people with CFS/ME which includes avoiding or cutting down on caffeine containing drinks particularly in an evening (McKenzie, 2014; NICE, 2007).
7. Coeliac disease is initially identified by taking a blood sample to test for antibodies. Recommended first choice for blood test is IgA tissue transglutaminase (tTGA) (NICE, 2009) via the GP. If the result is positive the GP will refer to a gastrointestinal specialist for intestinal biopsy to confirm or exclude coeliac disease. It is essential that a gluten-containing diet is continued before tests are carried out (NICE, 2009) ideally more than 1 meal daily for at least 6 weeks prior to testing. As Melissa had felt better and no longer experienced stomach pain and diarrhoea, she did not wish to feel unwell again and declined to have the test (Fraser-Mayall, 2014; NICE, 2009).
8. There is no evidence CFS/ME has a greater incidence of IgE mediated food allergy than the general population (McIntosh, 2014) and exclusion diets are generally not recommended for managing CFS/ME however they can be helpful with symptom management, especially with IBS symptoms (NICE, 2008;

McKenzie *et al.*, 2012). When eliminating certain food for example gluten or lactose free, patients should be provided with advice from a dietitian to ensure the diet remains balanced (NICE, 2007, 2008). Advice for a gluten free diet would be provided, taking into account the patients likes and dislikes and barriers to change, for example, Melissa feeling nauseous, having poor appetite and dietary intake. Regarding the reported lactose intolerance, this often occurs in association with the gluten intolerance as the gut inflammation can cause a deficiency in lactase. This associated lactose intolerance usually resolves as the gut heals over a period of time. Advice on non-dairy sources of calcium will be required during period of lactose elimination and when trialling the reintroduction of lactose at a later stage (McIntosh, 2012; Skypala & Ventner, 2014).

9. Nausea can be a common symptom of CFS/ME. When people experience nausea, advice should be provided such as avoiding drinking with meals, eating little and often, to opt for savoury, dry or cold foods dependent on what the individual finds benefit from and to avoid fatty or fried foods. If nausea is severe GP may consider anti-emetic drugs (NICE, 2007). For Melissa, if the nausea can be better managed, she will be more likely to increase dietary intake.

Answers to further questions

10. Dietary supplements are often used by CFS/ME patients and often high doses have been reported with a number of different nutritional supplements. The current advice is that there is no conclusive evidence to support the use of vitamin and mineral supplements to manage CFS/ME symptoms (NICE, 1993). Many vitamins provide very high or 'mega' doses and can be very expensive. A multivitamin and mineral supplement providing 100% RDA may be recommended and for individuals following a restricted diet, for example, those excluding milk and dairy foods may require an additional supplement such as calcium. Plus an EFA supplement such as evening primrose oil (up to 1000 mg/d) and fish oils (1000 mg/d). In those patients who may be housebound it would also be good practice to assess vitamin D and if required vitamin D supplementation to prevent osteoporosis 5–10 μg (NICE, 2007; Berkovitz *et al.*, 2009).
11. Amitriptyline is a tricyclic antidepressant which blocks the uptake of brain chemicals noradrenaline and serotonin. In CFS/ME this is often used to improve sleep and reduce muscle pain (NICE, 2007; McIntosh, 2014).
12. Often patients will wish to trial alternative therapies to manage CFS/ME symptoms and it is important to be sensitive to patients' decisions. Some patients may report a benefit from this but there is insufficient evidence that complementary therapies such as homeopathy are effective and therefore would not be recommended (Gandy, 2014; NICE, 2007).
13. Any telephone message that you leave should not include advice. There is potential for a telephone message to breech confidentiality if it is picked up by another member of Melissa's household. It is also possible that a message could be misinterpreted either by Melissa or by a third party.

CASE STUDY 17

Refsum's disease

Answers

1. Assessment

Domain	
Anthropometry, body composition and functional	Weight 76 kg Height 1.75 m BMI 25 kg/m^2
Biochemical and haematological	Normal blood biochemistry except plasma phytanic acid level which is highly abnormal at 800 µmol/L (normal range usually <30 µmol/L)
Clinical	Icthyosis, peripheral neuropathy, retinitis pigmentosa, shortened third fingers
Diet	*Breakfast* Bran flakes (30 g) with semi skimmed milk (100 g), orange juice (160 g), toast (27 g) with high polyunsaturated fat spread(7 g) and jam (15 g) *Mid-morning* Cappuccino(170 g) from machine with sugar (5 g) and chocolate chip cookies (2 × 13 g) *Lunch* Cheese and ham toasted sandwich (165 g), can of coke (330 mL), crisps (40 g) and an apple (112 g) *Evening meal* Spaghetti bolognaise (470 g) with parmesan cheese (10 g), bananas (100 g) and ice-cream (75 g) *Supper* Cheese (30 g) and crackers (2 × 5 g), can of lager (444 g)

Dietetic and Nutrition Case Studies, First Edition.
Edited by Judy Lawrence, Pauline Douglas, and Joan Gandy.

Companion Website: http://www.manualofdieteticpractice.com/

Assessment (*continued*)

Domain	
	Food frequency Sweets (100 g) and chocolates (40–65 g) – 2–3 × per week Crisps (40 g) and nuts (50 g) – daily *Alcohol* 2–6 units 3–4 × per week Cakes – 1–2 × per week typically doughnuts (75 g) or chocolate muffins (75 g) Biscuits (13 g each) – most days Take-aways – weekly, usually Indian (400 g) or Chinese (400 g) plus rice (300 g)
Environmental, behavioural and social	Married with a 3-year-old daughter, professional man, educated to at least A level standard

2. Impaired nutrient utilisation (phytanic acid) (problem) related to adult refsum's disease (aetiology), evidenced by elevated serum phytanic acid (signs) characterised by itchy scaly skin and neuropathy (symptoms).

3.
- Achieve weight maintenance and avoid weight loss or fasting.
- Reduce dietary phytanic acid intake to less than 10 mg a day to allow the minor pathway for degradation of phytanic acid to gradually reduce the plasma and tissue phytanic acid content.
- Reduce intake of adrenergic compounds and stimulants such as caffeine to a moderate intake.
- Avoid or correct nutritional deficiencies.

4. Phytanic acid is a fatty acid commonly found in the diet, derived mainly from the microbial breakdown of phytol component of chlorophyll. Rich sources include ruminant animal products such as beef, lamb, dairy products from these animals which contain fat, fish and fermented vegetable products.

Sources identified in food record: semi-skimmed milk (choose soya/skimmed), cappuccino (coffee with skimmed or soya milk), chocolate chip cookie (biscuit free from butter and chocolate containing milk as a fat source), cheese and ham toasted sandwich (choose ham sandwich or soya cheese and ham sandwich with no butter, use vegetable based spreading fat instead), bolognaise sauce (make with minced pork, chicken or turkey), parmesan (use vegan parmazano), ice-cream (use dairy free ice-cream), cheese and crackers (use soya cheese or soya cheese spread, check crackers do not contain butter or cheese), chocolates (choose dairy free), nuts (may contain phytanic acid, choose popcorn or crisps without cheese), cakes (choose cakes that do not contain butter or milk fat), biscuits (choose biscuits that do not contain butter or milk fat), takeaways (ensure avoid beef, fish, shellfish, lamb and dishes containing ghee or butter).

5. • Improvements in skin and neuropathy.
   • Prevent development of full clinical syndrome.
   • Slow down deterioration in vision and hearing.
6. Alan has a regular meal pattern and has maintained his weight. Fasting or weight loss will result in an increase in serum phytanic acid level and deterioration in his clinical state due to the release of phytanic acid from adipose tissue, the liver and other fat containing tissues.
7. Monitor weight and ensure no weight loss. Some weight gain is tolerable but not necessarily desirable.

   Monitor change in clinical symptoms – vision, neuropathy, gait, hearing, sense of smell, itchy skin. Vision, hearing and smell are not likely to improve, but any further deterioration should be noted and the referring clinician notified. Itchy skin, neuropathy and gait show improvement after a reduction in serum phytanic acid.

   Monitor change in serum phytanic acid concentration.

   Monitor dietary intake to ensure vitamin and mineral status do not deteriorate. Particular nutrients to assess are sodium (may increase if eats more pork products), calcium, iron, fat soluble vitamins, $n-3$ fatty acids.

   Outcome measures:
   - Weight stability
   - Improvement in clinical symptoms as described above
   - Reduction in phytanic acid levels
   - No nutritional deficiencies.

Answers to further questions

8. Phytanic acid (3,7,11,15 tetramethyl hexadecanoic acid) is a branched chain fatty acid that is common in the diet. Like other branch chained fatty acids it is rapidly metabolised by alpha-oxidation and plasma levels are usually less than 10 μmol/L (normal range 0–30 μmol/L). In adult Refsum's disease, there is an enzyme deficiency (phytanoyl CoA hydroxylase) in the alpha oxidation process and therefore cannot metabolise phytanic acid. The alternative metabolic pathway, omega oxidation, has a much lower capacity. This results in raised levels of plasma phytanic acid; this can be 100–6000 μmol/L at presentation.
9. Adult Refsum's disease is a genetically heterogeneous, rare autosomal recessive disorder. Two genes have been identified; PAHX which codes for phytanoyl CoA hydroxylase and peroxin 7 (PEX7), which codes for the peroxisomal target signal (PTS2) receptor (Jansen *et al.*, 2004).

   There are two identified breaks in the alpha oxidation pathway, which affect the activity of phytanoyl coA hydroxylase. Heritability is unlikely as the disease is recessive and Alan's would have to be homozygous to develop symptoms. Genetic counselling is available for affected families. Men and women are at equal risk of developing the disease.

CASE STUDY 18

Adult phenylketonuria

Answers

1. Impaired nutrient utilisation, requiring maintenance of normal low phenylalanine diet related to metabolic disorder characterised by phenylketonuria when low phenylalanine diet is not adhered to.
2. Aim: Anne to continue her low phenylalanine diet while in hospital. Objectives:
   - To provide a 2-day low phenylalanine menu for the hospital chefs for Anne's admission; and
   - To ensure Anne has the right low protein products to provide her low protein diet.
3. - Discuss her usual diet at home prior to admission, what she likes and dislikes, what low protein foods she may require, will she bring her own XP Maxamum and low protein food into hospital or do you need to order it in?
   - Devise a 2-day menu plan to give to the diet kitchen. Discuss with diet chef what a low phenylalanine diet is and the menu plan.
   - Once Anne is admitted, speak to ward and explain what PKU is and what a low phenylalanine diet is to ensure she receives the correct foods and that she takes XP Maxamum in the correct doses. May need to get XP Maxamum prescribed.
4. PKU is an inherited genetic condition where the body cannot break down phenylalanine into tyrosine because of loss of activity of the enzyme phenylalanine hydroxylase (Blau *et al.*, 2010). Untreated high levels in the blood can cause brain damage in babies and young children (Blau *et al.*, 2010). It is recommended that the diet be followed for life in adults (Trefz *et al.*, 2011; Medical Research Council, 1993).

   High phenylalanine concentrations in adults can affect executive functioning, concentration and organisation skills (Gentile *et al.*, 2010; Christ *et al.*, 2010), tiredness, headaches, mood swings (ten Hoedt *et al.*, 2011; Anjema *et al.*, 2011) and increased chance of depression and anxiety (Trefz *et al.*, 2011).

   Phenylalanine is an amino acid, therefore high protein foods are not allowed. Natural protein is giving in measured exchanges from medium protein foods and protein is giving in the form of protein substitutes that contain all the amino acids except phenylalanine (Blau *et al.*, 2010).

Dietetic and Nutrition Case Studies, First Edition.
Edited by Judy Lawrence, Pauline Douglas, and Joan Gandy.

Companion Website: http://www.manualofdieteticpractice.com/

5. • Breakfast: LP bread or toast, margarine, jam, marmalade/LP cereal and LP milk.
   • Lunch/dinner: LP pasta or rice with vegetable sauce/LP bread, toast, crackers/vegetables/salad.
   • Exchanges: cereal, peas, sweetcorn, potato, cereal bars, crisps, soup, baked beans, rice.
6. Include a brief sentence to summarise initial phone calls and further sentence to summarise feedback to referring dietitian. All details of care should be in one place. Sign and date each entry.
7. • Talk to patient and ward staff to ensure Anne is receiving her low phenylalanine diet.
   • Prescription chart to check XP Maxamum has been prescribed and taken.
   • Patients usually monitor phenylalanine by blood spots at home. Obtaining a phenylalanine reading in hospital would not be accurate/appropriate.
8. • Has Anne received a low phenylalanine diet while in hospital? Check with ward staff.
   • Has the kitchen provided meals as suggested? Ask Anne what food she has been provided with.
9. Call Anne before admission to introduce yourself and discuss her diet for hospital.
10. Speak to Anne and her metabolic dietitian to ascertain if Anne was happy with the service provided and whether or not she received the foods she asked for.

Answers to further questions

11. • PKU Lophlex LQ 20 (Nutricia), PKU Cooler 20 (Vitaflo International), PKU Lophlex Sensation (Nutricia), PKU Lophlex Powder (Nutricia), PKU Express 20 (Vitaflo International). All 20 g protein equivalent.
    • Cooler, Lophlex LQ and Lophlex Sensation are ready to drink/eat and therefore aid compliance. Easy to transport and take out of the home. If drunk straight from packet can't see colour or smell it. Lophlex Powder and Express are in pre measured sachets, just add required water.
    • All contain vitamins and minerals, aids compliance of vitamins and minerals.
    • Coolers contain omega 3 fatty acids, which are restricted in a low phenylalanine diet.
    • Powders and liquids come in a variety of flavours to aid compliance.
    • Phlexy-10 tablets (Nutricia) – tablets instead of a drink, but have to take around 75/day plus extra vitamins and minerals.
12. • Monitor phenylalanine concentrations at least monthly.
    • Use blood spot cards at home.
    • Phenylalanine between 120 and 480 μmol/L, values up to 700 can be accepted as dietary compliance becomes more difficult (NSPKU, 2004).
13. Maternal PKU syndrome – foetuses that are exposed to high levels of phenylalanine in the womb are at risk of learning difficulties, congenital heart disease, microcephaly and small birth weight. Pregnancy must be planned and phenylalanine levels kept between 120 and 250 μmol/L to reduce these risks. This involves following a very strict low-phenylalanine diet (Maillot *et al.*, 2007).

14. - Advised that diet for life is current recommendations, although it is the choice of the patient to follow the diet or not (MRC, 1993; Trefz *et al.*, 2011).
    - To discuss evidence for diet for life and the symptoms of high phenylalanine concentrations (Trefz *et al.*, 2011).
    - The patient may want to try a low phenylalanine diet again with your help to see if reduces symptoms.
    - If patient does not wish to follow diet, full diet history is needed to check if their diet is nutritionally complete as they often self-restrict protein in their diets. This may lead to a diet lacking in protein, iron, B_{12} and other vitamins and minerals (Das *et al.*, 2013). Extra vitamin and minerals and protein may be advised to complete diet.
    - Patients off diet still need to attend clinic annually to be monitored and nutritional bloods checked (NSPKU, 2004).
15. Post-operative levels of phenylalanine may be elevated. However this is usually transient and therefore does not require intervention.

CASE STUDY 19
Osteoporosis

Answers

1. Inadequate energy intake (problem) related to reduced appetite and pain (aetiology) characterised by 6.5 kg weight loss over a period of 4 months (signs and symptoms).
2. Mary's weight loss and her low BMI would be the first concern. She has lost 6.5 kg in 4 months, which is 13.7% of her initial body weight. Anything >10% in the last 6 months is considered severe (Blackburn *et al.*, 1977). She is not meeting her energy needs, there is a deficit of >500 kcal.

   Mary's protein intake is low. Evidence suggests that protein intake greater than the RDI can improve muscle mass, strength and function in the elderly and that it may improve bone health (Dawson-Hughes, 2003). Many studies have been carried out on the relationship between protein and various parameters of bone health including fractures, BMD and bone strength. Results are conflicting, with some studies suggesting a beneficial effect of protein on bone (Delmi *et al.*, 1990; Rizzoli *et al.*, 2001), and others showing a positive correlation between protein intake and bone loss (Huang *et al.*, 1996; Johnell *et al.*, 1995; Munger *et al.*, 1999). In some cases it appears that an intake of 1.5 g protein per kg body weight per day may be required in elderly individuals to be beneficial for health and function (Wolfe *et al.*, 2008).

   Mary is not compliant with her calcium and vitamin D supplements and her dietary intake of calcium is low. Mary's serum 25 (OH)D is very low at 23 nmol/L.

   Mary's fat intake is very high (48% total energy intake) and saturated fat intake is 25% of total energy intake. This needs to be taken into consideration because of her hypercholesterolaemia.
3. Mary's BMI is 16.9 kg/m^2 when using knee heel height, which would put Mary in the underweight category. When using stadiometer height, her BMI is significantly higher at 18.2 kg/m^2. As a result of the loss of height associated with osteoporosis particularly with vertebral fractures, stadiometer height may not be the most accurate method of measuring height. Patients recalled height must also be taken into consideration, or other methods such as knee to heel height, demispan, or ulna length. The current literature does not allow a BMI cut-off value for

Dietetic and Nutrition Case Studies, First Edition.
Edited by Judy Lawrence, Pauline Douglas, and Joan Gandy.

Companion Website: http://www.manualofdieteticpractice.com/

osteoporosis risk, but generally a BMI < 22–24 kg/m^2 is associated with less bone density throughout the body compared with a BMI > 26–28 kg/m^2. However, an increased body weight has no advantage to skeletal health when this increase becomes excessive (BMI > 30 kg/m^2) as this can lead to immobility, osteoarthritis and an increased risk of fall (Wardlaw, 1996).

4. Increase Mary's energy and protein intake to promote weight gain by increasing portions of carbohydrate at lunch and dinner; introduce snacks between meals; increase portion size of lean protein and choose healthy fats by increasing intake of nuts, seeds, olive oil, rapeseed oil, avocados, olives.

   Increase calcium intake by increasing low-fat dairy products (yoghurt, low fat cheese, glass of milk, milky drinks, rice pudding, frozen yoghurt, grated cheese on potato or vegetables). Encourage Mary to take calcium and vitamin D supplements as prescribed and encourage food sources of vitamin D, for example, oily fish, fortified milk and cereals.

   Reduce saturated fat and salt content and encourage Mary to eat unprocessed food with high fibre and vitamin and mineral content.
5. Outcome measures would include weight, serum 25 (OH)D and urinary calcium.
6. It is important to document all aspects of Mary's care. The records should include details of what has been assessed and details of what has been done and why. If informed consent was required for any aspect of care this should be obtained and documented.
7. Mary's fat mass and fat free mass are both below the 10th percentile for healthy women of her age (Kyle *et al.*, 2001) indicating that loss of muscle mass is possibly a result of protein energy malnutrition (PEM). Loss of muscle mass and therefore power will put her at risk of falls and possible fractures. The probability of PEM is confirmed by the results of the handgrip strength test. Mary's result of 13.3 kg is significantly below 23 kg which is 85% of normal, which is indicative of PEM.
8. The DXA scan shows significantly diminished total bone mineral density (BMD) and diminished BMD in the spine and femur. This is diagnostic of osteoporosis; Mary is therefore at risk of fractures associated with osteoporosis.
9. Besides protein, energy, calcium and vitamin D, phosphorus, magnesium, zinc and vitamins K and C are also important in osteoporosis.
10. The other AHPs that should be involved are:
    - A physiotherapist – weight bearing exercise can help maintain bone tissue in adults and improve posture, balance and muscle power, which help prevent falls.
    - An occupational therapist will be able to advise Mary on adaptations to her home that can reduce the risk of falls and aid her in her everyday activities.
11. The metabolic stress, and therefore increase in requirements, of such surgery is often underestimated. A stress factor of 20% should be added to BMR to account for the increase in energy requirements. A high protein, high energy diet, provided in small, frequent portions, should be prescribed.

CASE STUDY 20

Eating disorder associated with obesity

Answers

1. Height, weight and body mass index, as weight reduction is likely to be part of the intervention. As Maggie is sensitive about her body, measuring her waist may be unacceptably intrusive and distressing for her at this early stage. She may be taught to do it herself as a way of monitoring progress at a later stage.
2. Maggie has some elements of metabolic syndrome, so others should be investigated; namely, full lipid screen and random blood glucose.
3. The dietitian should also investigate other health problems, especially those that may be associated with obesity, for example joint or back pain, as improvements may help with maintaining motivation. Any current medication should be noted.
4. When Maggie's weight became a problem: age at first diet; history of dieting and weight cycling; links with life events such as pregnancies; how this relates to the development of disordered eating. Maggie may be able to remember her weight at particular points in her life, and her highest and lowest weight ever. This will help determine the progress of the disorder, and the maintaining factors that need to be addressed in treatment.

   Detailed history of weight and eating. It is helpful to take a history at least from the beginning of eating disorder symptoms, and sometimes from infancy, to consider early feeding difficulties. The history should seek to identify periods of low or high weight, and the degree of abnormality, weight cycling and instability, and any times when weight has been normal and stable. This can help to develop a shared understanding of the way eating, body weight, psychological factors and life events relate to each other.

   The following information about eating and drinking should be elicited:
   - Meal pattern, timing and frequency of eating, and variability of meal pattern.
   - Binge eating, grazing or other uncontrolled overeating; foods used for binge eating.
   - Emotional responses to food and eating, such as anxiety or disgust.
   - The social context of eating.
   - Fluid and alcohol intake.

Dietetic and Nutrition Case Studies, First Edition.
Edited by Judy Lawrence, Pauline Douglas, and Joan Gandy.

Companion Website: http://www.manualofdieteticpractice.com/

5. Maggie's responsibilities related to family eating; her own family and social eating; work, and how she manages eating at work. Pressures on Maggie's time, demands of family and work, and how these impact on her eating. Who knows about Maggie's eating problems and who might be supportive to her efforts with change. Where the barriers to change may lie.
6. Maggie's high BMI and history of weight cycling should be enough to prompt further investigation of the possibility of disordered eating. The context of a life with many responsibilities, and some distress during the assessment meeting that may indicate some stress, might be further indications.
7. There are brief screening tools for eating disorders that were developed to use in primary care (Cotton *et al.*, 2003; Morgan *et al.*, 1999). Although the complete screen would not be appropriate, the questions relating to uncontrolled eating could provide an opening to a discussion with Maggie about loss of control of eating.
8. • Uncontrolled eating and binge eating.
   • Obesity resulting from overall excessive energy intake.
   • Hypertension, which may be related to body weight and sodium intake.
   • Dyslipidaemia, which may be related to obesity and specific food choices.
9. Uncontrolled eating and binge eating.
10. Disordered eating pattern (problem) related to excessive hunger associated with strict dieting (aetiology) characterised by recurrent episodes of uncontrolled eating and binge eating (signs/symptoms).
11. Maggie has shown some sensitivity and distress. To help her to feel safe to discuss it she needs to feel she can trust the dietitian. Techniques of person-centred counselling can be helpful in this situation; in particular a warm, empathic, non-judgmental and collaborative presentation (Miller & Rollnick, 2007; Gable, 2007).
12. Techniques of motivational interviewing can elicit the information needed and foster trust, in particular the fundamentals of open questions, affirmations, reflections and summary (OARS).
13. Excessive hunger, possibly arising from strict dieting, is one driver of binge eating, so it may be useful to consider a period to stabilise eating and restore control before attempting weight reduction. An eating diary is a very useful tool to discover the context and drivers of binge eating, and consider strategies to establish better control of eating. Weight reduction may need to be at a modest rate, perhaps 1–2 kg/month, to prevent excessive hunger.
14. • Reduction in or abolition of binge eating.
    • Reduction in distress related to eating.
    • Reduction in body weight.
    • Improvement in blood lipids.
    • Reduction in blood pressure.
15. Maggie can be helped to agree SMART goals that will move her towards her aims. Before dietary management of any condition can be effective and sustained, Maggie needs to be able to control her eating. To help Maggie establish more control of her eating she needs to plan regular meals with a healthy mixture of foods in

amounts that will meet her present needs. This should stabilise her weight and reduce hunger as a binge driver. She should use a food diary to self-monitor her progress, and identify trigger events and barriers to change so that they can be managed effectively.

Over the longer term she can be given information about appropriate food choices to help reduce energy intake at a sustainable rate; to adjust fat intake to improve lipid profile; and to reduce sodium intake to help reduce blood pressure. She may also need to learn healthy ways to manage stress, so that she relies less on food as a comfort.

Answers to further questions

16. Supporting 'change talk' by eliciting positive discussion of Maggie's successes in all areas of her life, giving examples of people in similar situations who have done well, creating realistic expectations and offering a different approach for her try can begin to suggest to Maggie that she may be successful (Miller & Rollnick, 2007).

17. Maggie needs to learn about healthy eating to manage her weight and metabolic syndrome, and practise integrating it into her life. She can be encouraged to monitor her weight and have regular checks of blood pressure and lipids. She will need support to develop skills to achieve the changes she needs to make, and to identify and solve problems that may arise. For example, if she finds an eating diary useful, she can return to using it if she is aware that her weight is increasing.

18. Brief interventions from psychology workers are widely available in primary care through the Increasing Access to Psychological Therapies (IAPT) (2014) programme.

The dietetic assessment should seek indications of issues that the IAPT psychologist could helpfully address, such as mild to moderate depression or anxiety, or low self-esteem. This may be revealed from a history of previous episodes of depression or anxiety, or a current diagnosis of a mood disorder, or symptoms such as feeling unhappy, lack of enjoyment in usual sources of pleasure, poor concentration, or difficulties with sleep.

Reducing reliance on binge eating as a way of dealing with the stress of low mood may reveal these underlying psychological drivers, and if they are not addressed the binge eating may relapse as her habitual response, and the only one available to her. This may emerge during the dietitian's treatment programme, and it is therefore essential for her to get help to improve her mood, and develop healthy ways to manage stress, so that she can safely progress with her recovery from binge eating. Collaboration with the psychologist also provides a source of support with issues that may arise during the dietetic intervention, as barriers to change or sources of distress, for example bereavement or low self-esteem.

The dietitian may therefore need to refer to the IAPT service immediately after assessment, or a little later during the recovery journey. Awareness of waiting times for the IAPT service may also help the dietitian to decide on when to refer.

Close collaboration with the psychologist will help to provide the optimal support for Maggie.

19. The psychologist should be kept informed of progress at each dietetic review as assessed by the following:

- Goals successfully met;
- Difficulties that present barriers to progress;
- Factors that support change; and
- Goals Maggie has agreed to continue to work on.

You should ask Maggie for her permission to share this information with the psychologist. The assessment and progress reports made by the psychologist will help the dietitian to negotiate SMART goals, and find the right pace of change for Maggie.

CASE STUDY 21

Forensic mental health

Answers

1. BMI = 40 kg/m^2
   He is at high risk of developing several co-morbidities (Foresight, 2007) including:
   - Hypertension;
   - Type 2 diabetes mellitus – there will be significant insulin resistance at this degree of obesity making it harder to control. Poorly controlled diabetes will result in diabetic complications, such as peripheral neuropathy, retinopathy;
   - Cardiovascular disease;
   - Some cancers, for example, breast;
   - Liver disease;
   - Gastrointestinal diseases, for example, gall stones; and
   - Psychological and social problems, for example, low self-esteem.
2. Obesity class III (problem) caused by a combination of over-consumption of high-calorie foods, reduced opportunity for exercise and medication (aetiology) characterised by a BMI of 40 kg/m^2 (signs/symptoms).
3. The responsibility of assessing the stage of change could lie with the referring professional; that is, to determine if the patient wants a consultation with the dietitian prior to referring. However, given the health concerns of obesity-related co-morbidity of this patient, the referrer was correct in alerting the dietitian. This allowed the dietitian to introduce the dietetic service, establish a professional rapport, give evidenced-based health improvement information and ultimately left the 'door open' for further intervention. The integrity of the therapeutic relationship was still intact when the duty of care was closed. This will facilitate the ongoing relationship once the patient re-engages.
4. Barriers to change:
   - Mental ill health – mentally unable to make the decision to prioritise his health;
   - Medication – increases his appetite, causes lethargy;
   - Motivation – lacks motivation to change as in his perception his current large size provides security against threats from other patients; and
   - Environment – peer pressure, easy access to unhealthy foods, lack of exercise.

Dietetic and Nutrition Case Studies, First Edition.
Edited by Judy Lawrence, Pauline Douglas, and Joan Gandy.

Companion Website: http://www.manualofdieteticpractice.com/

5. The dietitian was correct to discharge the duty of care. The BDA statement of conduct states, '*Service users have a right to refuse intervention, and should be offered the opportunity to refuse it. Any such refusal should be respected and recorded in writing*'. (BDA, 2008)
6. Yes, a dietitian must respect the wishes of a patient. If the patient does not wish to engage with dietary change then it is ethical for a dietitian to discharge the patient.
7. Documentation should state the reason for discharge and be dated and signed.
8. The objectives of the intervention were to:
   - stabilise weight and halt weight gain;
   - educate on the importance of a balanced diet for wellbeing;
   - provide information on the function of the food groups;
   - inform on the health consequences of over eating;
   - provide information on portion sizes; and
   - stress the importance of reducing sedentary behaviour and increase activity.
9. A good outcome would be that the patient:
   - engaged with services;
   - agreed to the care plan to optimise nutritional wellbeing;
   - understood the need to change diet behaviour;
   - understood how to change his diet intake and lifestyle behaviour and was confident in doing so; and
   - followed the care plan.
10. - Knowledge gained;
    - Food/nutrient intake change;
    - Positive change in attitude and behaviour relating to diet and lifestyle;
    - Biochemistry, that is, reduced cholesterol, reduced blood glucose;
    - Reduced weight;
    - Reduced blood pressure;
    - Patient related outcomes such as better quality of life, better sleep and less abdominal pain from reduced constipation episodes; and
    - Medication change, for example, less laxative use.
11. The MDT would include the following:
    - The speech and language therapist to assess communication skills to ensure that the information is accessible to the patient, that is, the patient understands the terminology/vocabulary used when discussing eating behaviour and body weight; and to assist the dietitian with resources and the best methods of communication that the patient will understand;
    - The psychologist to work with the patient on motivation skills and cognitive behavioural therapy;
    - The patient's named nurses, who are with the patient 24 h and would be best placed to offer continual support and encouragement;
    - The occupational therapist who would reinforce the health messages while working with the patient on his ADL (Activities of daily living, such as cooking, shopping);

- The hotel services, who supply the ward menu, need to be involved if there were any special requirements such as extra fruit, vegetables, diet yoghurts and so on made available for the patient;
- Exercise counsellors to encourage activity; and
- Smoking cessation nurse to provide brief interventions to help the patient consider the benefits of stopping smoking.

Answers to further questions

13. The Mifflin–St Jeor equation is often used when working with this client group as it gives lighter energy requirements. It is often preferable when working with this group of patients.

14. In line with the SIGN 131 guidance on schizophrenia, which states '*Metformin should be considered for service users who are experiencing weight gain on antipsychotic medications*'.

15. Clozapine, increases the patient's appetite and disturbs glucose and lipid metabolism (Philpot, 2014).

CASE STUDY 22

Food allergy

Answers

1. Incomplete knowledge (problem) of dietary regimen related to the inability to identify situations that would cause exposure to allergens (aetiology) characterised by itchy mouth and symptoms associated with allergic reaction when eating (signs/symptoms).
2. Food allergy affects 8% of children, but milk and egg allergy, the two most common food allergies in children, are most likely to remit by adult life, which might explain why only 3.7% of adults are likely to have a food allergy. Not all food allergies remit so readily; over 90% of tree nut allergic children and 80% of peanut allergic children will remain sensitised and symptomatic into adulthood. There is no reliable data on the remission rates of seafood allergy.
3. Eggs are one of the most frequent causes of food allergy in children worldwide, but it commonly remits in childhood, although many remain unable to tolerate raw egg. Egg allergy in adults is therefore rare, and it is likely, given the negative skin prick and specific IgE test results, that Michael no longer has an egg allergy, or might be able to tolerate cooked egg. In addition, Michael is eating sponge cake, Christmas cake and desserts, all of which may contain cooked egg. Christmas cake might also contain raw egg in the form of Royal icing.
4. A food allergy generally manifests in symptoms usually within 30 min of eating. Symptoms can include itching, redness, flushing, swelling, urticaria or other rash, dysphonia as a result of swelling of the larynx, gastrointestinal disturbance, difficulty swallowing, breathing difficulties and hypotension. The reaction to the peanuts, apple and peach are typical allergic reactions, so too was the reaction to the scampi. The other two reactions or isolated nausea (rice pudding) and chest pain two hours after eating (fried chicken) and not typical of a food allergic reaction.
5. Egg, milk, rice, chicken, wheat, celery or spices (in the breadcrumbed chicken) and scampi. He is eating milk, chicken, wheat and rice regularly; hence, there is no need to test for these. If he was allergic to celery or a spice, he would have had considerably more reactions. There are no other allergens that needed to be tested.

Dietetic and Nutrition Case Studies, First Edition.
Edited by Judy Lawrence, Pauline Douglas, and Joan Gandy.

Companion Website: http://www.manualofdieteticpractice.com/

6. Peanut and tree nut allergies most commonly present in childhood; only 8–10% of cases are diagnosed in adolescence or adulthood. Michael's positive test to raw peanuts but not to roasted peanuts shows clearly that his reaction was most likely because of pollen-food syndrome (PFS) and not a nut allergy. The borderline positive blood test is a reflection of this, although less clear cut. Peanuts are often involved in PFS, but not as frequently as tree nuts, especially hazelnut and almond. The fact that he only had oral symptoms, which quickly resolved is also an indication that this is PFS.
7. If Michael has PFS, there is no need to stop eating other nuts that are not provoking symptoms. He can also tolerate chocolate bars, which often contain nuts, and is tolerating almonds in marzipan, so he is not at risk of a reaction when eating products that state they may contain nuts. Usually, it is consumption of the raw nut on its own that triggers a reaction, roasting it or coating it in chocolate usually renders it safe to eat.
8. The fresh apple will contain the PR10 allergens responsible for reactions in PFS. When the apple is cooked, these allergens are altered and so are not recognised by the birch pollen antibodies. The fact that Michael can eat apple pie is due to this phenomenon. The reagents used in the blood test are heat treated and therefore unlikely to contain these labile allergens, unlike the raw apple that will contain them in abundance, especially in the skin.
9. There is no need for Michael to avoid any fruit or vegetable unless it is provoking symptoms.
10. Avoidance of a single food or type of food (such as citrus fruit) will be of little significance if nutritionally similar foods (e.g. other fruit and vegetables) can be eaten instead. Michael's diet is varied and his negative egg challenge means he can add to the foods he can eat. The most common nutrient at risk is likely to be vitamin C, but his consumption of potatoes and other fruits and vegetables will mitigate for his lower intake. Many people with allergies have low vitamin D levels, so it might be helpful to check his levels to make sure they are optimum.

Answers to further questions

11. The gold standard test for diagnosis is an oral food challenge. In adults, this would be undertaken by the consumption first of sponge cake if not already eaten. Then moving on to well-cooked egg in the form of a hard boiled egg, giving the yolk first and then the white. Finally, loosely cooked egg in the form of scrambled egg is given. Prior to the challenge, skin prick tests to raw egg white can be undertaken to determine the likelihood of reaction to loosely cooked egg. New molecular allergy test can also be undertaken if available to Gal d 1 and Gal d 2. Gal d 1 is not destroyed on heating and is the allergen most associated with egg allergy that has not remitted. Gal d 2 is destroyed on heating and therefore people sensitised to Gal d 2 can usually tolerate baked egg. In Michael's case, the skin prick test to raw egg white was 5 mm but that for Gal d 1 and 2 were negative. He passed both the cooked and loosely cooked egg challenge.

12. Shellfish have a pan allergen called tropomyosin, which is a common allergenic component of shrimps, prawns, lobster, crab, mussels, oysters and even house dust mite. Therefore, it is a good test for scampi, although the low level of positivity makes an allergy less likely but does not rule it out. Even if Michael does not like shellfish and is not likely to eat them again, it is important to know whether he has an allergy to shellfish. The reason for this is because shellfish are not thermo-labile and remain potent allergens even after cooking. Thus, Michael is at risk from reactions due to contamination. Given that his reactions to the scampi were very severe, cross-contamination could be a major issue. A food challenge is not advisable given the dislike for shellfish and the nature of his reaction to scampi, but skin prick testing to different types of prawns, including scampi, might yield further useful information. This is because not everyone who is allergic to shellfish are allergic to tropomyosin, but may be allergic occasionally to other allergens in different species. Given his history and low levels of positivity to shrimp, Michael was skin prick test positive to several fresh prawns including a very large positive test to scampi (30 mm). This test confirmed that the reaction to scampi was most likely due to an allergy to scampi and he was advised to rigorously avoid all shellfish.
13. Generally, they are at a low risk unless there are many different fruits and vegetables involved, but even then, they can usually tolerate cooked fruits and vegetables. Some berries such as blackcurrants and cranberries rarely cause this problem and so are useful to suggest as alternatives. In addition, pasteurised fruit juices are also usually fine. Fruit smoothies need to be avoided as they can contain large quantities of allergen that can provoke more severe reactions.
14. This responsibility usually lies with the first person to review the patient during an encounter or with any health professional who subsequently diagnoses or confirms an allergy, hypersensitivities, intolerance or adverse drug reactions. Check with the local policy.

CASE STUDY 23
HIV/AIDS

Answers

1. The patients will be coming to terms with their HIV diagnosis, and the implications this brings. They may be upset or shocked, and be worried about disclosure, given the fear about HIV stigma. They may have questions about their future, and it is important to allow newly diagnosed patients the opportunity to ask any questions about their health. The dietitian should know who the patient can be referred to locally for emotional support.
2. All patients should be afforded the same degree of confidentiality with regard to record keeping, but the dietitian should reassure the patient about confidentiality, be mindful that the patient may not wish to take home written materials regarding HIV.
3. Andy's BMI is 29 k/m^2, and it would appear that he is currently gaining weight from his usual, stable body mass. His waist and waist-to-hip ratio both indicate increased risk for cardiovascular disease. It is recommended within the British HIV Association guidelines (Asboe *et al.*, 2012) to perform a full set of anthropometry measurements annually in order to assess for onset of lipodystrophy (antiretroviral-associated body shape changes). It is good dietetic practice to perform a subjective global assessment.
4. The CD4 and HIV viral load are indicative of late presentation with HIV: it is likely that Andy has been unknowingly living with HIV for some time. At this level of immunosuppression, assessment should be made for the presence of oral or gastrointestinal opportunistic infections, and increased likelihood of loss of lean body mass. A CD4 count below 200 is indicative of a higher risk for water and food borne infection.
5. Electrolytes and renal function appear normal. A slightly low haemoglobin level is relatively common in advanced HIV infection, although this could also reflect anaemia. Liver function is normal apart from a raised GGT, which may be associated with stress from chronic alcohol consumption. Lipids and glucose are all elevated, although the phlebotomy was not fasting. The vitamin D level is suboptimal.

Dietetic and Nutrition Case Studies, First Edition.
Edited by Judy Lawrence, Pauline Douglas, and Joan Gandy.

Companion Website: http://www.manualofdieteticpractice.com/

6. Andy reports feeling tired all the time. This is a fairly non-specific symptom that requires further investigation if it persists. His blood pressure is raised, and this measurement should be repeated.
7. The lethargy may be because of a wide variety of causes. An HIV-specific aetiology includes general immunosuppression, HIV-related anaemia, malabsorption, and low testosterone levels (hypogonadism). General causes of tiredness include depression, anaemia and thyroid disorders.
8. To maintain correct blood levels and prevent HIV viral resistance, antiretrovirals should be taken at the same time every day, and certain medicines must be taken with food. Food–drug interactions can be checked online (University of Liverpool, 2015). Darunavir must be taken with food for adequate absorption; however, the other antiretrovirals in Andy's regimen can be taken with or without food. The four medicines are all taken together once daily, and so should be taken with a meal. Andy works shifts, and the potential for a negative impact of this on meal patterns and adherence to his medications should be fully explored.
9. Andy eats regularly. However, his diet is lacking in wholegrains, fruits and vegetables. He consumes a large amount of sugar.
10. His alcohol consumption is excessive, and his use of recreational drugs is frequent. Together, these will be having a major impact on his health and wellbeing, and a potentially negative impact on adherence to antiretrovirals. In terms of diet, his use of drugs and alcohol during the weekend results in irregular nutritional intake. This may have a negative impact on adequate food that needs to be eaten for absorption of Darunavir.
11. Imbalanced dietary intake of carbohydrates (problem) related to lifestyle factors (aetiology), characterised by weight gain, raised triglycerides and glucose levels (signs/symptoms).
12. Food safety should be discussed given his low CD4 count. Healthy heart advice combined with a modest energy restriction would be appropriate at this stage given the raised BMI, lipids and glucose. Dietary sources of vitamin D should be advised, together with advice on safe sun exposure.
13. A fasting phlebotomy should be recommended, with glucose and a full lipid panel measured. Further tests for anaemia may be warranted. Referral for support for alcohol and drugs advice should be discussed with Andy, as should the referral for exercise advice.
14. If blood pressure remains raised, salt reduction should be discussed. If adequate food intake combined with Darunavir proves problematic, this should be discussed with the MDT. Ten year disease risk calculators could be considered, including those for cardiovascular disease, diabetes and osteoporosis.
15. In addition to usual dietary outcome measures, you may wish to monitor BMI and waist in particular with the aim to reduce both towards the normal range. Adherence to his antiretroviral therapy is key, as well as quality of life. Patient-reported outcome measures may be useful to help engage the patient with setting their own goals.

Answers to further questions

16. Antiretroviral must be taken correctly 95% of the time to prevent viral resistance developing. Assessing timing and compliance with food–drug interactions is a key component of care given by dietitians. Extended diet histories, with care taken to record timings and patterns, may help the wider MDT monitor to address any potential difficulties with respect to adherence.

17. You may wish to consider adding stress factors for opportunistic infections, and for HIV itself in those patients who are immunocompromised and acutely unwell. However, activity levels are likely to be reduced in those who are unwell, and there is a lack of evidence for raised energy expenditure in those stable on antiretroviral therapy with an undetectable HIV viral load.

18. In addition to height and weight, a wide range of circumferences and skinfolds are used, in order to monitor lipodystrophy (fat re-distribution syndrome). DEXA scans can be used either for body composition analysis, or bone mineral density.

19. Newly diagnosed patients should be assessed by a dietitian for the following:

- The need for food safety advice.
- Dietary adequacy and the potential need for micronutrient supplementation.
- Anthropometry and advice to achieve a normal BMI.

Those commencing antiretroviral therapy should be assessed for the following:

- Ability to adhere to drug regimens.
- Anthropometry baseline for monitoring for lipodystrophy.
- Achievement or maintenance of a normal BMI.

20. You should consider those patients experiencing side effects of HIV or antiretroviral therapy, and those at risk of or experiencing metabolic change. In pregnancy, HIV positive mothers should be supported with respect to infant feeding choices.

CASE STUDY 24

Type 1 diabetes mellitus

Answers

1. Degree and frequency of hypoglycaemia (hypos), hypo awareness, symptoms of hyperglycaemia, presence of diabetes complications and so on.
2. Approximately 5% weight loss; BMI 22.4 kg/m^2 5/12 ago and currently 21.3 kg/m^2.
3. Unintentional weight loss is a possible symptom of hyperglycaemia – Harry may be unaware of the significance of this.
4. It is likely that young adults, particularly males, who lose weight unintentionally, will be unhappy with this weight loss. Anecdotal experience suggests they frequently report a desire to gain weight, particular lean muscle mass. Male patients are likely to be motivated by the prospect of improvements in their strength and fitness levels, as well as aesthetic changes. Helping the patient to understand the relationship between blood glucose control, insulin, weight and body composition may improve motivation to improve blood glucose control. This is because a very high HbA1c suggests insufficient insulin, which in turn will inhibit the ability to build muscle or to maintain body weight.
5. Lypohypertrophy is a common problem that occurs from repeated use of the same injection site, also known as 'Lypos'. It is the accumulation of fat and possibly some scar tissue under the skin in response to tissue damage, which then resembles a lump. Lumps can vary in size. Injection into these lumps may affect the absorption of the insulin, resulting in a time action profile of the insulin that does not match that expected, thereby leading to unpredictable effects on blood glucose. Lypohypertrophy can be avoided by regularly rotating the injection site. Once the area affected is no longer used for injection, the lumps will resolve although this can take many months.
6. 19–26 Carbohydrate portions (10 g), depending on whether Harry has the crisps, chocolate bar and the snack before bed.
7. Harry's diet does not meet current health eating guidelines as it is high in fat and sugar and low in vegetables and fruit. Whilst advice to improve the quality of his diet is important, the effectiveness of this advice alone in controlling blood glucose in type 1 diabetes, that is, without concomitant advice on matching insulin

Dietetic and Nutrition Case Studies, First Edition.
Edited by Judy Lawrence, Pauline Douglas, and Joan Gandy.

Companion Website: http://www.manualofdieteticpractice.com/

doses, is limited. The knowledge and skills required to implement carbohydrate estimation and insulin dose adjustment should be prioritised at this stage. Dietary quality can be addressed at a later stage, depending on the patient's own priorities.

8. Harry's insulin regimen means that snacking should be a choice, rather than a necessity. Snacks may be needed to manage exercise, or occasionally to correct blood glucose before bed; however, if occurring regularly that may indicate the need to adjust the insulin dose.
9. Patients stop engaging with services for a wide range of reasons. Perhaps, Jack has found it too challenging to undertake the self-monitoring activities that were discussed in the clinic. Alternatively, he may find his social life has had an impact on his diabetes and his interest in engaging with all the necessary self-care activities. Jack may have changed jobs and may be unable to attend clinic appointments. Patients often have pre-conceived ideas about what health professionals will 'demand' of them and perceive too many barriers to an effective therapeutic relationship. The solutions to these problems are as varied as the issues themselves; however, at the root of all effective relationships with patients is counselling and communication skills. Advanced listening skills, a thorough and effective assessment that explores the patient's wishes, fears and understanding of the situation are all vital. In this case, encouraging Jack to attend a structured education programme could have a huge impact through the contact he would have with other people with type 1 diabetes. Besides the education element of the course, the emotional support and vicarious learning that takes place in the scenarios are hugely valuable in motivating patients. A telephone call rather than a standard letter may have more impact and can help Jack to feel supported to connect with the service. Finally, ensuring that the services are flexible and accessible may help avoid some patients from disengaging. Are there clinics at the right times, in the right locations? Are we able to offer support by email, telephone or text message?
10. A structured education programme aims to improve a patient's knowledge, skills and confidence so that they can increasingly take care of their own condition. It should cover all aspects of diabetes such as diet, carbohydrate counting, insulin doses and foot care. NICE recommends that all newly diagnosed diabetics should be offered such a programme. Dose Adjustment for Normal Eating (DAFNE) is an example of a programme for type 1 diabetes. Evidence suggests an improvement in HbA1c of approximately 1% and significant improvements in quality of life is achievable following attendance (DAFNE Study Group, 2002). An example of a programme for type 2 diabetes is the Diabetes Education and Self-management for Ongoing and Newly Diagnosed (DESMOND).
11. Healthy lifestyle programme declined (problem) related to poor transfer from child services (aetiology) evidenced by repeated cancellation of appointments (signs and symptoms).
12. Outcome measures could include weight and BMI changes, HbA1C and patient engagement with services as monitored by attendance records.

Answers to further questions

13. Transition care should be planned, structured and age-appropriate. Summary of NICE Recommendations for transition:
    - Regular attendance at clinic (3–4 × year);
    - Time to familiarise with practicalities of transition;
    - Agree local protocols;
    - Timing depends on individual's physical development, emotional maturity and local circumstances;
    - Transfer at time of relative stability;
    - Organise age-banded clinics jointly with adult colleagues; and
    - Inform young people of changes in diabetes care – BG targets and screening for complications.

    There is an increased risk of diabetes-related hospitalisation during the transition period. Those transferred to a new health care team with no change in physician were 77% less likely to be hospitalised. Young people who have less than 1 appointment per year after transition have higher HbA1c values, increased hospitalisation and higher rates of diabetic complications.
14. The time action profile of insulin detemir suggests its duration is up to 18 h. The purpose of a background insulin is to provide a basal supply of insulin across 24 h. Audit data from the DAFNE programme suggests that people with type 1 diabetes who inject background insulin twice a day will achieve a better HbA1c.
15. Yes, a dated and signed record of all contacts with Harry should be kept.

CASE STUDY 25

Type 2 diabetes mellitus – Kosher diet

Answers

1. Rebekah's BMI = 37 kg/m^2.
2. Ideal waist circumference (WC) for Caucasian women is <80 cm (International Diabetes Federation (IDF), 2006).
3. Rebekah's BMI shows that she is obese (National Obesity Observatory, 2009) and therefore at risk of associated health problems including cardiovascular disease. Her obesity would have also contributed to the development of insulin resistance and Type 2 diabetes. Rebekah's WC is above the ideal value and indicates that she has excess visceral adipose tissue (central obesity). This also indicates that she is at risk of developing other associated conditions. Her central obesity, hypertension and Type 2 diabetes show that she fulfils the criteria for the presence of metabolic syndrome (IDF, 2006).
4. Inconsistent carbohydrate intake (problem) related to an inability to combine diabetes education with strict dietary laws (cause) characterised by high random blood glucose levels.
5. To make diabetes education culturally appropriate for Rebekah, facilitating her to make appropriate changes to her diet to reduce her weight and improve her diabetes control thereby reducing her HbA1c level.
6. An energy deficit of 500 kcal/day is an achievable restriction to Rebekah's diet and would result in a weight loss of 0.5 kg (1lb) per week.
7. SACN (2008) recommend that an adult diet should contain <35% of food energy as total fat of which <11% should be saturated fat. Carbohydrate should be 55% of total energy and protein the remainder.
8. Rebekah should be encouraged to develop her own meal plan based on the dietary advice provided by the dietitian on food choices and portions.
9. The dietary laws (Kashrut) date from the old testament and detail the selection, preparation and consumption of foods; only certain foods (Kosher) are permitted. The laws include the following:
   - Milk and milk products must not be cooked or served for the same meal as meat or poultry. All items used for the preparation or serving of meat and milk

Dietetic and Nutrition Case Studies, First Edition.
Edited by Judy Lawrence, Pauline Douglas, and Joan Gandy.

Companion Website: http://www.manualofdieteticpractice.com/

must be cleaned and stored separately. People wait 3–6 h between having a meat meal and having milk.

- Milk products and meat must be bought from kosher shops and must have kosher labels.
- Four legged animals with cloven hoofs that chew the cud, for example, sheep, goats and cattle are permitted. All others, including pig, are forbidden.
- Poultry such as chicken, goose, turkey, and duck are allowed but most others are not.
- Animals must be slaughtered by shechita, a slaughtering method that must be carried out by a trained and authorised person. A sharp knife is used to quickly cut the throat, which severes the jugular vein and carotid artery. The blood is drained from the carcass that is then salted and soaked in water to remove any remaining blood. Meat prepared in this manner is kosher.
- Only scaly fish with fins, such as cod, plaice, trout, tuna are permitted to be eaten. Other fish including eels and shellfish are forbidden.

10. Some of the traditional foods are high in fat/sugar; pastry dishes, meat stews (cholent), potato bake, vermicelli bake (high carbohydrates/sugar) stewed carrots with honey, schnitzel, cakes/biscuits, kreplach (pastry savoury in chicken soup), chicken fat fried, egg with mayonnaise and tuna with mayonnaise. Few low-fat or low-energy foods are available; kosher foods may not have nutrition labelling.

11. Obesity co-morbidities include (Foresight, 2007):

- Hypertension.
- Type 2 diabetes mellitus – there will be significant insulin resistance with this degree of obesity making it harder to control. Poorly controlled diabetes will result in diabetic complications such as peripheral neuropathy, retinopathy.
- Cardiovascular disease.
- Some cancers, for example, breast.
- Liver disease.
- Gastrointestinal diseases, for example, gall stones.
- Psychological and social problems such as low self-esteem.

12. Six sessions are optimum although this will vary depending on resources and Rebekah's needs. The dietary intervention would centre around reducing energy and fat intake. The following topics need to be discussed.

- Regular meals that are more balanced (carbohydrates, protein, fruit and vegetables).
- Traditional foods and how they may be cooked differently to reduce fats and sugars.
- Portion sizes.
- Cooking methods and use of oil.
- Drinks and snacks.
- Discuss increasing physical activity; acceptable ideas could be; going to a female gym, going to female classes which may be given in the local area, going for walks with friends either in evening or in the day when most children are at school or nursery.

13. • Encourage Rebekah to consider her biggest weakness and how she might enjoy the many meals and courses but still eat healthily.
• If she is having all her meals at home, she can choose more freely what to make and cook.
• If going out for meals, encourage a high vegetable intakes and less carbohydrates moderate protein.
• When eating dairy food choose lower fat varieties or eat less of the regular variety.

14. • Agree on nutrition/dietetic goals (e.g. in the next weeks will try to have regular, balanced meals).
• Aim for an average weight loss of 2 kg/month.
• Reduce sugar and fat content of her diet while adhering to a strict kosher regimen depending on patient's motivation.
• Prepare and cook foods with less oil and fats.
• Cut down on high fat/sugar foods that are not mandatory to be eaten.
• Eat less of higher fat foods.

15. • Lack of understanding of the implications of being overweight, diabetic complications and hypertensio.n
• Lethargy and lack of motivation to change lifestyle.
• Being busy with the children and not finding time to look after her self.
• Lack of support from husband and/or family to make changes.

16. • Explain the complications of obesity, DM and hypertension.
• Educate on how to structure meals and portions.
• Be as supportive as possible within clinic limits and consultation agreements.
• Give her a lot of encouragement, tell her it is possible and you have seen this to be possible previously.

17. • Changes in dietary habits.
• Increased level of physical activity.
• Blood glucose levels.
• Lipid profile levels.
• BMI.
• Waist circumference.

CASE STUDY 26

Type 2 diabetes mellitus – private patient

Answers

1. This pathway is privately funded by the client and not paid for by the NHS. In addition, for clinical competence, freelance dietitians need good business skills. Fees must reflect overheads such as room hire, travel, time, CPD, insurance and other professional fees. The Freelance Dietitians Group (FDG) of the BDA provides members with guidance on all aspects of setting up private practice, including charging of fees.
2. Elizabeth has an excessive energy intake (problem) related to lack of exercise and food consumption (aetiology) as shown by her weight and glycosylated haemoglobin (signs/symptoms).
3. Dietitians may take self-referrals for medical problems provided a diagnosis has been made and sufficient background information is available. Given the complexity of Elizabeth's problems (type 2 diabetes, hyperlipdaemia and hypertension) a medical diagnosis, as in this instance, is the safest practice.
4.
   - Assume that the information provided by the GP is accurate. Anthropometric measurements (weight, height and BMI) should be repeated at the initial consultation. Consider when the GP's measurements were taken. Has there been any significant change in this time period? Were the blood tests done within the last 3 months? Is the patient doing any self-monitoring? What are the results?
   - The initial absence of information on medication is unfortunate. You need to know what oral medications are prescribed for all her conditions, and whether she is taking insulin. Are all medications being taken as prescribed? Can the patient be relied upon to give accurate details, or should the GP be contacted?
   - A diet history is required. This can be from a 24 h recall at the consultation, or a 3-day food diary could be completed in advance. Although this lady is Afro-Caribbean, we cannot assume that she is following an Afro-Caribbean diet.

Dietetic and Nutrition Case Studies, First Edition.
Edited by Judy Lawrence, Pauline Douglas, and Joan Gandy.

Companion Website: http://www.manualofdieteticpractice.com/

- There is limited information on the client's environmental, cultural and social situation. It is important to gain an understanding of the client's lifestyle. As a freelance dietitian, especially when dealing with self-referrals, it is useful to obtain further information prior to the initial consultation. This can be done by telephone, email or face to face.

5. Even though referred by her GP, it is still important to gain the client's consent to share or request information, for example, a summary letter or request for further medical information. Unauthorised contact could be seen as a breach of confidentiality, particularly by self-referred patients.

   Writing a summary of your consultation for the GP is not just a courtesy. It enables other health care professionals to reinforce key messages. It also advertises your services. Sending a copy to the patient gives them a clear summary of what was agreed with you in the treatment plan.

6. Private medical insurance for dietetics is generally restricted to patients referred by a medical consultant and limited to 2 or 3 consultations. The current exception in the United Kingdom is BUPA, who in April 2014 started to recognise GP referrals to dietitians registered with the BUPA Network.

   Many insurance policies will cover only acute problems or diagnosis. Type 2 diabetes is considered a chronic condition and Elizabeth was diagnosed 12 years ago.

   In all cases, if patients are seeking to pay for their consultation with medical insurance, they must be advised to contact their insurance company ahead of the appointment to obtain authorisation. The dietitian will then invoice the insurance company.

   The dietitian must make it clear that if an authorisation number is not available, the patient will be invoiced. The patient may decide not to proceed with the appointment.

7. The patient has come at the GP's suggestion but she is prepared to pay, which implies reasonable motivation. Try to establish why she did not engage with previous interventions. Taking this, and her reasons for accepting the private referral into account, will give insight into the patient's expectations and assist in planning appropriate ways to motivate behaviour change.

   The patient will expect provision of detailed, personalised advice that was not given to her previously.

   Fees should be discussed prior to the consultation. Explain clearly what is and is not covered by them. Written scales of fees can help. Can you offer a discount for prepayment for a package of consultations? Check that the client is willing to accept this. Consider a written agreement as part of a signed registration form.

   You need confident, clear answers, particularly regarding potential costs.

8. - Know your limitations and do not be afraid to admit you need to check a fact before giving an answer.
   - All dietitians must maintain adequate CPD/Life Long Learning. Freelance dietitians are often working in isolation and so need to make good use of BDA resources, BDA specialist groups and branches, maintaining contact with colleagues, reading journals and using online CPD opportunities.

- Remember you must develop both business as well as clinical skills.
- The HCPC standards are designed to protect the client. Practicing within it minimises risk but freelance dietitians must also maintain adequate professional indemnity, public liability insurance and registration for data protection.

9. Records should be maintained of the consultation and any other communication with the client, by post, telephone or emails, as you would in an NHS setting. Refer to the HCPC Standards of conduct performance and ethics and the HCPC Standards of Proficiency and BDA Process for Nutrition and Dietetic Practice supported by BDA Guidance for Dietitians for records and record keeping. Then register with the Information Commissioner's Office (ICO) for data protection. https://ico.org.uk/for-organisations/register/.

10.
- Produce your own or purchase from other sources. If producing your own, it is advisable to ask for peer review from a colleague.
- You should not use NHS dietetic department materials without permission, payment and acknowledgement.
- There are many sources of reliable leaflets such as NDRUK, BDA food facts, BDA specialist groups, Diabetes UK.
- Your contact details should be on all material you provide to clients.

11.
- Try to determine this information prior to the initial consultation as it can help with planning your nutrition and dietetic intervention.
- Make sure expectations are realistic and achievable within the Professional code of practice. The patient's budget may be a limitation. With chronic conditions such as diabetes, long-term NHS monitoring and care will ultimately be required. The freelance dietitian has a duty of care to ensure that the patient is aware of this and is encouraged to re-engage with appropriate NHS care pathways.

12. The freelance dietitian has the advantage of being outside the usual care pathway and may be perceived as providing a fresh start. Paying for the service can greatly aid motivation. The patient may benefit considerably from feeling that they are receiving very personalised care. In addition, there are more direct lines of communication. There is scope for monitoring and follow up by various routes such as telephone, email or Skype. Reasons may be purely practical, for example, location or timing of clinics.

13.
- Elizabeth clearly has poorly controlled diabetes and will need lifelong, ongoing monitoring and support, which private insurance will not cover (chronic disease management exclusions) and the patient may not be able to self-fund for an extended, or life-long period.
- In a limited number of consultations (possibly two or three), the freelance dietitian has a duty of care not only to motivate and re-educate the patients to manage their diabetes better, but also to encourage them to work more closely with their GP and NHS diabetes services.
- This case study illustrates the benefits of a freelance dietitian complementing the usual NHS care pathways.

14. The components of the dietetic care process are identical to all dietetic interventions, both NHS and private and comprise the following:

- Identification of nutrition and dietetic diagnosis diagnosis.
- Plan nutrition/dietetic intervention.
- Implement nutrition/dietetic intervention.
  As in NHS practice, remember to
- Monitor and review.
- Evaluate and develop your service.

CASE STUDY 27

Gestational diabetes mellitus

Answers

1. Imbalanced dietary intake of carbohydrate (problem) related to intake of sweetened tea and carbonated drinks (aetiology) characterised by elevated blood glucose levels (signs/symptoms).
2. Hormones produced during pregnancy, for example, progesterone, oestrogen and human placental lactogen are needed to ensure that the foetus is supplied with extra glucose and nutrient needed for growth. This results in an increased need for insulin. However, some women can not produce enough insulin or there is insulin resistance which, results in hyperglycaemia. This is known as gestational diabetes mellitus (GDM) and is usually diagnosed during the second trimester. In other women, GDM may be diagnosed during the first trimester of pregnancy. In these women, the condition most likely existed before the pregnancy.
3. The risk factors are:
   - Obesity (BMI > 30 kg/m^2).
   - Family history of diabetes (parent, sibling).
   - An unexplained stillbirth or neonatal death in a previous pregnancy, and/or a very large infant in a previous pregnancy – ≥4 kg (8.8 lb).
   - Gestation DM in previous pregnancy.
   - Pre-eclampsia in previous pregnancy.
   - South Asian, Black Caribbean or Middle Eastern ethnicity.

   Badra is at risk for GDM as she was obese before conceiving (BMI 30 kg/m^2), was diagnosed with pre-eclampsia in previous pregnancy and she is South Asian.
4. Complications include:
   - Miscarriage.
   - Stillbirth.
   - Macrosomia (high birth weight) – increases the risk of assisted (e.g. forceps) or caesarean delivery, induced labour, birth problems such as shoulder dystocia (obstructed labour), which may impede or stop the baby's breathing during birth.

Dietetic and Nutrition Case Studies, First Edition.
Edited by Judy Lawrence, Pauline Douglas, and Joan Gandy.

Companion Website: http://www.manualofdieteticpractice.com/

- Premature delivery – associated with many complications including respiratory distress and jaundice.
- Postnatal problems in the baby, for example, hypoglycemia.
- Foetal distress during labour.
- Increased risk of the mother developing GDM in later pregnancies and type 2 DM later in life.
- The baby is at increased risk of developing diabetes and/or obesity later in life.

5. An oral glucose tolerance test (OGTT) is performed. A fasting blood glucose level is measured and then repeated 2 h after the woman has had a glucose drink (75 g glucose). The most frequently used diagnostic criteria are the WHO/IDF (2006) criteria:
   Fasting venous plasma glucose (VPG) $\geq$ 7 mmol/L (this test is not diagnostic in GDM)
   VPG $\geq$ 7.8 mmol/L 2 h after the glucose load.
   While WHO also recommends using HbA1c as a diagnostic tool for DM it does not recommend its use as a diagnostic tool in GDM (WHO, 2013).
6. Current diet

Nutrient	Current diet	Comments
Energy (kcal/d)	2084 kcal/day (Henry, 2005) + 40% physical activity + 200 kcal as Badra is in third trimester	As patient is obese >30 kg/m^2 BMI Energy prescription: 75%
Protein (g)	78 g	As per PENG guidelines: 75% of daily requirements (0.17 g Nitrogen/kg/day)
Fat (g)	74 g	As per PENG guidelines: 75% of daily requirements (1 g/kg/day)
Carbohydrates (g)	130–225 g/day	Moderate carbohydrate intake (Diabetes UK, 2011)
Iron (mg)	14.8	RNI
Calcium (mg)	700	RNI
Zinc (mg)	7	RNI
Folate (μg)	300	RNI
Vitamin C (mg)	50	RNI
Vitamin A (μg)	700	RNI

Source: SACN (2011) and DH (1991).

Badra's diet is high in added sugar, alcohol, fat, mainly in saturated fat, and is low in fruits. She is not always managing five fruit and vegetables every day and therefore not managing her vitamin, minerals and fibre requirements. She is also exceeding her daily recommended total of carbohydrates and salt intake (6 g/day) as her current diet may provide salt between 8 and 10 g/day.

7. Aims of the dietary intervention are as follows:
   - Tighter blood glucose control as per NICE (2015) – fasting 3.5–5.9 and <7.8 mmol/L 1 h postprandial;
   - Prevent further weight gain; and
   - Establish healthy eating pattern and food choices.
8. Intervention:
   - Start consultation with clarifying understanding of health risks. This lady is at high risk of developing type 2 diabetes and CHD. Discuss the significant benefits of losing 5–10% body weight and consider weight loss after delivery. This would reduce her risk of progressing onto type 2 diabetes and improve her lipid profile and BP.
   - Suggest three regular meals with some starch in each meal/not to skip meals.
   - Eating a healthy breakfast would also reduce snacking between meals.
   - Swap biscuits for fruit and improve fibre/micronutrient intake of diet and stop adding sugar to drinks and consider sweeteners (try different brands).
   - Avoid very large intakes of carbohydrates if causing post-prandial hyperglycaemia, for example, 12 in. baguette.
   - Reduce added sugar intake.
   - Take packed healthy lunch to work.
   - Consider using less salt in cooking and swap it with herb and spices.
   - Discuss healthier choices of foods/drinks and portion control when eating out.
   - Consider reducing fat in curries and swap with healthier fats; choose monounsaturated fats.
   - Explore ways to include exercise in daily routine.
9. The glycaemic index (GI) is a ranking of carbohydrate-containing foods based on the overall effect on blood glucose levels. Foods that are absorbed slowly have a low GI rating, while foods that are more quickly absorbed have a higher rating. High GI foods raises post-prandial glucose levels quicker than low GI foods.
   - Choosing slowly absorbed carbohydrates, instead of quickly absorbed carbohydrates, can help even out blood glucose levels when you have diabetes.
   - Glycemic load is a measure that takes into account the amount of carbohydrate in a portion of food together with how quickly it raises blood glucose levels (Diabetes UK, 2011).
   - Badra's diet is a mixture of high/medium GI carbohydrates, for example, white toast, baguette, whole meal chapatti flour. Badra has high glycaemic load meals, for example, 12 in. baguette and crisps (about 80 g carbohydrates) or large jacket potato and regular cola (about 100 g carbohydrates).
   - Badra should be choosing whole grain carbohydrates source, for example, granary bread, mixed grain chapatti flour and should be thinking of reducing her carbohydrate portions to about 50 g/meal and include more low-fat protein options, vegetables and salads in her meals.

10. Outcome measures
- Blood glucose levels.
- HbA1c.
- Weight.
- Pregnancy outcome.

11. Barriers to change include the following:
- Lack of basic knowledge of healthy diet. To provide tips on cardio protective mediterranean diet based on vegetables, fruits, beans, whole grains, olive oil and fish. Maybe Badra needs to bring her mother-in-law and her husband to the diet consultation to improve their understanding of healthy diet and life style.
  - Not enough understanding about the change and lack of vision, direction and priority. Badra needs to understand the importance of diet and tight blood glucose control from the perspective of her pregnancy.
  - Well-established habits are difficult to change. To use 'Motivation Interview' technique for behaviour change.
  - Lack of time to cook healthy foods; Badra will need to be more organised; for example, prepare healthy lunch in advance for the next day, involve mother-in-law and husband help in shopping and in preparation of healthy evening meals.

12.
- Traditional Asian beliefs of high fat/energy intake during and after pregnancy may help with the delivery and lactation. Obese women are more likely to be delivered by caesarean section than women in the normal BMI category. As Badra is obese, a healthy diet with good fats such as olive oil in moderation will help to maintain her weight and a healthy diet and good hydration would help during lactation.
- Asian diet is generally high in salt. As Badra is on medication for blood pressure, advice on low/moderate salt should be provided during consultation.
- Her understanding of the importance of exercise and old Asian beliefs in relation to pregnancy should be addressed. If Badra was not doing any exercise before the pregnancy, then taking up strenuous exercise would not be advisable. Walking for 15 min twice daily, five times a week can be advised.
- Iron, vitamin D deficiency among South East Asians: to give advice and to check if Badra is on any supplements. To check if Badra is on any vitamin A supplements as too much vitamin A could harm the baby.

13. Explain the following:
- Hypoglycaemia is caused by low blood glucose levels (usually <4 mmol/L).
- Causes could be missed or delayed meals, not enough starchy food, insulin tablet dose too high, excessive exercise or drinking alcohol on an empty stomach.
- Symptoms are trembling, sweating, weakness, headache, tingling lips or tongue, irritability, slurred speech, numbness or blurred vision.

- Treatment is to take 3 glucose tablets/1/2 glass of Lucozade or sweet fizzy drink/2 tsp of sugar. Check blood glucose levels in 15–20 min, if still low then repeat treatment. Follow up with a complex carbohydrate snack such as a slice of bread/small banana/digestive biscuit.

14. As Badra is on insulin (long acting) she will need good education on injection technique, storage of insulin, hypoglycaemia and home monitoring.

Answers to further questions

15. Alcohol passes and crosses the blood placental barrier to the baby. A baby's liver is one of the last organs to develop fully and does not mature until the later stages of pregnancy. Therefore, babies cannot metabolise alcohol and exposure to alcohol can seriously affect development. The Department of Health recommends that pregnant women should avoid alcohol altogether. And if you do opt to have a drink, it recommends that you stick to one or two units of alcohol (equivalent to one small glass of wine) once or twice a week to minimise the risk to your baby.

High levels of caffeine during pregnancy can result in babies having a low birth weight, which can increase the risk of health problems in later life. Too much caffeine can also cause a miscarriage. Caffeine should be limited to no more than 200 mg a day. Decaffeinated tea and coffee are useful alternatives. Cola and high-energy drinks also contain caffeine and should be avoided.

16. Food safety

Cheese that use mould in ripening such as camembert, brie or as a rind such as goat's cheese and soft blue veined chesses such as gorgonzola may contain listeria bacteria, which causes listeriosis. Listeriosis is rare but even a mild infection can cause a miscarriage, stillbirth or illness in the neonate.

Eggs should be well cooked (solid yolk and white) to prevent salmonella poisoning. Raw and undercooked eggs and egg products such as mayonnaise should be avoided.

Unpasteurised (raw/green top) milk and milk products should be avoided. If no other milk is available unpasteurised should be boiled before consuming.

All pâté, including vegetable pâtés, should be avoided as they can contain listeria.

CASE STUDY 28

Polycystic ovary syndrome

Answers

1. Excessive energy intake (problem) related to frequent consumption of high fat foods (aetiology) characterised by obesity (signs/symptoms).
2. The presence of two or more of the following: (ESHRE & ASRM, 2004):
   - Oligo-ovulation leading to oligomenorrhoea (<9 menses/year), or anovulation leading to amenorrhoea.
   - Hyperandrogenism: clinically (hirsutism, male pattern alopecia, acne) or biochemically.
   - Polycystic ovaries.

   Other endocrine disorders should be excluded. A woman can be diagnosed with PCOS without polycystic ovaries; a woman with polycystic ovaries but no other symptoms should not be diagnosed with PCOS.
3. - Insulin resistance and type 2 diabetes – oral glucose tolerance test.
   - Cardiovascular disease – full lipid profile, blood pressure.
4. Reduced energy diet to facilitate weight loss:
   - Spread carbohydrate intake throughout the day and promote inclusion of lower GI sources.
   - Reduce refined sugar and higher GI sources.
   - Reduce saturated fat intake from shallow fried breads in ghee/butter such as thepla and paratha and avoid cheese.
   - Reduce total fat intake – reduce intake of cheese. Promote alternative vegetarian choices such as low-fat hummus; use a non-stick pan and minimal oil when cooking.
   - Try to increase intake of fruit and vegetables; use as snacks and to bulk up meals.
   - Include protein in meals.
   - Include a folic acid supplement as planning to conceive.
5. Short term – weight loss
   - If insulin resistance or type 2 diabetes is present, improve glycaemic control.
   - If hyperlipidaemic, improve lipid profile.

   Long term – continue and maintain weight loss.

Dietetic and Nutrition Case Studies, First Edition.
Edited by Judy Lawrence, Pauline Douglas, and Joan Gandy.

Companion Website: http://www.manualofdieteticpractice.com/

6. She may have barriers to change such as feeling that she cannot have input into what food is bought and cooked, as she is living in an extended family.
7. This patient currently feels she is motivated but does not feel she has adequate support to make changes. Consider asking if her husband would like to accompany her to consultations. If he agrees then he may be a useful source of support.
   - Highlight that weight loss is likely to help her conceive.
   - She also feels that she has inadequate time to eat regularly.
   - Strategies could be discussed regarding planning meals and snacks when at work to avoid the pattern of missed meals and then having large snacks later. In addition, the patient could consider helping with the shopping, cooking and planning meals as leftovers can be used for lunch.
8. - Ovo-lacto vegetarian – does not eat eggs, meat and fish; particularly avoiding beef and beef products.
   - Ghee is used in cooking.
   - Although alcohol is forbidden, it depends how strictly they abide to religion. Some second- and third-generation Hindus may consume some alcohol and eggs but are unlikely to do so during religious festival periods. Always useful to ask younger patients rather than assume dietary habits.
   - Special sweet and savoury dishes may be eaten during festivals; these are often deep fried.
9. Several validated PA questionnaires are available. The general practitioner physical activity questionnaire (GPPAQ) was commissioned by the Department of Health (2009) for use in the NHS.
10. Discuss with Nisha and agree on a SMART aim, for example, increase regular moderate exercise; initially, aim for 30 min 5 days/week and increase to 1 h/day. Using an exercise diary can monitor this.
11. - Mother-in-law does all the cooking and shopping. Nisha feels that she may be unable to influence cooking choices.
    - She misses her breakfast, as her journey to work is much further now and so needs to leave earlier.
    - Finds that she is snacking in the day because she is getting hungry as the day passes and then in the evening eats a much larger meal than she did previously.
    - Used to take food from home prior to getting married but now tends to buy whilst at work, as she does not do the food shopping.
    - Finds vegetarian lunch choices limited when buying readymade foods.
    - Limited support.

    These barriers can be overcome by encouraging Nisha to discuss her dietary needs with her mother-in-law, and suggesting quick and easy breakfasts such as microwavable porridge, low-energy, healthy snacks such as fruit and suitable lunches. Encourage Nisha to discuss PCOS and its treatment with her husband and mother-in-law explaining how the dietary intervention will help her lose weight and improve the chances of her to conceive.

Answers to further questions

12. Most women with PCOS will have some degree of insulin resistance and metformin reduces insulin levels. Metformin has also been shown to improve fertility (Tang *et al.*, 2010).

13. Hyperinsulinaemia promotes hyperandrogenism in the ovaries and reduces production of sex hormone binding globulin, which leads to increased testosterone. High levels of insulin and testosterone result in irregular menstruation, anovulation and accumulation of immature follicles resulting in reduced fertility.

14. Many women with PCOS report taking supplements (Jeannes *et al.*, 2009). There is no conclusive evidence to support their use in the management of PCOS. However, it is important not to be dismissive of Nisha's interest in supplements. It is important to discuss the importance of evidence and to respect her opinions.

CASE STUDY 29

Obesity – specialist management

A specialist community weight management service for severe and complex obesity (NHS tier 3)

Answers

1. $52\,kg/m^2$
   She is at high risk of developing several co-morbidities (Foresight, 2007) including
   - Hypertension.
   - Type 2 diabetes mellitus – there will be significant insulin resistance with this degree of obesity making it harder to control. Poorly controlled diabetes will result in diabetic complications such as peripheral neuropathy, retinopathy.
   - Cardiovascular disease.
   - Some cancers, for example, breast.
   - Liver disease.
   - Gastrointestinal diseases, for example, gall stones.
   - Psychological and social problems, for example, low self-esteem.
2. Although NICE (2006) guidance CG43 states that waist circumference may be used in addition to BMI, there are practical difficulties in people with a BMI of over $35\,kg/m^2$. It may be difficult to locate the correct position for the tape measure due to skin folds. In addition, at BMI greater than $35\,kg/m^2$, the waist circumference does not add to the predictive power of disease risk.
3. Susan's HbA1c is diagnostic of type 2 diabetes, which increases her risk of cardiovascular disease; however, her lipid profile is normal apart from HDL cholesterol (NICE, 2008).

Dietetic and Nutrition Case Studies, First Edition.
Edited by Judy Lawrence, Pauline Douglas, and Joan Gandy.

Companion Website: http://www.manualofdieteticpractice.com/

Parameter	Normal	Actual	Comment
Total cholesterol (mmol/L)	<4.0	3.8	Normal
HDL cholesterol (mmol/L)	≥1.0	0.91	Low
LDL cholesterol (mmol/L)	<2.0	1.49	Normal
Triglycerides (mmol/L)	<4.5	3.08	Normal

4. Other blood tests might be the following:
   - Thyroid function.
   - Vitamin D levels due to link between low vitamin D and obesity.
5. - Sleep study due to Epworth sleep score.
   - Diabetes/endocrinology clinic depending on previous and current input.
6. Obese class III (problem) associated with anxiety and depression (aetiology) characterised by BMI of 52 kg/m^2 and PHQ and GHD7 scores (sign/symptom).
7. Ascertain what Susan would like to achieve and what would she regard as a successful outcome. Involve her in setting outcome measures and targets.
8. - Overcoming barriers to weight loss.
   - Energy balance.
   - Eatwell plate and food groups.
   - Appropriate portion sizes for weight loss.
   - Healthy snacking.
   - Appropriate drinks and fluids.
   - Reading food labels.
   - Low energy eating plans.
   - Healthy cooking techniques.
9. - Reduction in portion sizes.
   - Reduction in number of takeaways per week.
   - Reduction in sugar-sweetened soft drink consumption.
   - Increased level of daily activity.
10. - Encourage her to save the money she would spend on takeaways towards a treat, for example, holiday, manicure.
    - Quick easy lunch or meal ideas.
    - Education on healthy takeaway ideas.
11. - Carbs and Cals book and application (Chevette & Balolia, 2013).
    - Plate models.
    - Food models.
    - Weighing food.
    - Practical portions, for example, meat, the portion of palm of hand.
12. - Food diary or online recording application.
    - Exercise diary.
    - Weighing herself.

13. • Susan has been unsuccessful in maintaining weight loss in the past; lack of belief in one's ability is a major barrier to success.
  • Positive feedback from behaviour change may be slow to emerge, it is important that Susan's expectations are realistic.
  • Initial rate of weight loss will slow, which may be discouraging.
  • As Susan looses weight, she will need to make further changes to her behaviour to continue to lose weight, which may be increasingly difficult.

14. • Documentation in the medical notes should be timely, accurate, signed and dated.
  • Communication between the dietitian, physiotherapist and psychologist should occur regularly at, say, team meetings, by email and documentation in the medical notes, etc.
  • It is important to communicate with the GP on patient progress and also if more local support is needed, changes or additions to medication, that is, required and so on.

15. • Weight.
  • HbA1c.
  • Improvements in the following:
    ◦ PHQ score.
    ◦ GAD score.
    ◦ Epworth sleep score.
  • Decrease in blood pressure.
  • Increased physical activity – assessed by questionnaire or diary.

CASE STUDY 30

Obesity – Prader–Willi syndrome

Answers

1. The most appropriate assessment would be to use PWS-specific charts in combination with the standard growth charts. Several PWS-specific growth charts have been proposed and produced from Japan (Nagai *et al.*, 2000), Germany (Hauffa *et al.*, 2000) and the United States (Butler & Meaney, 1991) although no charts exist from UK data.
2. On the standard UK growth charts, Shelley's weight is between the 91st and 98th centiles, which considered in isolation is not an extreme measurement. Height is below the 0.4th centile, which is an extreme measurement. There is a large discrepancy between height and weight centiles. Short stature is typical in Prader–Willi Syndrome; therefore, she was given growth hormone until the age of 13. If Shelley's measurements are plotted on the German PWS-specific charts her weight is on the 50th centile and height on the 25th centile suggesting a very different picture to that suggested by standard charts and less of a discrepancy.
3. BMI should be calculated and plotted on a gender-specific chart. There is a very significant increase since the growth hormone stopped. The BMI chart should make the changes more obvious and allow comparison to the distance from the centile lines.

   There is considerable difference in the body composition of PWS patients compared with non-PWS individuals, which will have an impact on true BMI evaluation. Therefore, BMI is only to show comparisons for individual progress, not for comparison to the general population. As there are no existing current published standards, comparisons with other data such as the recent GOSH body composition data are inappropriate. Changes in body composition may occur since stopping the growth hormone, as it affects body composition (NICE, 2010).
4. Raised glucose was suggestive of type 2 diabetes, which was confirmed by GTT. Abnormal lipid profile (raised triglycerides, total cholesterol, raised LDL and slightly low HDL). Liver function tests were normal.
5. Excessive energy intake (problem) related to over consumption of food (aetiology) characterised by diet history and high BMI (sign/symptom).

Dietetic and Nutrition Case Studies, First Edition.
Edited by Judy Lawrence, Pauline Douglas, and Joan Gandy.

Companion Website: http://www.manualofdieteticpractice.com/

6. It is more useful to use BMI than weight as it gives a better perspective on growth. As Shelley is 16 years old and no longer on growth hormones she is unlikely to grow any taller. Shelley has not gained height over the past year; therefore, to achieve improvements in BMI weight loss will be required. BMI maintenance may be more realistic initially as her BMI has been increasing over the past year. An additional goal may be to improve glucose control. Improving BMI should also improve other biochemical parameters such as lipid profile and HbA1c. Aim for a stable BMI, for example, for 6 months. Then once achieved set target of moving towards the next centile BMI line, that is, the 99.6th centile. It may be sensible to aim for the 99.6th centile (BMI 32.5 kg/m^2) over the following year, although you may need to be slower.

Short-term aims should be focussed around small behaviour changes that are acceptable to Shelley, for example, to swap squash with water for no added sugar squash or to switch from 2 digestive biscuits to 1 rich tea biscuit or swap muesli bars with vegetable sticks. Routine is important and therefore swaps work better than stopping things. Using tools with visual measures such as the pedometer to increase activity, can work well.

Outcome measures could include micronutrient and macronutrient adequacy, improved BMI, improved biochemistry, improved body composition, and may be cardiovascular fitness if you have the tools to measure.

7. There is uncertainty on the energy requirements for PWS; they are typically lower due to low tone and high fat mass. Several authors have suggested using kcal/cm (6–8 kcal/cm of height for weight loss and 10–12 kcal/cm height for maintenance) but most of the literature agrees that requirements are approximately 60% energy for age (Butler *et al.*, 2006). The EAR for a 16-year-old girl is 2110 kcal/day; 60% = 1266 kcal/day (SACN, 2011).

The US PWS association have proposed energy guidelines (Borgie *et al.*, 1994) but these are not based on prospective data and care is recommended if using these.

It is important to check for dietary adequacy; particularly micronutrients, essential fatty acids and fibre, as such restricted energy intakes make it harder to achieve recommended intakes. Micronutrient requirements have not been observed to be any different. A small study suggests that body composition in PWS can be significantly positively affected by the macronutrient composition of the diet and level of fibre. The change of focus towards lower carbohydrate (45% total energy) is similar to that for diabetes management (Miller *et al.*, 2013).

8. The impact of having a brother with Asperger's could include communication difficulties, limited likes and dislikes of food, especially different textures and smells as sensory difficulties are common. Meal time routines could be very important to both Shelley and her brother and any disruption may be upsetting. He may like a set pattern of certain foods on specific days or may prefer a particular order in which food is eaten, for example, vegetables to be eaten separately. This could be tortuous for someone with PWS as food is continually tempting and there could be a lack of understanding between both brother and sister at meal times.

An athletic, active brother will have a higher energy requirement. He is likely to be within a normal BMI range but may be eating larger portions than other family members as well as regular snacks. Someone with PWS may find others having additional food very unjust.

9. Shelley has started to become more involved with her dietetic care by keeping her photo food diary. The main responsibility is likely to remain with her parents and carers for some time, but Shelley should still be encouraged to be involved by using the communication tools such as the Makaton app (www.makaton.org) on her iPad. She will need support from family, respite, health professionals and school/college. Although she should be involved in planning her meals and activities and encouraged to take some responsibility this is likely to be a slow process and its success should be closely monitored. Structure and routine will be important aspects.
10. Barriers to change may include difficulties in implementing self-control around food, lack of understanding, motivation and little support from home as her mother is unwell and father away. Are there other professionals/services working with the family that may be able to help implement plans? Clinic appointments may not be given a high priority as life is busy with the family having differing needs. Are there safe guarding concerns? The differing needs of the three children and mother are also a potential barrier to change. Other barriers to change include respite and the carers' views on and/or understanding of the need for a consistent approach and routine. Sedentary activities where additional food is likely to be consumed such as going to the cinema need to be carefully managed.
11. Collaborative working would include the wider MDT:
    - Consultant – to monitor Shelley's general health/condition.
    - Clinical nurse specialist – facilitator between different health/social professionals and may be the first person to contact.
    - Speech therapist – speech and swallow issues.
    - Physiotherapist – muscle tone and physical exercises to maximise muscle power and general fitness.
    - Occupational therapist – activities of daily living.
    - Psychologist – emotional and cognitive needs and assessments.
    - Dietitian – nutritional needs.
    - GP – awareness of wider family issues.
    - Social services – care needs.
    - Mental health services – mother's depression. Without help her mental health is very likely to impact on Shelley's care.

    The family will have many professionals involved with her brother and so it is important to remember the impact of having so many professionals involved with a family. It is good to attend a child's Team Around the Child (TAC) meeting to ensure that your plan fits with those of the wider team.
12. Over the next couple of years Shelley's care will start to transition across to adult services. This is likely to affect all of her health and social care services. When Shelley finishes college and may be looking for employment it is likely that it would be of benefit if she can be guided into the non-food sector. Shelley may also

move out of the family home and start to live more independently; this is likely to be in the form of some sort of supported housing. Routine and consistency will remain important to help her to manage these changes.

13. Little change to dietetic aims, but important enough to ensure that the family understand the link between carbohydrates (refined and unrefined) and blood glucose levels. This is a chance to re-emphasise these. The diagnosis of type 2 diabetes can be a strong motivator for change so it is important to use this. It is also a lot for a family to digest and should therefore be considered when looking at appropriateness of goals being set.

Answer to further question

14. People aged 16 years and over are entitled to consent to their own treatment as they are presumed to have sufficient capacity, that is, the ability to use and understand information to make a decision, and communicate any decision made. This can be overruled if there is significant evidence to suggest otherwise. If the health care team feels that a person does not have the capacity to give consent, and there is no advanced decision or there is no formal appointment with anyone who could make decisions for the person, then they will need to carefully consider what is in the person's best interests. The decision should be on an individual basis dependent on the medical and mental abilities (see Case study 4 for further details).

CASE STUDY 31
Bariatric surgery

Answers

1. NICE Guidance CG 43 (2006) states that surgery can be considered provided the following conditions have been met:
   - Aged 18 and over and children who have reached physiological maturity.
   - BMI > 40 kg/m^2 without co-morbidities.
   - BMI > 35 kg/m^2 with co-morbidities.
   - First line treatment with BMI > 50 kg/m^2.
   - All non-surgical measures have been tried (see below).
   - There should be no clinical or psychological contraindication for surgery.
   - Comprehensive multi-disciplinary assessment.
   - Commit to long-term follow-up.

   This patient does meet NICE criteria for surgery but has chosen to pay for surgery abroad. NHS England Clinical Commissioning Policy: Complex and Specialised Obesity Surgery (2014) requires patients to spend a period of time (usually 12–24 months) in a tier 3 weight management service. Although Abi has attempted to lose weight in the past she will still be required to engage with a tier 3 weight management service before being considered for surgery. Demand for surgery exceeds capacity in many areas resulting in long delays locally. Abi wants to get pregnant and is no doubt concerned about her age. She may have been concerned that the tier 3 service would be a delay to obtaining surgery.
2. Patients need a comprehensive assessment prior to surgery and long-term follow-up (with the dietitian) in order to avoid nutritional deficiencies.

   Key members of the multi-disciplinary team are:
   - Specialist bariatric dietitian.
   - Bariatric surgeon.
   - Bariatric physician.

   If needed there should also be access to other health care professionals such as:
   - Psychologist.
   - Cardiologist.
   - Respiratory physician.

Dietetic and Nutrition Case Studies, First Edition.
Edited by Judy Lawrence, Pauline Douglas, and Joan Gandy.

Companion Website: http://www.manualofdieteticpractice.com/

3. - How often does she vomit?
   - Does she have any nausea or pain?
   - Are her bowels open regularly?
   - What other medications does she take?
   - Does she take a vitamin and mineral supplement?
   - Has she returned work? If so:
     - What times are her meal breaks?
     - How long does she get for each break?
4. - What is her understanding about her diet after surgery?
   - What food texture has she struggled with and what can she cope with?
   - What size portions does she have?
   - How fast does she eat?
   - Does she eat regular meals?
   - Does she eat and drink at the same time?
   - What is her understanding about vitamin and mineral supplements?
   - Is she aware of dumping syndrome and its possible causes?
   - Does she have a strong support network from family and friends?
   - Other influences on food choices and cooking such as cultural, religious family or financial influences.
5. Inadequate dietary intake of protein (problem) related to restricted food intake (aetiology) characterised by food intolerances and regurgitation (signs/symptoms).
6. - Patients may not have been appropriately assessed and prepared for surgery.
   - Patients may not have sufficient information about the procedure they have had.
   - Dietary information and advice in a foreign language or poorly translated.
   - There may be no follow-up included in the package.
   - If follow-up is available it may be too difficult to access because of the distance.
7. To improve nutritional intake by:
   - providing information about appropriate food textures and portion sizes for this stage after surgery;
   - discussing practical tips on how to improve the quality of her diet;
   - discussing the gastric bypass and how it impacts on nutrition;
   - discussing appropriate eating behaviours such as:
     - eating slowly;
     - chewing food well;
     - stopping before she feels full;
     - not eating and drinking at the same time; and
     - having a regular meal pattern.
   - discussing and addressing barriers to change such as how to fit meals and drinks into her working day; and
   - negotiating and agreeing dietary changes.
8. Her current diet is of poor nutritional quality.
   - Offer practical advice on the type of foods and meals with the appropriate texture for this stage after surgery.

- Offer advice on increasing the protein intake of her diet.
- Discuss alternative sources of protein that may be better tolerated at this stage.
- Focus on regular meals.
- Explain why it is preferable not to eat and drink at the same.
- Discuss portion sizes.
- Discuss the risk of having 'soft calories' that are easily tolerated.
- Discuss the benefits of increasing her physical activity.
- Discuss fluid intake and appropriate drinks.

9. Rates of weight loss vary considerably depending on initial weight, type of surgical procedure, age, gender and level of activity/mobility. In addition, patients will have periods when weight loss plateaux and they can become quite anxious. It is much better to get patients to think of their weight loss over a prolonged period of time; 'it took them a long time to gain weight and they won't lose it overnight!' Patients should be encouraged to focus on the quality of their diet (including protein), their portions' sizes, new eating behaviours, mindful eating and being as physically active as possible.
10. - Does she have her operation notes or any information about her surgical procedure?
    - What advice has she been given about her diet after surgery?
    - What is her current eating pattern?
    - Is her fluid intake adequate?
    - How often does she vomit/regurgitate and is it associated with anything in particular?
    - What medication is she taking?
    - Does she check her blood glucose levels?
    - Is she taking any vitamin and mineral supplements?
    - Is she using any contraception?
11. Currently, she is unlikely to be meeting her micronutrient requirements.
    - She needs to improve the overall quality of her diet and paying special attention to protein and calcium foods as well as fruit and vegetables.
    - She should start taking a complete multivitamin and mineral supplement.
    - She may also need to take additional iron, calcium and vitamin D supplements and regular vitamin B_{12} injections.
12. - A small pouch is made at the top of the upper stomach, which is then anastomosed to the proximal jejunum bypassing the duodenum as shown in Figure 31.1.
    - Malabsorption of calcium, iron, vitamin B_{12} and vitamin D may occur.
    - There is some debate about the absorption of medicines after surgery and patients are advised not to rely on the oral contraceptive pill alone but to use additional forms of contraception such as the barrier method and so on.
13. Surgical complications are possible in the short term (anastomotic leak, incisional hernia, bleeding, etc.) and the long term (stricture, obstruction, anastomotic ulcer) and require immediate referral back to the bariatric centre.

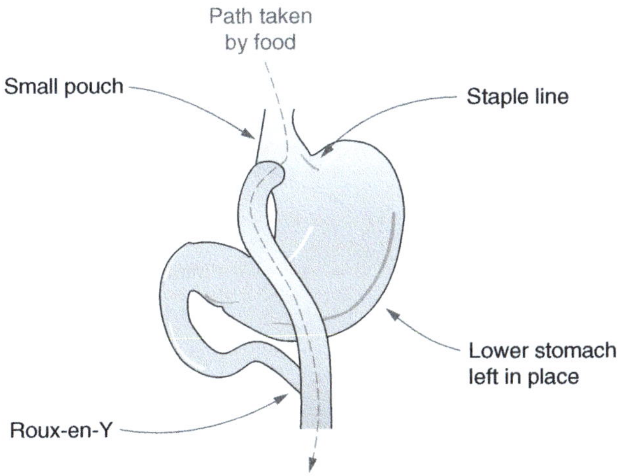

Figure 31.1 Roux-En-Y-Gastric bypass. The National Bariatric Surgery Register: First report 2010 – Dendrite Clincial Systems Ltd

Nutritional complications are possible usually as a consequence of poor quality diet, food intolerances and reduced intake. For example:

- Protein malnutrition (if continual low protein intake).
- Risk of iron deficiency anaemia.
- Vitamin B_{12} and vitamin D deficiency.
- Thiamine deficiency (with persistent vomiting).
- Smaller risk of zinc and copper deficiencies.

14. Intragastric balloon (Figure 31.2), adjustable gastric band (Figure 31.3), sleeve gastrectomy (Figure 31.4), duodenal switch (Figure 31.5).

15. A change in some gut hormones (e.g. glucagon like peptide 1) following this procedure may induce remission of type II diabetes

- Weight loss will improve diabetes control.
- Patient may be able to reduce or stop metformin.
- Patient should be encouraged to follow a healthy balanced diet.

16. Make use of the dietitian's counselling skills such as:

- Being non-judgemental.
- Displaying empathy.
- Building rapport.

17.
- Fear of not losing weight or re-gaining weight.
- Fear of eating because of vomiting/regurgitation.
- Not having had a good experience with dietitians in the past.

  Can overcome barriers by:
  - Being non-judgemental and displaying empathy.
  - Building rapport.
  - Offering practical and objective advice.
  - Using behaviour change skills.

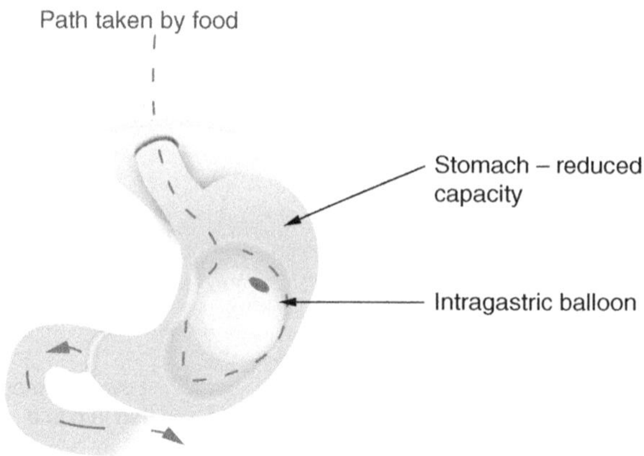

Figure 31.2 Intragastric balloon. The National Bariatric Surgery Register: First report 2010 – Dendrite Clincial Systems Ltd

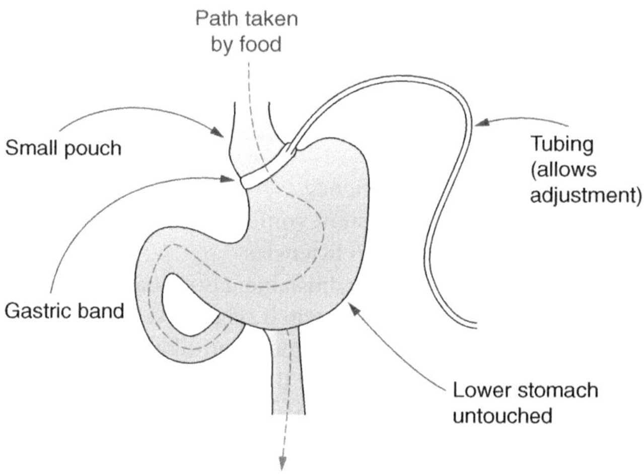

Figure 31.3 Adjustable gastric band. The National Bariatric Surgery Register: First report 2010 – Dendrite Clincial Systems Ltd

18. • Follow-up appointment for one month:
- Contact details so Abi can get in touch if her symptoms become worse or she has increasing difficulties with eating and drinking.
- Encourage her to keep a food and symptom diary and bring it to the next appointment.
- Arrange appropriate blood tests if they have not been done for sometime.

19. • Ask Abi what she would like to achieve in the short and long term.
- Discuss realistic weight loss.
- Pregnancy and improvement in diabetes are likely to be raised.

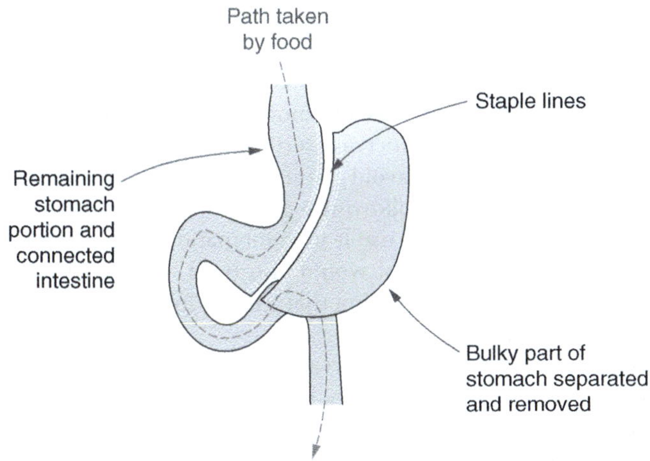

Figure 31.4 Sleeve gastrectomy. The National Bariatric Surgery Register: First report 2010 – Dendrite Clincial Systems Ltd

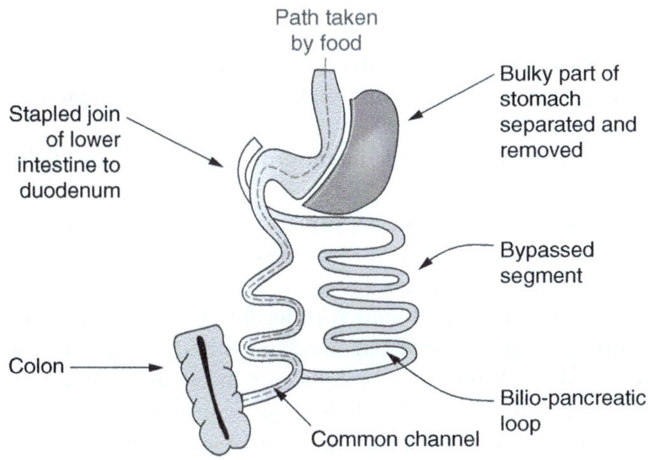

Figure 31.5 Duodenal switch. The National Bariatric Surgery Register: First report 2010 – Dendrite Clincial Systems Ltd

20. Commissioning of bariatric surgery requires patients to be discharged back to their GP's care 2 years after surgery. GPs need to ensure that these patients have regular blood test (6 monthly) in order to exclude any nutritional deficiencies. GPs also need to monitor the patient's weight and ensure that they are taking a complete multivitamin and mineral supplement. Any problems that are thought to be related to bariatric surgery warrant a referral back to the bariatric service.

Long-term follow-up with a specialist bariatric dietitian is essential; follow-up with bariatric physician if needed.

Answers to further questions

21. Pregnancy is not encouraged within the first 18 months after surgery because this is the period of fastest weight loss and mother and baby could be compromised nutritionally. Weight loss can increase fertility and it is important that Abi uses some form of contraception to avoid getting pregnant. There is some debate about the absorption of medication following a gastric bypass and if Abi is using an oral contraceptive then she should use it in combination with other contraceptives such as the barrier method. Abi would also need to take additional folic acid pre-conception. There is a suggestion that 5 mg of folic acid may be required but the evidence base is poor.
22. There is some evidence that the 'starvation phase' of weight loss that occurs in the early stages after bariatric surgery increases the risk of small for gestational age (SGA) infants. There is also a suggestion that there is an increased risk of pre-term birth. Poor nutritional status of the mother (if non-compliant with supplements) may also impact the nutritional status of the foetus (Abeezar *et. al.*, 2012; CMACE/RCOG, 2010; Kaska *et.al.*, ; Norgaard *et. al.*, 2014; Siega-Riz *et.al.*, 2009).
23.
   - Abi would need general advice on her overall diet with particular attention to protein, iron and calcium intake.
   - She should be given practical advice to ensure she gets sufficient calories.
   - Abi will need to change to a multivitamin and mineral supplement specific for pregnancy.
   - She should periodically check foetal growth and consider liaising with her obstetric team.
   - Small, frequent meals or snacks can usually help alleviate the nausea that accompanies morning sickness. Dry foods in particular are quite good. Some women respond well to ginger (as in plain ginger biscuits or ginger tea).
24. Obese women often have problems with fertility mainly because of disturbances in ovulation (anovulation and oligoovulation) and an increased risk of PCOS (Jeannes, 2014). As little as 5% weight loss in obese PCOS patients improves spontaneous ovulation rates. The following factors are thought to be involved: reduced insulin resistance, decreasing levels of androgens and stabilising levels of sex hormones (NICE, 2010).
25. Bariatric surgery is an effective treatment option, which aids weight loss, reduces co-morbidities and mortality and improves quality of life. Patients who have undergone bariatric surgery experience improvements in diabetes and lipid profiles and are more physically active when compared with an obese control group (Abeezar *et.al.*, 2012; Buchwald *et. al.*, 2004; O'Brien *et. al.*, 2013; Sjostrom *et.al.*, 2004, 2007).
26. As morbid obesity is associated with co-morbidities such as diabetes and sleep apnoea, there are high costs to the health service economy; therefore, preventing and/or treating obesity-related co-morbidities results in cost savings. When considering the appropriateness of a patient's case for bariatric surgery, the MDT will consider the associated health benefits of such surgery against the risks of either going ahead or not with surgery (NICE, 2006; NHS England, 2013; Office for Health Statistics, 2010; Picot *et. al.*, 2009).

CASE STUDY 32
Stroke and dysphagia

Answers

1. Smoking, high blood pressure, obesity BMI > 30, raised total cholesterol and total cholesterol: HDL ratio >4.
2. Acquired swallowing difficulty (problem) related to cardiovascular accident (aetiology) characterised by inadequate dietary intake (signs and symptoms).
3. To provide a textured modified diet that meets Anne's nutritional and hydration requirements in a safe way.
4. Ensure that high risks foods are not served. Ensure that the appropriate texture of food is served. Ensure that the patient remains hydrated. Ensure that small frequent meals and snacks are served. Educate Anne and her family and any other health care professional as to the appropriate foods to eat and how to fortify dishes to increase the energy density and nutrient intake in small volumes, the appropriate use of thickener and the importance of maintaining a posture that ensures safe feeding.
5. Coming to terms with the modified texture, how the food is presented, food choice as it may be limited because of being in an acute setting and may not fully take into account Anne's likes and dislikes, reduced appetite because of medical condition, patient taking food they know they can eat safely and getting used to foods and fluids thickened to the correct consistency. What are the alternatives to foods Anne would normally consume, for example, bread can be soaked in milk or other liquid.
6. Thicken fluids to the appropriate consistency, ensure that fruit and vegetables are included in the meal plan and that thickened drinks are available between meals.
7. Essential to record in-patients records at time of initial intervention, at regular intervals and when any change to the original plan (either because of change in persons medical condition or as nutritional intake improves).
8. Initially, changes to her swallowing ability; changes in anthropometric measurements; food and fluid intake.

   Longer term – anthropometric measurements, biochemistry.
9. Not initially but when/if her swallow returns to normal then re-assess.

Dietetic and Nutrition Case Studies, First Edition.
Edited by Judy Lawrence, Pauline Douglas, and Joan Gandy.

Companion Website: http://www.manualofdieteticpractice.com/

10. Team work is essential to optimise outcomes. To monitor any changes in swallow, to ensure rehabilitation happens around meals times, to ensure correct tools to optimise nutritional intake, for example, non-slip mats, drinking cups. Be involved in ward rounds, multidisciplinary team meetings, case conferences and so on as relevant. Ensure that all dietetic interventions are recorded in the patient's care notes. Ensure continuity of care both in acute and community care settings. Other relevant health care professional staff include speech and language therapist, physiotherapist, occupational therapist, radiographer, social services, nursing and medical teams (both acute and community).
11. Food shopping – reduced mobility therefore difficulties with shopping.

    Identification of appropriate foods to modify to the correct texture, Meal preparation of energy-dense foods – how to make foods more nourishing, freezing and storage, reheating,
    - Cooking facilities.
    - Cooking skills – how to overcome the difficulties in preparing food.
    - Potential difficulties self-feeding.

Answers to further questions

12. Stop smoking, consume more than five portions of fruit and vegetable, moderate blood pressure by reducing salt intake, achieve a healthy weight, increase the intake of $n-3$ fats by consuming 1–2 portions of oily fish per week.
13. Yes, grapefruit should be avoided when taking simvastatin but not other statins (BNF, 2014).

CASE STUDY 33
Hypertension

Answers

1. Excessive dietary intake of sodium (problem) related to over consumption of salted and processed foods (aetiology) characterised by raised blood pressure. (signs and symptoms).
2. 26.8 kg/m^2.
3. In Stage 1 hypertension, clinical blood pressure is 140–159 mmHg systolic blood pressure and 80–99 mmHg diastolic blood pressure, subsequent average blood pressure measured at home is 135/85 mmHg or higher. In Stage 2 hypertension, clinical blood pressure is 160–179 mmHg systolic blood pressure and 100–109 mmHg diastolic blood pressure, and subsequent average blood pressure measured at home is 150/95 mmHg or higher.
4. Cardiovascular disease is a leading cause of death for people with diabetes. Diabetes doubles the risk of cardiovascular disease, causing nearly 60% of deaths in patients with diabetes.
5. A waist circumference of greater than or equal to 94 cm is associated with increased risk of morbidity and a waist circumference of greater than or equal to 102 cm is associated with a substantially increased risk of morbidity for men. The figures for women are 80 and 88 cm, respectively. For Asian men, a waist circumference of greater than or equal to 90 cm is associated with a substantially increased risk of morbidity, for Asian women a waist circumference greater than 80 cm is associated with substantially increased risk of morbidity.
6. Poorly managed high blood pressure is associated with stroke and heart disease. People with hypertension are twice as likely to die from stroke and heart disease as people whose blood pressure remains within normal levels. Reducing blood pressure by just 10 mmHg reduces stroke risk by 41%.
7. The aims of the dietary intervention are to reduce John's blood pressure by reducing sodium intake and increasing potassium intake. Lifestyle intervention would include reducing alcohol intake and potentially increasing exercise levels. SMART aims should be negotiated with John but might include:

Dietetic and Nutrition Case Studies, First Edition.
Edited by Judy Lawrence, Pauline Douglas, and Joan Gandy.

Companion Website: http://www.manualofdieteticpractice.com/

- Swapping cheese for fruit for all desserts by the next appointment;
- Increasing fruit and vegetable consumption to four portions daily by the next appointment;
- Eliminating bar snacks by the next appointment;
- Not adding salt to food in restaurants by the end of next month and not adding it at home by the end of the following month (if appropriate);
- Reducing alcohol consumption by $1/3^{rd}$ by the 3-month mark; and
- Reducing blood pressure by 10 mmHg within 6 months.

8. The exact nature of the intervention should be agreed with John. It is likely that swapping cheese for a fruit-based dessert and avoiding bar snacks would be the easiest changes to make. If salt is being added at the table, it would be good to target this when John is feeling confident about his ability to change his habit, potentially after being successful with the first two changes.
9. Lifestyle changes that help prevent and manage hypertension include reduction of alcohol intake and increased exercise. Alcohol should be taken with food to reduce its effect on blood pressure. A small intake of alcohol may be cardio-protective. John may find it helpful to keep a diary to monitor his intake of alcohol. No assessment has been made of John's activity levels, although it is likely that he is active as his BMI is not as high as might be expected from the diet history. Activity levels should be addressed at a future appointment. The DASH diet used increased consumption of fruit and vegetables, low-fat dairy food, wholegrain cereals, nuts and seeds to increase levels of potassium, calcium, magnesium, protein and fibre, whilst restricting sugar and saturated fats to manage hypertension.
10. The main sources of salt in John's diet appear to be the cheese, crisps, nuts and bar snacks and the ham sandwiches; his high consumption of restaurant food is likely to contribute to his salt intake as well. No assessment has been made regarding the use of added salt at the table; this would need to be evaluated as it could be a big contributor to John's sodium levels.
11. Repeated diet history and blood pressure measurement could be used to monitor and evaluate the intervention.
12. Barriers to change would include the work-related nature of John's food consumption and the potential lack of control over the amount of salt added to restaurant food. John could be helped to overcome these barriers by discussing potential alternatives to lunch-based meetings and alternatives to restaurant meals in the evening when travelling. If John is adding salt at the table then it would be helpful to discuss the time taken for taste preferences to alter, strategies for adding alternative flavour to foods and re-shaping habitual behaviours.
13. The referral letter should include enough information from your assessment and intervention to enable a new dietitian to take over the treatment. John's permission must be obtained before disclosing details. It would be good practice to copy both John and his GP into the letter.

CASE STUDY 34
Coronary heart disease

Answers

1. Male gender, positive family history of CHD, smoker, hypercholesterolemia, overweight with abdominal obesity, hypertension and alcohol.
2. The main considerations of a cardio-protective diet are fruit and vegetables, saturated fat, salt, carbohydrates, stanols and sterols, nuts, soluble fibre, soya protein, dietary cholesterol and alcohol.
3. Troponin T and I are proteins released into the blood when the cardiac muscle is damaged during a myocardial infarction (MI). Levels are negligible in a non-MI patient. Troponin increases gradually after an MI and is repeated 6–12 h after onset of symptoms. The level is related directly to the amount of muscle damage.
4. Additional information:
   - How easy will it be to introduce changes in cooking and meal preparation?
   - Does Jonathan add milk and sugar to his tea and coffee?
   - Saturated fat – there is no information about dairy products currently in his diet history. For example, what type of spread does Jonathan use, What type of milk (if any) does he use?
   - What type of fat is used in cooking?
   - What type of meat does he eat – does he use lean cuts, cut fat off, take skin off chicken and so on?
   - Fruit and vegetables – explore whether Jonathan eats any additional fruit and vegetables in his diet – for example does he add vegetables when cooking curry/bolognaise, how many portions of vegetables does he eat with an evening meal of meat, potatoes and vegetables?
   - Wholegrains – does Jonathan use any wholegrain options such as wholemeal pasta or brown rice?
   - Salt – when cooking meals, are stock cubes or salty sauces and so on used?
5. Excessive dietary intake of fat (problem) related to lack of information about a cardio-protective diet (aetiology) characterised by abdominal obesity (signs and symptoms)

Dietetic and Nutrition Case Studies, First Edition.
Edited by Judy Lawrence, Pauline Douglas, and Joan Gandy.

Companion Website: http://www.manualofdieteticpractice.com/

6. • Reduce waist circumference by 5 cm in 2 months.
   • Reduce intake of saturated fat.
   • Reduce salt intake.
7. Jonathan may be apprehensive regarding the perceived restrictions of a cardio-protective diet and may feel that changing or reducing foods and drinks he is used to and enjoys could leave him feeling deprived. He may be concerned that it will take longer to shop and cook, or it may be more expensive to choose healthier options. His wife does the cooking and he may be concerned with whether or not she will support dietary changes.
8. Weight loss would be encouraged as Jonathon's BMI puts him in the overweight category. He also has a waist circumference in the high-risk category, which is a strong indication of cardiovascular risk. The benefits of weight loss include improvements in lipid profile, reduced blood pressure, lowered all-cause, cancer and diabetes mortality, improved glycaemic control, reduced risk of type 2 diabetes and reduced osteoarthritis-related disability (SIGN, 2010). These factors should be discussed with Jonathan and his motivation for making changes to achieve weight loss should be explored.
9. Gather information regarding cooking methods and check intake of foods high in salt. Discuss aims to decrease salt intake to less than 6 g/day.
   • Common sources of salt include processed foods, sauces, cheese and salty snacks such as crisps and nuts.
   • Discuss choosing lower salt alternatives for packaged food, aim to stop adding salt during cooking and at the table.
   • Discuss alternative flavouring such as herbs and spices that can be used.
   • Discuss adaptation of taste buds to a reduction in salt intake.
10. It is recommended to reduce salt intake as salt is composed of sodium chloride, which contributes towards high blood pressure. Both rock/sea salts and table salt are approximately 100% sodium chloride and therefore rock salt should not be used as an alternative to table salt. It is better to try and gradually adjust to the taste of food without salt, and use other herbs and spices for flavour (CASH, 2014).
11. Moderate alcohol intake (1–2 units/day) is thought to help protect CHD in men over 40 years and post-menopausal women. However, it is known that women who persistently drink over three units of alcohol per day and men who drink more than four units are more likely to suffer from conditions such as hypertension, which is an independent risk factor for cardiovascular disease. It is therefore advisable for Jonathan to reduce his alcohol intake.

    The current government guidelines are given as daily, rather than weekly amounts, for example, over the weekend, to limit excessively heavy drinking. This type of excessive drinking, binge drinking, is known to be harmful and can cause problems such as abnormal heart rhythms or an enlarged heart (cardiomyopathy). The current recommendations are no more than 3–4 units/day for men and no more than 2–3 units/day for women. Two to three alcohol-free days are also encouraged.

As Jonathan should be encouraged with losing weight, it would be beneficial to discuss the energy content of alcohol and how reducing his intake would also help in weight loss.

12. Jonathan is taking atorvastatin, which interacts with grapefruit juice. He should therefore be advised to avoid grapefruit and its juices (Hinchliffe and Green, 2014; BNF, 2014).

13. After taking of the diet history you should discuss his diet and his weight and what the benefits of change would be. Ask Jonathan to consider his motivation to make changes. Jonathan chooses to focus on losing weight, reducing salt intake and reducing alcohol intake as he feels these are the most important to him.

14. Depending on the frequency that you can review Jonathan within your services, it would be useful to promote self-monitoring of his goals, for example, keeping food diaries and self-reviewing these. Encourage Jonathan to self-monitor his weight and waist circumference. You may wish to discuss with Jonathan if there are any local slimming groups or dietetic services that he could self-refer to or that you could refer him to, if he would find this type of support beneficial. Encouraging Jonathan to discuss his goals with his wife and friends and family to gain social support can help compliance. Suitable outcome measures might include waist circumference, BMI, lipid profile and blood pressure.

Answers for further questions

15. Discuss with Jonathan that studies of supplementation with high doses of folic acid (Hinchliffe & Green, 2014), vitamin E (Kris-Etherton *et al.*, 2004) and garlic (Rahman & Lowe, 2006) have not shown reductions in cardiovascular disease incidence; however, a healthy balanced diet high in vitamins and minerals should be encouraged (Hinchliffe & Green, 2014).

CASE STUDY 35
Haematological cancer

Answers

1. On admission, Terry had a BMI of 20 kg/m^2. According to PENG guidelines, this is borderline between underweight and desirable (Todorovic & Micklewright, 2011). Based on his usual weight of 68 kg and his admission weight of 61 kg he has a clinically significant weight loss of 10.4% in less than 2 months (Todorovic & Micklewright, 2011). His current weight of 70 kg was not taken into consideration because of the likelihood that he is fluid overloaded as medications include furosemide. Terry's weight has increased by 9 kg during admission. Weight shifts are common in this patient group because of large intravenous infusions given during treatment as well as changes in organ function. The dietitian would need to consider loss of lean body mass and how to measure this for future reviews. Consider the use of other anthropometric measurements like grip strength (Beckerson, 2014).
2. As a standard practice, energy requirements should be calculated using predictive equations, which are adjusted for stress and activity factor.
   Basal metabolic rate is calculated using the Henry (2005) equations as recommended by PENG (Todorovic & Micklewright, 2011). Estimated dry weight is used; therefore, in this case admission weight was used.
   $11.4 \times 61 + 313 \times 1.75 + 113 = 2198\,\text{kcal}$
   Using current PENG guidelines the current stress factor to add for leukaemia is 25–34%.
   In addition, an activity factor is added. This will differ between patients depending on how mobile they are. Point to consider is that these patients are in isolation, which may limit their activity levels even if mobile.
   Calculating nitrogen requirements as recommended by PENG (Todorovic & Micklewright, 2011). Patient is as hypermetabolic, therefore use a nitrogen range of 0.2–0.3 g N/kg/day.
   Therefore, requirements are 12–18 g N/day.

Dietetic and Nutrition Case Studies, First Edition.
Edited by Judy Lawrence, Pauline Douglas, and Joan Gandy.

Companion Website: http://www.manualofdieteticpractice.com/

3. Risks specific to this patient group:
   - Infection.
   - Bleeding.
   - Malnutrition.
   - Psychological.
   - Mucositis.
   - Gastrointestinal side effects.
   - Dysgeusia.
   - Anorexia/satiety.
   - Electrolyte and fluid imbalances.
   - Organ failure.

   It is essential to consider the risks associated with the diagnosis of AML, the impact of high dose chemotherapy, further medical intervention as well as the psychological factors during active treatment. Subsequently, this will affect nutritional status and potentially increase the risk of malnutrition and impact nutritional interventions.

   Some specific risk factors to be considered are:
   - Organ toxicity – high dose chemotherapy can cause gastrointestinal, renal, bladder, pulmonary, cardiac, neurological and hepatic complications, which can lead to organ failure.
   - Neutropenia and persistent infectious complications – increased risk of bacterial sepsis, pneumonia and fungal infections having effect on morbidity and mortality, and consequently impacting nutritional requirements further. Consider side effects of antimicrobial, antifungal and antiviral medication, which may further hinder oral intake. Increased isolation and hospital institutionalisation if prolonged and multiple hospital admissions, may affect psychological well-being. Implications of neutropenic dietary restrictions on a diet that is already nutritionally compromised also need to be considered.
   - Electrolyte and fluid imbalances – commonly exacerbated by chemotherapy, antimicrobials, antiviral, corticosteroids medication, additional intravenous fluids, increased output secondary to vomiting and diarrhoea, and malnutrition with minimised oral intake.
   - Fatigue and bleeding – caused by anaemia caused by reduced red blood cells or increased bruising and bleeding resulting from thrombocytopenia (low platelets). Repeated blood and platelet replacement may be required via intravenous infusions. Consider meal pattern on reflection of sleep patterns if heightened fatigue. In addition, if considering enteral nutritional intervention, liaise with medical teams regarding the appropriate baseline range of platelets required prior to inserting nasogastric or nasojejunal feeding tubes.
   - Dietary related side effects – mucositis affecting any part of the gastrointestinal tract resulting in mouth or throat pain, ulceration, abdominal pain, nausea vomiting and diarrhoea. Dysgeusia, anorexia and early satiety can further compromise and impact overall nutritional intake resulting in malnutrition.

4. Inadequate energy intake (problem) related to reduced food consumption secondary to chemotherapy (aetiology) evidenced by clinically significant weight loss of 10.4% weight in less than 2 months (signs/symptoms).
5. The dietary aim is to optimise nutritional intake, minimise the risk of malnutrition and significant weight loss during active treatment.
6. To provide therapeutic dietary advice according to dietary-related side effects and neutropenic dietary advice during neutropenic periods.
   - Answer should include a discussion of the rational for optimising nutritional intake with focus on calorific and protein-dense oral intake with the patient, as well as the consideration of the role of oral nutritional supplements to meet increased nutritional demands. Realistic goal setting with consideration to patient's dietary and beverage preferences. Also focusing neutropenic dietary advice around this, providing suitable practical alternative options to include and prevent further restriction of oral intake.
   - Explore causes and trends for dysgeusia, anorexia and early satiety. Discuss practical dietary strategies to enhance oral intake.
   - Liaise with catering staff, nursing staff and family/friends as appropriate to support oral intake.
   - Summarise SMART aims, goals and dietary advice with patient and set follow-up plans to assess and review advice and compliance.
7. The important biochemical results are:
   - Albumin – the patient's albumin levels are below the normal range. A decrease in albumin levels may be the result of decreased synthesis, increased catabolism (use and loss), or a combination of these. Albumin cannot be used as an independent indicator of nutritional status. The most common cause of decreased plasma albumin levels is related to the inflammatory processes (i.e. acute-phase response and chronic inflammatory disorders).
   - CRP – the patient's CRP is raised. CRP is an acute-phase protein and the levels of CRP will fluctuate during treatment. From examining the biochemistry and the patient's clinical status, the patient also has a low neutrophil count and raised temperature. Using these clinical parameters along with CRP value it would indicate that the patient has neutropenic sepsis.
   - Magnesium and phosphate – these two minerals are below the normal range. Mineral losses are common and can be exacerbated by antimicrobials and immune-suppressive drugs. Terry is on two antimicrobials. Tumourlysis syndrome in which cells are destroyed in response to chemotherapy causes potassium and phosphorous to move into the vascular space. Diarrhoea can also contribute to losses of fluid, sodium, magnesium and potassium. Terry is on Loperamide, which would indicate possible diarrhoea which in turn could have also contributed to low electrolytes and minerals. Chemotherapy is likely to be the main reason to contribute to shifts in electrolytes and minerals.
   - Platelets, neutrophils, haemoglobin, white cell count – all are below the normal reference range. Chemotherapy drugs work by attacking cells that are dividing quickly; this has an effect on non-cancer cells in the body including the bone marrow. This therefore leads to increased risk of infection as a result of low

white blood cell count and low neutrophils, easy bruising or bleeding because of low blood platelets and fatigue because of low red blood cells.

8. Acute myeloid leukaemia (AML) is a rare type of cancer. It is more common in people over 65 years. In AML, too many early myeloid cells are produced. In most types of AML, the leukaemia cells are immature white blood cells. In some less common types of AML, too many immature platelets or immature red blood cells are produced. For more information on AML and treatment implications see Beckerson, 2014).
9. Points to consider (Beckerson, 2014):
   - Young family.
   - Travel distance for friends and family.
   - Being in isolation.
   - Unable to provide income for family.
   - Future family plans.
   - Fertility.
   - Weight loss and body image.
   - Hair loss.
   - Spiritual needs.
10. The patient has identified concern around neutropenia, therefore establish current understanding of neutropenia and specific queries regarding diet. Ensure dietary advice is tailored to patient's needs, addressing all the concerns raised.
    Discuss rationale for neutropenic diet, dietary restrictions are recommended to reduce the risk of infection without significantly compromising nutritional intake. Provide written information on neutropenic dietary advice for patient's reference and to discuss with family/relatives as required. Discuss hospital and catering provision for neutropenic diet.
    Terry's diet is currently nutritionally inadequate and includes foods that are not advised during neutropenia such as salad and probiotic yoghurt. Discuss practical alternatives with patient to replace food and beverages according to dietary preferences to ensure that oral intake is not further compromised.

Answers to further questions

11. The side effects from transplant conditioning protocols can be more severe and last longer than those experienced during induction chemotherapy this is dependent on (see Figure 35.1):
    The extent and severity of any side effects are dependent on:
    - Whether the transplant is autologous or from a donor.
    - Whether it is a related or an unrelated donor.
    - The type of conditioning used in particular for donor transplants whether the conditioning regimen is myeloablative or reduced intensity.
      A reduced intensity conditioning protocol is less likely to cause mucositis.
    - Consider advising a prophylactic NGT prior to the development of severe mucositis if a myeloablative regimen is being used.

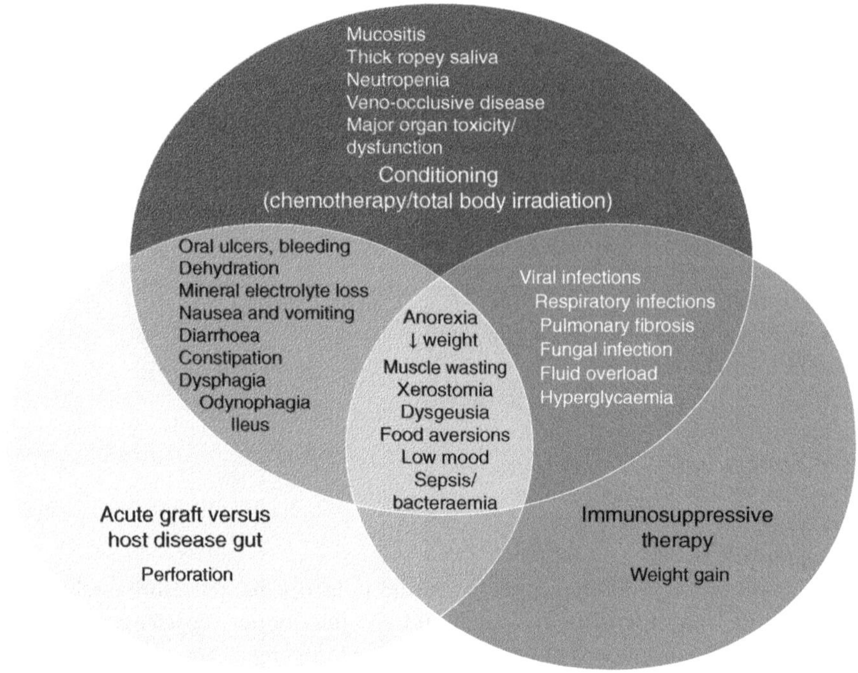

Figure 35.1 Side effects of stem cell transplant impacting nutritional status. (Gandy (2014, Figure 7.15.2). Reproduced with permission from Wiley Blackwell.)

- Consider how emetogenic the proposed conditioning regimen is. A naso-jejunal tube may be more appropriate if significant vomiting is a risk.
- An explanation of parenteral nutrition may be appropriate for patients having a myeloablative donor transplant.

  Side effects of SCT impacting nutritional status are shown in Figure 35.1.

12. Additional points to be considered:
    - Platelet counts – local practice will vary but many clinicians will not insert NG tubes when platelets are below 50. In some centres a platelet count of 20 and a top-up infusion of platelets is acceptable.
    - Mucositis – if present, mucositis may prevent NGT insertion due to the risk of pain, bleeding or further damage to the inflamed or ulcerated mucosa. However, mucositis to grade 2–3 will not prevent placement as long as the patient agrees to placement and the platelets are at an acceptable level.
    - GI side effects – will inform the choice of feed in terms of its composition, volume and rate.
    - Choice of tube – post-pyloric feeding may be preferred if the patient is experiencing nausea and/or vomiting. NGTs may be placed in patients who are struggling with loss of appetite and poor intake, who are not vomiting.
      - Choice of feed – standard, elemental, semi-elemental according to GI symptoms.

- Treatment plans – you will need to alter your feed regimen to allow for scans or radiotherapy. Overnight feeding may have fewer interruptions.
- Drug–nutrient interactions;
  - Will the feed time affect any of the medications the patient is taking.
  - Bisphosphonates – food and feed reduces absorption, therefore give the dose at least 2 h after feed or food and allow at least 30 min before re-starting the feed.
  - Penicillin – most commonly prescribed penicillins are unaffected with the exception of phenoxymethylpenicillins and ampicillin.
  - Phenytoin – absorption significantly reduced by enteral feeds. Use alternative anti-epileptic or allow a 2-h break before and after phenytoin dose. Monitor levels closely.
  - Quinolone antibiotics, for example, ciprofloxacin – bind to divalent ions in enteral feed to varying degrees. Ciprofloxacin has the most pronounced interaction with a 60% reduction in peak levels if co-administered with feed. Where possible, use an alternative antibiotic. Administer the dose during a break in the feed. Quinolones are usually administered twice daily.
  - Tetracyclines – absorption reduced by 70–80% in the presence of milk or dairy products. Stop feed an hour before and after administered.

13. Low magnesium is likely to be multifactorial. Any discussion should include the following:
    - GI side effects – in particular, malabsorption and diarrhoea.
    - Inadequate oral intake – Note many foods rich in magnesium are limited by neutropenic dietary advice (e.g. leafy vegetables, nuts and seeds). Patients requiring a soft diet are also likely to be eating less fibrous foods and more processed foods both of which are likely to lower dietary magnesium intakes.
    - Oral magnesium supplements are poorly tolerated; hence, IV supplementation required.
    - Medications
      - That decrease Mg absorption, for example, proton pump inhibitors, antibiotics.
      - That increase its excretion, for example, diuretics, immunosuppressants, particularly cyclosporine, antifungals particularly ambisome and laxatives.

CASE STUDY 36

Head and neck cancer

Answers

1. Other assessments required:
    - Current medical management of symptoms.
    - Support John will receive at home with enteral feeding (family and district nursing as appropriate).
    - John's dexterity.
    - Estimated nutrient intake.
    - Body mass index (BMI).
    - percentage of weight loss.
    - Anthropometrics, such as grip strength dynamometry.
    - Speech and language therapist review.
2. Biochemistry:
    - Urea – assess hydration.
    - Phosphate, magnesium, potassium – assess refeeding risk.
    - Low haemoglobin – possible cause of fatigue.
    - Other tests
        - C-reactive protein as albumin is low;
        - HbA1C and blood glucose.
3. Henry (2005) or Clinical Oncological Society of Australia (COSA) (Findlay *et al.*, 2011) can be used as long as the practitioner is able to justify their use.

    Use COSA if BMI in normal range:
    - Energy 30 kcal/kg;
    - Protein 1.2 g/kg; and
    - Fluid 30 mL/kg.

    If the BMI is outside the normal range, Henry or Schofield equations can be used. A stress factor would need to be added although these are always an estimate.
4. Reduced oral intake and alcohol abuse.
5. Medical interventions
    - Mouth washes and mouth care advice, for example, salt water mouth washes, difflam, lidocaine gel.
    - Analgesia.

Dietetic and Nutrition Case Studies, First Edition.
Edited by Judy Lawrence, Pauline Douglas, and Joan Gandy.

Companion Website: http://www.manualofdieteticpractice.com/

- Secretion management, for example, carbocysteine, nebuliser, H_2O_2.
- Skin care.
- Fluids.
- Blood transfusion to ensure haemoglobin above 120 g/L.

6. Inadequate oral intake (problem) related to side effects of radiochemotharapy (aetiology), characterised by 19.8% weight loss in past 3 months (7.2% weight loss in past month) – signs and symptoms.
7. Aims
   - Prevent further weight loss and maintain present weight.
   - Maintain and improve nutritional status with adequate fluids, energy, protein.
   - Reduce risk of refeeding syndrome.
   - Meet daily nutritional requirements.
   - Maintain oral intake.
   - Swallow exercises.
   - Ensure John understands the importance of continuing to take food/fluids orally.
   - Good blood sugar control.
8. The aims could be achieved with nasogastric tube (NGT) feeding and encouraging oral intake (Nugent, 2010). The following would implement the intervention:
   - Liaise with medical team, recommend NGT placement, provide justification;
   - Discuss this with John and obtain consent for nasogastric tube placement;
   - Liaise with ward nursing staff to place NGT;
   - Calculate nutritional requirements;
   - Discuss feeds with John and provide enteral feeding regimen for ward staff;
   - Liaise with ward doctor to discuss risk of refeeding and initiate hospital refeeding policy;
   - Request 4 h glucose monitoring whilst enteral feed is established; and
   - Document intervention.
9. To meet Health & Care Professions Council requirements of professional practice and to ensure that everyone involved in John's care are aware of the implementation.
10. Liaise with the following HCPs (Talwar & Donnelly, 2011):
    - Community dietitian – dietetic care after hospital discharge.
    - Pump company nurse – training for John on tube care and use of the infusion pump.
    - Nursing staff – training on medication and liaison with district nurses for support at home.
    - Clinical nurse specialists – support at home.
    - Speech and language therapist – assess swallow and ensure patient has swallowing exercises.
    - Medical team – adequate management of symptoms.
    - Physiotherapy and occupational therapist – fatigue management.
    - District nursing team – support with enteral feeding at home.
11. Swallowing exercises should start at the beginning of radiotherapy as they become critical when a patient is unable to manage adequate or any solid food.

12. Potential barriers
    - Inadequate home support
    - Colour blindness and ability to undertake pH testing safely
    - Ensuring adequate district nursing support.
13. Outcome measures
    - Weight, grip strength – to assess nutritional status.
    - Quantity of enteral and oral nutrition consumed to ensure patient meets nutrition prescription.
    - Frequency of swallowing exercises.
    - Documentation of oral diet/fluids consumed.
    - Biochemistry to evaluate hydration status and electrolyte levels.
    - General condition.
    - Tolerance to enteral nutrition.
    - Stool charts.
    - Urine output.
    - Position of nasogastric tube.
    - Condition of nasogastric tube and nasal passages.
    - Oral intake – solids.
    - Fluid balance charts.
    - Blood results U&Es.
    - Weight, grip strength.
    - Volume of feed given.
    - Name of feed given.
    - Medication.
    - Blood sugars and onward referral to diabetes team if required.
    - Frequency of swallowing exercises.
14. Minimum of fortnightly (Findlay *et al.*, 2011)

Answers to further questions

15. Both Carboplatin and radiotherapy may reduce haemoglobin and cause anaemia. Carboplatin may reduce platelets, increase urea, creatinine and lower magnesium and potassium. Sometimes it is difficult to determine if a patient has refeeding syndrome as a result of chemotherapy-induced deranged electrolytes.
16. There are a number of toxicity scoring systems available including RTOG, (Radiation Therapy Oncology Group, 2014) WHO and CTCAE (Cancer Therapy Evaluation Program, 2010). All have limitations particularly when evaluating nutrition problems. CTCAE is the most comprehensive system and probably can be tailored to head and neck cancer treatment related toxicity.
17. Enteral feeding should commence when a patient is at risk of malnutrition and has an inadequate oral intake (National Institute for Health and Clinical Excellence, 2006; Talwar & Findlay, 2012). In practice, this is open to interpretation. ESPEN guidelines state oral intake of 60% and predicted continued poor oral intake for >10 days. In practice, <75% of requirements is used as a measure of inadequacy as this would equate to about 0.5–1 kg (1–2 lbs) of weight loss per week.

18. Some clinicians advocate that patients with adequate pre-treatment swallow function and oral intake have pre-treatment gastrostomy tubes and continue with oral diet during treatment until they are no longer able to take adequate amounts of oral diet to maintain nutritional status. Others offer patients with adequate pre-treatment swallow function the option of continued oral feeding, until they are unable to take adequate oral nutrition to maintain nutritional status and then proceed with (reactive) passage of an NG tube.

Systematic reviews have failed to demonstrate evidence for functional, nutritional, quality of life or health economic benefit of either approach; UK practice is variable. The NIHR TUBE trial started in 2014. This feasibility trial randomises patients to prophylactic gastrostomy or reactive nasogastric feeding. This two-year study will provide further information on the most appropriate method of enteral feeding in this patient population.

19. As a result of previous heavy alcohol intake John may need gastroenterology assessment to ensure that there was no evidence of liver damage and associated complications such as portal hypertension and varices.

John would need appropriate, timely management of warfarin (anticoagulant) to ensure his international normalised ratio (INR) (a monitor of anticoagulation effectiveness) is at an appropriate level for gastrostomy insertion.

20. Discuss prophylactic gastrostomy placement at time of diagnosis and place prior to commencement of oncological treatment.

Explain benefits of gastrostomy and when enteral nutrition is planned to start.

Work closely with speech and language therapist to ensure that swallowing exercises are implemented, thereby reducing risk of tube dependency post radiation therapy (RT).

21. Set up specialised service for this patient group involving HNC dietitian and nutrition nurse.

Regular monitoring and review by HNC dietitian in the community.

Ensuring good communication between HNC dietitian with primary and tertiary services.

22. Regular *Back to eating* groups promoting rehabilitation post RT treatment. Work with speech and language therapists, clinical nurse specialist and clinical psychologist.

23. Long term side effects are as follows:
- Management of xerostomia;
- Dental decay and the importance of good oral hygiene;
- Lymphedema; and
- Monitoring swallow.

24. Health and well-being sessions.

25. Your discussion should include the following issues:
- Nutritional status;
- Effect of treatment;
- Body image;
- Medication;
- Quality of life;
- Tube dependency;

- Complications;
- Community support; and
- Financial implications.

  Table 36.1 gives information about gastrostomy and nasogastric feeding tubes to help with decision making (NB: This table is not exhaustive).

26. Risk factors (Talwar, 2011):
    - Patient factors including previous alcohol intake and risk of portal hypertension.
    - Patient's ability to care for feeding tube.
    - Nutritional factors including degree of malnutrition.
    - TNM factors.
    - Treatment modality.
    - Radiation/chemoradiation, dose and field size and expected duration of enteral tube use.
    - Surgery including impact on ability to eat as well as any further proposed treatment.

Table 36.1 Information about gastrostomy and nasogastric feeding to help with decision making.

	Gastrostomy	Nasogastric
Nutritional status	Less degree of weight loss	Greater degree of weight loss
Effect on treatment	Patients have fewer hospital admissions and continue their treatment uninterrupted Associated with reduced set up variations whilst receiving radiotherapy	Easy and quick to place so may lead to less interruptions during treatment Less likely to cause an infection which may delay chemotherapy
Body image	Hidden away and concealed beneath clothing	More visable
Medication	Easy to administer	Difficult to administer and more likely to block; so unable to administer feed
Quality of life	Can improve physical well-being, ability to meet nutritional needs as well as providing relief of pressure when experiencing fatigue	More inconvenient, uncomfortable and has a greater impact on family life and social activities
Tube dependency	May lead to higher risk of tube dependency as less motivated to return to oral intake	Some studies have shown a reduction in number of days fed
Complications	Procedure complications of mortality, bleeding, peritonitis, sepsis, abscess, tumour seeding from PEG Ongoing complications of site infection, buried bumper, damaged tubes	Tube displacement Tube blockage Tube placement into the lung and risk of death
Community support	Many patients are able to self-care with a gastrostomy as it requires less aftercare	More community support required
Financial	Expensive to insert	Cost of caring for tube including district nurse support, replacement tubes and X-rays not calculated

27. Most NHS trusts have adopted a trust wide policy for refeeding syndrome; these guidelines should always be followed.
28. It is very difficult to differentiate and therefore it is best to treat the patient as if they are suffering from refeeding syndrome (particularly if the patient has risk factors such as reduced or intake, etc.) in the preceding few days and be mindful that chemotherapy may also be a contributing factor.

CASE STUDY 37
Critical care

Answers

1. The metabolic response to critical illness involves muscle breakdown to amino acids for gluconeogenesis and protein synthesis for the immune response and tissue repair. There is an increased demand for energy, proteins, and micronutrients. These mechanisms are mediated by cytokines and the counter regulatory hormones catecholamines, glucagon and cortisol. This results in a loss of body mass; most notably body protein.
2. Inadequate oral food and fluid intake (problem) related to inability to eat and drink (aetiology) as evidenced by intubation and sedation (sign/symptom).
3. An individualised enteral feeding plan was provided to meet her nutrient and fluid needs. A commercial feed, for example, Jevity Plus providing 1.2 kcal/mL with fibre should be used at an infusion rate of 63 mL/h. Over 24 h, this provides 1800 kcal, 84 g protein, 70.5 mmol sodium and 71.1 mmol potassium.
4. International guidelines (Kreymann *et al.*, 2006; Singer *et al.*, 2009; McClave *et al.*, 2009). recommend using 25 kcal/kg – 25 kcal × 65 kg – 1625 kcal. However, this does not reflect her age, gender or illness severity. Therefore, it may be more accurate to use the Henry (2005) equation to predict basal metabolic rate (BMR) adding a factor for stress (SF) and activity (AF) to make it more specific.

   Daily energy requirements (Henry, 2005)

$$\text{BMR } 9.7 \times 65 \text{ kg} + 694 = 1325 \text{ kcal} + 10\% \text{ AF} + 20\text{–}30\% \text{ SF for TBI}$$

$$= 1722\text{–}1855 \text{ kcal}$$

   Protein

   Can be calculated using the (McClave *et al.*, 2009; Singer *et al.*, 2009) recommendation

$$1.2\text{–}1.3 \text{ g/kg} - 78\text{–}85 \text{ g protein/day}$$

$$\text{Or } 0.2 \text{ g N2} \times 65 \text{ kg} - 13 \text{ g N2} \times 6.25 - 81 \text{ g protein/day}$$

Dietetic and Nutrition Case Studies, First Edition.
Edited by Judy Lawrence, Pauline Douglas, and Joan Gandy.

Companion Website: http://www.manualofdieteticpractice.com/

5. • Disease state;
   • Surgery;
   • Infection;
   • Sedation;
   • Paralysis; and
   • Inactivity.
6. • Hypernatraemia is common in critically ill patients especially those with a TBI. It is highly unlikely to be caused or influenced by the sodium content of enteral feeds. Reasons for hypernatraemia in TBI include:
   • Large insensible losses such as sweating.
   • Diabetes insipidus.
   • Osmotic diuretics to treat cerebral oedema.
   • Diarrhoea, vomiting, large GI aspirates.
   • Hypertonic saline administration.
   • Primarily need to treat the cause of the hypernatraemia; that is, if there is fluid depletion give additional water via the NGT or IV fluids. There is a relatively small difference in the sodium content of normal feeds versus low sodium feeds, which will not have a significant bearing on plasma sodium levels; therefore, changing the enteral feed sodium content is not recommended.
7. • Most admissions to ICU are emergencies with no known weight or height.
   • Patients are bedbound and immobile, so obtaining an accurate weight and height is challenging. Some ICU beds have an ability to weigh but these weights need to be interpreted with caution due to oedema, fluid retention and ICU equipment on the bed.
   • If present, fluid accumulation in upper limbs will make MUAC inaccurate.
   • Surrogate measures have not been validated for use with critically ill patients and are therefore best used as a guide only.
   • Sedated patients would be unable to use handgrip strength, and patients are often too weak or confused on waking from sedation to perform this.
8. • Gastrointestinal intolerance such as large gastric aspirates, diarrhoea or vomiting.
   • Fasting for extubation or tracheostomy, surgery, diagnostic tests, physiotherapy, NGT pulled out.
9. The most commonly accepted method is to measure gastric residual volumes (GRVs) or large gastric aspirates. These are used as a marker of gastric emptying and assumed to reflect enteral feed intolerance. In addition, monitoring nausea, vomiting, abdominal distension and discomfort. Not all patients in ICU are heavily sedated and some, if lightly sedated, can indicate that they are in abdominal discomfort or pain.
10. Regular administration of prokinetic agents, which increase gastrointestinal motility. Metoclopramide and erythromycin are the most frequently used. Both drugs in the intravascular format have been found to promote gastric emptying (Dhaliwal *et al.*, 2014). Post-pyloric enteral feeding is considered an effective way of overcoming large GRVs, reducing the risk of aspiration. However, it can be a challenge to get these tubes successfully inserted (Dhaliwal *et al.*, 2014).

11. • To review gastrointestinal tolerance to feeding.
    • To monitor gastric residual volumes, episodes of vomiting (sedated, paralysed and ventilated patients are all able to vomit).
    • To re-visit predicted equations for energy on next review. Patients on ICU change clinical conditions hour by hour and therefore it is very important to re-visit energy predictions at least twice a week. Clinical parameters that would influence energy expenditure, that is, stress factors and activity, needs to be considered. If using the Penn State equation, as many ICU dietitians now do, you should definitely do this a few times a week.
    • To review in 2 days.
    • Volume of feed delivered.

Answers to further questions

12. • International societies (Kreymann *et al.*, 2006; Singer *et al.*, 2009; McClave *et al.*, 2009) have recommended 25 kcal/kg (Cerra *et al.*, 1997; Singer *et al.*, 2009). It is quick and easy to use; however, it is not age-, gender-, or condition-specific and there is ambiguity over which weight to use. As a result of these factors it has a very low accuracy rate when compared with measured energy expenditure (MEE) (Frankenfield *et al.*, 2009).
    • Henry (2005) with stress factors (SF) has the advantages of being familiar and also gender-, age-, disease- and activity-specific. Devised from data from healthy individuals and relies on the use of SFs to make it clinically applicable. The SFs for ICU are based on outdated ICU practices that have improved considerably and therefore the SF may not reflect the current impact on metabolic rate. This predictive equation does not reflect clinically meaningful ICU parameters that are known to have an impact on EE.
    • Ireton-Jones (Ireton-Jones *et al.*, 1992) is probably the best known ICU-specific equation. It was developed on burns and trauma patients and includes factors for trauma and burns patients. It is gender- and age-specific. However, when validated against indirect calorimetry it has been shown to be inaccurate. It overestimates in non-obese and underestimates in obese patients (Frankenfield *et al.*, 2009).
    • The Penn State University equation (Frankenfield *et al.*, 2004) is gender-, age- and height-specific. It includes clinical parameters specific to ICU that have an impact on MEE (temperature and ventilation settings). It is significantly more accurate than other equations (Frankenfield *et al.*, 2009) but requires knowledge of mechanical ventilation and ventilator settings. However, it does not capture physical activity, so as patients recover it may be appropriate to add an activity factor.
    • The Harris & Benedict (1919) equation was derived from healthy individuals. It is widely used outside of the United Kingdom, despite the lack of evidence to support its use. There are different versions in use that incorporate factors for disease state and activity, aiming to make them clinically applicable. It has

not been shown to be accurate in critically ill patients and is not therefore recommended by the American Dietetic Association (Frankenfield *et al.*, 2007).

13. The Penn State equation is currently the best validated equation in critically ill (Frankenfield *et al.*, 2009) patients with the highest accuracy compared to other equations. It takes age, gender and clinical parameters into consideration.

14. Critical illness is associated with an acute state of insulin resistance and hyperglycaemia. It is believed to be related to the metabolic effects of sepsis and injury including the role of proinflammatory cytokines. It is thought to occur secondary to raised endogenous production or exogenous provision of insulin antagonists, such as noradrenaline, adrenaline, cortisol and glucagon (Bessey *et al.*, 1984).

15. Medications shown in Table 37.1

Table 37.1 Medication used in ICU.

Drug	Rationale for use on ICU	Nutritional considerations
Atracurium	Paralysing agent – used to allow better synchronisation with the ventilator in patients with severe respiratory failure. Also used to manage raised intracranial pressure in severe TBI	Decreases energy expenditure and gut motility
Propofol 250 mg/h	Sedation agent – used to keep the patient safe and comfortable whilst being ventilated. It can also treat pain Propofol is effective in TBI patients as it is fast acting but also wears off quickly; hence, neurological status can be assessed	Contributes additional energy of 1 kcal/mL Risk of fat overload
Fentanyl	Opioid analgesia and sedation agent	Can cause constipation and decrease gut motility resulting in reduced gastric emptying
Noradrenaline	Vasoconstrictor or vasopressor – used to increase blood pressure and increase heart rate by stimulating alpha receptors in walls of peripheral blood vessels to constrict and narrow	High doses cause a reduction of hepatic, renal and splanchnic blood flow Can lead to enteral feeding intolerance and risk of gut ischaemia
Insulin – sliding scale	To treat critical illness-associated insulin resistance and hyperglycaemia	Caution when enteral nutrition is held to avoid hypoglycaemia
Sodium docusate	Laxative used to treat constipation	Enteral nutrition is often considered a cause of diarrhoea. Therefore need to check that diarrhoea is not result of repeated doses of laxative
Lansoprazole	Proton pump inhibitor used to inhibit gastric acid secretion. Used for stress ulcer prophylaxis in critically ill patients	Alters pH and can make NG tube placement confirmation by pH paper unreliable
Phenytoin IV	Anticonvulsant	If given via the enteral route requires a break from feed for drug absorption

16. Propofol is in a lipid solution that provides 1 kcal/mL. It is provided as mg/h; therefore, you need to convert mg to mL (10 mg = 1 mL/h). Propofol comes in 1% and 2% solutions.

- In this case
  - 1% – 250 mg/h = 25 mL × 24 h = 600 mL/kcal
  - 2% – 250 mg/h = 12.5 mL/h × 24 h = 300 mL/kcal
- You need to decide how much energy from propofol you would consider detrimental and lead to overfeeding complications. There is no agreed standard and it may vary on a patient-to-patient basis. Most dietitians will take it into consideration especially if the amount exceeds 200 kcal/day for a prolonged period. If the propofol provides 200 or more kcal per day it may be appropriate to change to a feed that delivers a higher protein to energy ratio and reduce the energy delivered by the feed by 200 kcal.

17. There is no universally agreed definition for a large GRV; however, currently 250–500 mL is the accepted value for a large aspirate, instigating treatment. (Dhaliwal *et al.*, 2014). The REGANE study (Montejo *et al.*, 2010) compared GRV cut offs of 200 mL versus 500 mL (intervention group). The mean enteral feed delivery was significantly higher in the intervention group. The incidence of pneumonia, duration of mechanical ventilation and ICU length of stay was similar in both groups. Increasing the volume of the GRV cut-off to 500 mL was not associated with worse complications or outcomes and can be equally recommended as a normal limit for GRV.

CASE STUDY 38
Traumatic brain injury

Answers

1. Anthropometry
    - Mid-upper arm circumference (MUAC) and calf circumference (CC) – distribution of weight and nutritional status;
    - Body mass index – nutritional status;
    - Usual weight – pre-injury nutritional status;
    - Family reported height – compare ulna height accuracy Smith *et al.*, (2011).

   Biochemical/haematological
    - Urea – renal function, hydration status;
    - Haemoglobin – iron status, anaemia;
    - Calcium (corrected) – deficiencies, risk of refeeding syndrome (RS);
    - Magnesium – deficiencies, risk of RS;
    - Phosphate – deficiencies, risk of RS;
    - Estimated glomerular filtration rate – renal function NICE (2006).

   Clinical
    - Tracheostomy secretions – colour and viscosity can indicate infection/hydration Morris *et al.* (2013);
    - Medications dose and time – fluid required, drug–nutrient interactions, nutrients provision from medications;
    - Oedema – inaccurate weight.

   Dietary
    - Volume of IV fluids – fluid and electrolyte provision;
    - Religious or cultural beliefs – enteral feed choice;
    - Emergency NG feeding started – early nutrition provided;
    - Previous dietary intake – RS risk, nutritional adequacy pre-injury.
2. Day 1
    - Glucose and CRP high, albumin low – inflammatory response to TBI;
    - LFTs high – liver function may be affected by TBI (Sanfilippo *et al.*, 2014).

   Day 7
    - Sodium and urea upper limit of normal – possible dehydration. Note that one-off result should be repeated.

Dietetic and Nutrition Case Studies, First Edition.
Edited by Judy Lawrence, Pauline Douglas, and Joan Gandy.

Companion Website: http://www.manualofdieteticpractice.com/

Table 38.1 Outcome measures.

Outcome measure	Frequency	Justification
Weight	Weekly	Nutritional status, % weight loss (NICE, 2006)
MUAC	Fortnightly	
Consciousness	1–2 days	Alertness alters energy requirements
CRP, WCC	Daily	Inflammatory response, infection
Sodium, potassium, urea	Daily	Kidney function, hydration status
Glucose	Daily	Hyperglycaemia and hypoglycaemia is damaging for the brain (London Health Sciences Centre, 2012)
Tracheostomy secretions	Daily	Fluid losses, infection, (Morris *et al.*, 2013)
Gastric aspirates	Daily	Gastric motility, absorption of feed, (Stroud *et al.*, 2003)
Fluid balance	Daily	Hydration status
Temperature	Daily	Fluid and sodium requirements
Stool charts	Daily	Monitor for malabsorption and diarrhoea relating to antibiotic use and for any effect of antibiotic use
Perspiration episodes	1–2 days	Hydration status, autonomic storming (McLaughlin & Moore, 2014)
Skin integrity	2–3 days	Pressure ulcer increased nutritional requirements

- CRP high but trend reducing, albumin low but increasing – acute inflammation phase improving.

Day 14
- Sodium and urea high – dehydration, reduced kidney function;
- CRP increased further and WCC high – probable infection.

3. Inadequate enteral nutrition infusion (problem), related to starting the nutrition infusion (aetiology) characterised by weight loss (signs/symptoms) (McLaughlin & Moore, 2014).
4. The aim of the dietetic intervention is to minimise obligatory losses to LBM in the catabolic stage.

   Outcome measures – illustrated in Table 38.1
5. Enteral feeding regimen

   Energy

   Basal metabolic rate (BMR) (Henry, 2005)

   16×72 (weight) $+ 545 = 1697 + 509$ (30% stress factor) $+ 170$ (10% activity factor) $= 2376$ kcal/day

   Protein

   Nitrogen

   0.2×72 (weight) $= 14.4$ g/day $\rightarrow$ Total protein $= 14.4 \times 6.25 = 90$ g/day

   Fluid and electrolytes

   Fluid

   35×72 (weight) $= 2520$ mL/day $+$ (Pyrexia) 2×72 (weight) $= 144$ mL/day

Table 38.2 NG feeding regimen.

Day	Feed	Rate	Hours	Provides (24 h)
1	1.5 kcal/mL	25 mL/h 50 mL/h	10 10 Rest 4 (Phenytoin)	750 mL, 1125 kcal and 45 g protein (plus IV fluid)
2	1.5 kcal/mL + 1 × 25 mL 4.5 kcal/mL bolus	75 mL/h	20 Rest 4 (Phenytoin)	1525 mL, 2363 kcal and 90 g protein (plus IV fluid)

Total = 2664 mL/day

Sodium 1 × 72 (weight) = 72 mmol/day + (Pyrexia) 1.5 × 14 = 21 mmol/day = 93 mmol/day

Potassium 1 × 72 (weight) = 71 mmol/day

Minerals

Calcium – 17.5 mmol/day

Magnesium – 12.3 mmol/day

Phosphate – 17.5 mmol/day

Medication

- Interactions – feed needs to be stopped before and after phenytoin (BNF, 2014);
- Nutrient provision – sodium provided from IV fluids.

Treatment

- Therapy input and nursing care, for example, position changes, respiratory care;
- NG feeding regimen shown in Table 38.2.

6. Enteral nutrition not optimised to requirements (problem) related to increased perspiration, loose stools catabolism and autonomic storming from TBI (aetiology) characterised by raised sodium, urea, CRP and WCC 7.1% weight loss, cloudy urine of lower volume, (signs/symptoms).
   Changes to feeding regimen
   - Estimate nutritional requirements again with new weight and alter feeding regimen.
   - Increase fluid for a positive fluid balance and minimise further urinary infections.
7. - Medical – blood tests, fluid needs;
   - Nursing – feed provision, monitoring fluid, bowels, gastric aspirates, weight;
   - Speech and language therapy, physiotherapy, occupational therapy – time off feed for therapy sessions.
8. Consent
   - Day 1–13
     - Assess capacity (Department of Health, 2005);
     - Unlikely to have capacity to consent (Triebel *et al.*, 2012);
     - Every effort should be made to obtain the opinion of family and friends;
     - Treat in best interests.

- Day 14 onwards
  - May have capacity (Triebel *et al.*, 2012);
  - May respond to simple commands such as finger movement or blinking;
  - Assess capacity regularly to exclude coincidence responses;
  - Follow speech and language therapist's communication guidelines.
- Documentation is important with respect to the following:
- To demonstrate that you are working within the standards of conduct, performance and ethics (HCPC, 2008);
- Evidence that you fully assessed patient capacity;
- Evidence that you involved family/friends with the best interest decision in the absence of capacity;
- Possibility of intermittent capacity thus recording decision making process provides insight into TBI staging.

9.
- Reflect and assess progress using outcome measures detailed above.
- Weight – return to normal or not;
- Reflect on dietetic involvement and document in professional portfolio.
- Present as a case study.

10. For diagnosis – GCS categorises the severity of a brain injury (SIGN 2009). GCS score mild (13–15) moderate (9–12) or severe (<9) (Haydel *et al.*, 2013).

Prognosis – used alongside CT scan assessment (NICE, 2014) GCS predicts an inverse relationship between GCS and rate of mortality. Mild, moderate and severe TBI is 0.1%, 10% and 40% mortality, respectively (Haydel *et al.*, 2013). GCS can be used as a predictor of outcome (Ting *et al.*, 2010).

11. Transgastric post pyloric tube

There is evidence that TBI patients suffer gastrointestinal symptoms for example vomiting (Wang *et al.*, 2013; Pinto *et al.*, 2012). In rehabilitation TBI patients may progress to gastrostomy feeding (McLaughlin & Moore, 2014). Access to the small bowel and stomach with one stoma site is beneficial for the patient and cost-effective to the NHS. Alcohol is a contributory factor for TBI (NICE 2014). The causes of TBI in the UK are:

- Falls – 35%;
- Motor vehicle-related injury – 17%;
- Non-intentionally being struck by or against an object – 16%; and
- Assaults – 10%. (Haydel *et al.*, 2013)

12. Up to ⅔ of TBI patients have a history of alcohol abuse or high risk drinking and almost ½ of American TBIs are alcohol related (Bombardier & Turner, 2009). Therefore, nutrition education targeting alcohol related TBI risk may help to reduce its incidence if it was given similar precedent to smoking cessation legislation. Government funding and endorsement by national supermarkets would be essential to tackle one of the primary causes of TBI. However, the impact of nutrition education would be difficult to assess.

13. Acute

- Critical care nutrition assessment;
- Responding quickly to an unstable critical patient;
- Assist in preventing secondary brain injuries;

- Minimise significant lean body mass loss;
- Minimise gastrointestinal intolerances;
- Work with the complex care nutrition support multidisciplinary team (Consultant, Pharmacist, Nutrition Nurse);
- Establish an artificial nutrition feeding regimen;
- Transfer to a rehabilitation dietitian;
- Promote good nutrition care within critical care unit – policy, training, resources;
- Rehabilitation;
- Rehabilitation nutritional assessment;
- Review and manage the nutritional impact from ongoing TBI side effects, for example, spasticity/contractures, inhibition, autonomic dysfunction, ageusia/dysgeusia, memory impairment and personality changes;
- Facilitate transition from artificial nutrition support to oral diet in liaison with SLT;
- Promote a long-term eating for health plan, for example, healthy eating, nutrition support, weight reduction, enteral feeding and texture modification;
- Work with specialist rehabilitation multidisciplinary team (SLT, OT, Physiotherapy, Art and Music Therapists, Consultants, Psychology, Mental Health specialists, TBI charities) to promote independence and integration back into the community;
- Where necessary, employ modified communication under guidance from SLT, to include the TBI patient with decision making; and
- Promote good nutrition care within rehabilitation unit – policy, training, resources.

CASE STUDY 39

Spinal cord injury

Answers

1. • Tricep skinfold thicknesses can be measured but his high levels of upper body muscle mass prior to injury followed by enforced bed rest and denervation below the level of injury can produce deranged results that may not be associated with inadequate nutritional intake.
   • Blood zinc levels may be useful to ascertain whether supplementation is required to aid healing of the pressure ulcer.
   • Results of swallowing assessments would indicate if a reduction in enteral feed is possible.
2. Acquired swallowing difficulty (problem) related to traumatic brain injury (aetiology) as evidenced by rapid weight loss (sign/symptom).
3. • To ensure that nutritional requirements are met and rate of weight loss is reduced.
   • To ensure that the enteral feed contributes to improved bowel management with less frequent and more formed stools.
   • To ensure that times of feeds do not hinder rehabilitation.
4. • Discuss feeding times to ascertain whether he would prefer increased breaks in the feed, adding in boluses or an overnight feed.
   • Suitable longer term feeding routes should be discussed to seek his views on gastrostomy feeding.
5. • Documented feeding regimen.
   • Gradual introduction of an enteral feed that contains fibre with regular monitoring of bowel motions to ascertain the exact amount of fibre required.
   • Gradual increase of feeding rate to introduce increasing rest periods. By monitoring Stan's hunger he will be able to vocalise whether bolus feeds are required during the day or just an overnight feed.
6. Written feeding regimen should be provided for nursing staff. Full, signed and dated information should be provided in the medical notes and in dietetic records.
7. • Speech and language therapists to monitor ability to swallow and texture requirements for oral intake.

Dietetic and Nutrition Case Studies, First Edition.
Edited by Judy Lawrence, Pauline Douglas, and Joan Gandy.

Companion Website: http://www.manualofdieteticpractice.com/

- Physiotherapists to monitor chest secretions and levels of possible physical activity.
- Occupational therapists to help determine what adaptations may be required for future care.

8.
- Predictive equations have shown to over-estimate energy requirements by approximately 10% following spinal cord injury (Monroe *et al.*, 1998). If using Henry (2005) equations aim for a lower range, 10% stress and 10% activity factors would be the most to be added.
- As the patient is ventilated, if equipment is available, indirect calorimetry would be useful to identify exact nutritional requirements.

9.
- There is considered to be 9 kg obligatory weight loss with tetraplegia (Cox *et al.*, 1985). This is because of loss of possible muscle mass below the level of injury and may not be an indicator of malnutrition. It is associated with the denervation below the level of injury and enforced bed rest. It is important to check that nutrition is not a contributing factor.
- The weight loss for Stan could have been more dramatic as he had a heightened level of muscle mass prior to the injury.
- Evidence suggests that within a year post injury most spinal cord injured patients have increased their body weight above ideal weight (de Groot et al., 2010). Overfeeding in the acute phase may not be beneficial in the long term.

10. Bowel management is difficult in patients with spinal cord injuries. Transit times are reduced and over use of fibre containing feeds can increase transit times rather than reducing them (Cameron *et al.*, 1996). Whilst increasing the fibre content of the feed may be beneficial, it may be best to have some of the feed containing fibre and some not.

11. NICE guidelines state that evidence is not consistent for specific recommendations on additional protein to promote healing of pressure ulcers. Correction of any deficiency is required (NICE, 2014). American (ADA, 2013) guidelines indicate an increased need of protein, 0.2 g additional protein/kg body weight for a grade three pressure ulcer, but were based on consensus statements. Micronutrients such as vitamin C and zinc need consideration. However there is insufficient evidence for exact recommendations (NICE, 2014).

12.
- Changes in medical condition – monitor nausea, vomiting, bowel movements.
- Changes in psychological state as he copes with changing body shape.
- Changes in medication – For example antibiotics that may be introduced to treat an infection could affect his bowel management.
- Chest physiotherapy may require a rest in feeding and the frequency of which indicate whether there is any aspiration of feed that may require post pyloric feeding or changes in feeding position.
- Weekly weighing.
- Outcomes from swallow assessments.
- Healing of skin condition, frequency of turns in bed. If frequency increases it would indicate further deterioration in skin condition.

13. Platform scales that take a bed or a wheelchair (note that bed or chair need to be subtracted from weight) can be used. If appropriate, a weighing hoist can be used.

Answers to further questions

14. Long-term energy requirements for tetraplegics are low because of the lack of energy expenditure. Recommendations are for 22.7 kcal/kg/d (Cox *et al.*, 1985). This intake needs to be reduced further if weight loss is required.
15. Stan will have upper motor neurone (UMN) or reflexic bowel syndrome. This results in the loss or impairment of the sensory perception of the need to defecate and the loss or impairment of voluntary control of the external anal sphincter. Chemical stimulants are commonly used with UMN and therefore a softer stool is required. A high fibre intake with adequate fluids may therefore be helpful.

CASE STUDY 40

Burns

Non-ventilated scald injury in an elderly patient

Answers

1. Unintentional weight loss (problem) related to reduced intake and likely secondary to pre-admission acute and chronic illness (chest infection, confusion) and social circumstances, exacerbated by acute burn injury and medication side effects (aetiology) characterised by greater than 10% body weight loss over 4 months (signs/symptoms).
2. Oral intake of approximately 650 kcal, 25 g protein and 600 ml fluid.
3.
   - Specific overall goal is to provide a nutrition support intervention, which will preserve nutritional status and hydration as far as possible, thereby optimising wound healing and functional rehabilitation.
   - To minimise loss of lean body mass.
   - To optimise wound healing.
   - To provide longer term nutritional support beyond discharge.
4.
   - Maintenance of energy, protein and fluid intake against estimated nutritional and hydration requirements – analysis of food record charts and fluid balance charts.
   - Weight maintenance – whilst recognising the influence of presence and resolution of oedema in these patients.
   - Investigation to exclude anaemia as having a potential nutritional cause. If it is nutrition related (e.g. dietary folate or B12 deficiency) then treatment and monitoring of iron and vitamin levels long term, likely as an outpatient.
5. It is important to use the normal ranges of the laboratory where the measurements were taken. Although laboratories undergo extensive quality control there, will be some variation in the normal ranges. All biochemical and haematological measures should be interpreted using clinical judgement.
6. Raised urea suggests dehydration as a result of hypovolaemia secondary to burn exudates losses and pre-admission illness (reduced fluid intake)

Dietetic and Nutrition Case Studies, First Edition.
Edited by Judy Lawrence, Pauline Douglas, and Joan Gandy.

Companion Website: http://www.manualofdieteticpractice.com/

- Hypoalbuminaemia secondary to transcapillary escape and also burn exudate loss (protein rich) in a setting of inflammation.
- Raised WCC and CRP reflecting inflammatory response.
- Low Hb, high MCV (macrocytic anaemia) pre-admission – exclude dietary deficiency as the cause if history can be obtained from patient or proxy: folate, vitamin B12 deficiency or deficiency of both as a result of dietary inadequacy. The medical history as presented does not suggest other identified causes such as excess alcohol intake, Coeliac disease, pernicious anaemia or malignancy but these may require further investigation to be excluded. Anaemia may be a contributory or sole factor in her pre-admission confusion and would have contributed to her kettle scald accident.

7. • Patient is not sedated or on mechanical ventilation; therefore, use the Ireton-Jones equation for estimated energy expenditure for spontaneously breathing patients:
  - $IJEE = 629 - 11(A) + 25(W) - 609(0)$;
  - Where A = age (years), W = weight (kg), O = obesity (1 if present, 0 if absent);
  - Therefore: $629 - 11(80) + 25(69) - 609(0) = 1474$ kcal/day.

8. • Metabolic: Inflammatory response will increase energy and nitrogen requirements as a result of hormonal and cytokine-mediated effects leading to hypermetabolism and muscle proteolysis, even though this injury may not be classed as a major burn. Loss of micronutrients may occur via wound exudate. Secondary inflammatory hits are also possible from subsequent infection with the loss of skin barrier.
- Functional: on-going confusion, acute illness related anorexia, alien environment, injuries and dressings to arms limiting manual dexterity for eating/drinking.

9. • Ensure nursing staff are completing ongoing nutrition screening tool, food charts, fluid charts.
- Assistance with mealtimes via nursing staff.
- Functional assistance and input from occupational therapists to optimise activities of daily living, for example, cup and utensil modification.
- Physiotherapists to assist with mobilisation and weighing as part of monitoring.

10. All records should be completed as soon as possible after the consultation, at least by the end of the working day.

11. • Set up social services assessment through the MDT recommendations (dietitian, physiotherapist, occupational therapist) – as poor coping at home already identified pre-burn.
- Consider meals on wheels, frozen or microwave meals.
- Patient to be followed up in community by dietitian to ensure appropriate transition from a high protein–high energy approach to diet to longer term healthy eating to manage her chronic disease.

CASE STUDY 41

Telehealth and cystic fibrosis

Answers

1. Assessment

Anthropometry	Weight 58 kg Height 1.8 m BMI 18 kg/m^2
Biochemistry	Sodium 149 mmol/L Potassium 4 mmol/L Phosphate 0.73 mmol/L Corrected calcium 2.11 mmol/L Magnesium 0.8 mmol/L Albumin 25 g/L C reactive peptide 100 mg/L
Clinical	Cystic fibrosis Influenza Medication Creon Zantac Tobramycin Timentin Occasionally VITABDECK
Environmental	Student, shared house with friends

2. • Check compliance with enzymes and vitamins.
   • Undertake a thorough assessment of dietary intake and match this to his enzyme intake. The dietitian should focus on obtaining a detailed diet history and try to determine fat intake at each meal and snack and calculate the amount of lipase taken with each gram of fat. Poor distribution or omission of enzymes can increase malabsorption (Stapleton et al., 2006, CF Trust, 2002).

Dietetic and Nutrition Case Studies, First Edition.
Edited by Judy Lawrence, Pauline Douglas, and Joan Gandy.

Companion Website: http://www.manualofdieteticpractice.com/

- Check Justin's social circumstances to ensure he is able to access adequate nutritious foods and that he has the knowledge, time and facilities for meal preparation.

3. - As he has not attended the tertiary hospital, it is likely he has not had his annual screening for vitamin levels and glucose tolerance and bone mineral density.
   - Vitamin A, D, E and K – as CF patients malabsorb fat despite pancreatic enzyme replacement these vitamins may also be malabsorbed.
   - Numerous factors can affect biochemistry results for vitamins, including seasonal variations and illness and inflammation (Stapleton et al., 2006). Ideally, vitamin levels should be taken when the patient is clinically stable but as he is a poor attendee it would be good to suggest these, if possible.
   - Cystic fibrosis related diabetes mellitus is a frequent complication of CF as patients get older and is often associated with weight loss; hence, testing for glucose tolerance is essential during this illness.
   - An assessment of fat malabsorption could be made by testing the amount of fat in the stool, through faecal microscopy. Additional tests of malabsorption may be available.
   - Bone mineral density is also usually monitored annually as osteopenia and osteoporosis are common complications of CF due to malnutrition, vitamin D deficiency, lung disease and steroid use (Stapleton et al., 2006; CF Trust, 2002).
4. - The Henry (2005) equations could be used to estimate energy requirements.
   - Generally, it is thought that 120–150% of normal requirements are needed for people with CF. This is variable between individuals.
   - The reasons for this increase include a degree of malabsorption, increased work of breathing, anorexia and decreased intake during exacerbations, and an abnormal adaptive response to malnutrition (CF Trust, 2002).
5. - Unintentional weight loss (problem) related to CF and viral infection (aetiology) as characterised by BMI $< 19\,kg/m^2$ (signs/symptoms).
6. - Restore weight (check if using supplements and enzymes appropriately).
   - Weight is currently indicating a degree of malnutrition, and aggressive nutrition support is indicated to investigate the reasons and effective strategies to restore weight to a healthy range.
7. When considering a phone or Skype consult you must consider security and confidentiality. You would need to check with your employer regarding any issues with using Skype on the hospital systems including security of Internet-based services. When connecting to Justin you need to consider his privacy during the consultation and commence the consult by confirming his identity and ensuring you have his permission to conduct the consultation (Dietitians Association of Australia, 2014). Note that it is important to check guidelines in your country of practice. In addition, you will need to consider how you would document care and if your workplace has any relevant policies in place about this. The individual electronic health care record will make this simpler. Telephone support has been shown to be effective in reducing hospitalisations in some chronic illnesses (Dietitians of Canada, 2014).
8. It will be difficult to obtain any anthropometry or to check for any signs and symptoms of nutritional deficiency and malnutrition (Dietitians Association of

Australia, 2014). The consultation may be less free-flowing and hence the rapport may be difficult to build. In addition, if the client becomes emotional this is also challenging.

9. • Take time to re-establish a relationship with Justin.
   • Encourage Justin to express his goals for the consultation and discuss what you can do to help meet them.
   • Ask Justin if he feels there was a particular reason for his getting the flu and subsequent chest infection.
10. • Non-compliance with recommended nutrition plan (problem) because of changed social circumstances (aetiology) characterised by irregular enzyme usage and poor food choices.
11. • To support Justin to incorporate vitamin supplements as prescribed into his daily routine.
   • Ensure majority of foods consumed are nutrient and energy dense (Dietitians of Canada, 2011; Stapleton et al., 2006; Cystic Fibrosis Trust, 2002).
   • Encourage re-commencing nutritional supplements such as high-energy, high-protein drinks to assist in restoring weight in the short term. Justin may need assistance in accessing and purchasing these.
   • Providing a written record of agreed goals of management from the consultations and an agreed plan for follow-up with you.
12. Anticipatory guidance for travel would be valuable. This could include some discussion on the need for letters about the medications he usually takes, safe transport and storage of his enzymes in the heat, the need for increased salt if he is working in a hot and humid environment and how to incorporate this into his diet, and food safety and hygiene.
13. A team expert in the management of CF has been shown to give the best patient outcomes. The UK Standards of Care, from the CF trust recommend that all patients are cared for by a multidisciplinary team at a specialist CF centre. The team will have expert knowledge, have current practices, be peer reviewed, have access to diagnostic facilities, emergency care and in and outpatient services. The MDT will consist of specialist consultant paediatricians or adult physicians, medical support from trainee(s), clinical nurse specialists, physiotherapists, dietitians, occupational therapists, clinical psychologists, social workers, pharmacists, secretarial and administrative workers (CF Trust, 2011). Continuity of care is essential.

Answers to further questions

14. This is thought to be because of ongoing damage to the pancreas affecting insulin secretion. It can occur intermittently and is considered to be distinct from both type 1 and type 2 diabetes but has features of both (Moran *et al.*, 2010). Nutritional management focuses on maintaining blood sugars within the normal range and keeping a healthy weight. Hence the patients' diet may still include both high fat and high sugar foods. Advising on a regular consumption of carbohydrates with meals and snacks is necessary. Foods containing large amounts of sugars can be consumed as part of a meal with high fat foods slowing absorption. Patients may need to be taught to adjust insulin depending on food intake and exercise.

APPENDICES

APPENDIX A1
Dietary reference values

Energy

Table A1.1 **Estimated average requirements (EARs) for energy of children 0–18 years.**

Age	EAR [MJ/day (kcal/day)]	
	Boys	Girls
0–3 months	2.6	2.4
4–6 months	2.7	2.5
7–9 months	2.9	2.7
10–12 months	3.2	3.0
1–3 years	4.1	3.8
4–6 years	6.2	5.8
7–10 years	7.6	7.2
11–14 years	9.8	9.1
15–18 years	12.6	10.2

Source: Gandy 2014. Tab A3.1, p. 931. Reproduced with permission from Wiley Blackwell.

Table A1.2 **Estimated average requirements (MJ/day) according to height and weight at BMI = 22.5 kg/m² and assuming a physical activity level (PAL) of 1.63.**

Age (years)	Height (cm)	Weight (kg) BMI = 22.5 kg/m²	EAR (MJ/day)
Males			
19–24	178	71.5	11.6
25–34	178	71.0	11.5
35–44	176	69.7	11.0
45–54	175	68.8	10.8
55–64	174	68.3	10.8
65–74	173	67.0	9.8
75+	170	65.1	9.6

Source: Gandy 2014. Tab A3.1, p. 931. Reproduced with permission from Wiley Blackwell.

Dietetic and Nutrition Case Studies, First Edition.
Edited by Judy Lawrence, Pauline Douglas, and Joan Gandy.

Companion Website: http://www.manualofdieteticpractice.com/

Table A1.2 (*continued*)

Age (years)	Height (cm)	Weight (kg) BMI = 22.5 kg/m^2	EAR (MJ/day)
Females			
19–24	163	29.9	9.1
25–34	163	59.7	9.1
35–44	163	59.9	8.8
45–54	162	59.0	8.8
55–64	161	58.0	8.7
65–74	159	57.2	8.0
75+	155	54.3	7.7

Source: Gandy 2014. Tab A3.2, p. 931. Reproduced with permission from Wiley Blackwell.

Table A1.3 Reference nutrient intakes for protein.

Age	Weight (kg)	RNI (g/day)
0–3 months	5.9	12.5
4–6 months	7.7	12.7
7–9 months	8.8	13.7
10–12 months	9.7	14.9
1–3 years	12.5	14.5
4–6 years	17.8	19.7
7–10 years	28.3	28.3
Males		
11–14 years	43.0	42.1
15–18 years	64.5	55.2
19–50 years	74.0	55.5
50+ years	71.0	53.3
Females		
11–14 years	43.8	41.2
15–18 years	55.5	45.4
19–50 years	60.0	45.0
50+ years	62.0	46.5
Pregnancy		
Lactation		+6.0
0–4 months		+11.0
4+ months		+8.0

Source: Gandy 2014. Tab A3.3, p. 931. Reproduced with permission from Wiley Blackwell.

Table A1.4 Reference nutrient intakes (RNIs) for vitamins.

Age	Thiamin (mg/day)	Riboflavin (mg/day)	Niacin[1] (mg/day)	Vitamin B_6[2] (mg/day)	Vitamin B_{12} (µg/day)	Folate (µg/day)	Vitamin C (mg/day)	Vitamin A (µg/day)	Vitamin D (µg/day)
0–3 months	0.2	0.4	3	0.2	0.3	50	25	350	8.5
4–6 months	0.2	0.4	3	0.2	0.3	50	25	350	8.5
7–9 months	0.2	0.4	4	0.3	0.4	50	25	350	7
10–12 months	0.3	0.4	5	0.4	0.4	50	25	350	7
1–3 years	0.5	0.6	8	0.7	0.5	70	30	400	7
4–6 years	0.7	0.8	11	0.9	0.8	100	30	500	—
7–10 years	0.7	1.0	12	1.0	1.0	150	30	500	—
Males									
11–14 years	0.9	1.2	15	1.2	1.2	200	35	600	—
15–18 years	1.1	1.3	18	1.5	1.5	200	40	700	—
19–50 years	1.0	1.3	17	1.4	1.5	200	40	700	—
50+ years	0.9	1.3	16	1.4	1.5	200	40	700	—[3]
Females									
11–14 years	0.7	1.1	12	1.0	1.2	200	35	600	—
15–18 years	0.8	1.1	14	1.2	1.5	200	40	600	—
19–50 years	0.8	1.1	13	1.2	1.5	200	40	600	—
50+ years	0.8	1.1	12	1.2	1.5	200	40	600	—[3]
Pregnancy	+0.1[4]	+0.3	—[5]	—[5]	—[5]	+100	+10	+100	10
Lactation									
0–4 months	+0.2	+0.5	+2	—[5]	+0.5	+60	+30	+350	10
4+ months	+0.2	+0.5	+2	—[5]	+0.5	+60	+30	+350	10

Source: Gandy 2014. Tab A3.4, p. 932. Reproduced with permission from Wiley Blackwell.

[1]Nicotinic acid equivalent.

[2]Based on protein providing 14.7% of the estimated average requirement (EAR) for energy.

[3]After the age of 65 years the RNI is 10 µg/day for men and women.

[4]For the last trimester only.

[5]No increment.

Table A1.5 Reference nutrient intakes (RNIs) for minerals and trace elements.

Age	Calcium (mg/day)	Phosphorus[1] (mg/day)	Magnesium (mg/day)	Sodium[2] (mg/day)	Potassium[3] (mg/day)	Chloride[4] (mg/day)	Iron (mg/day)	Zinc (mg/day)	Copper (mg/day)	Selenium (µg/day)	Iodine (µg/day)
0–3 months	525	400	55	210	800	320	1.7	4.0	0.2	10	50
4–6 months	525	400	60	280	850	400	4.3	4.0	0.3	13	60
7–9 months	525	400	75	320	700	500	7.8	5.0	0.3	10	60
10–12 months	525	400	80	350	700	500	7.8	5.0	0.3	10	60
1–3 years	350	270	85	500	800	800	6.9	5.0	0.4	15	70
4–6 years	450	350	120	700	1100	1100	6.1	6.5	0.6	20	100
7–10 years	550	450	200	1200	2000	1800	8.7	7.0	0.7	30	110
Males											
11–14 years	1000	775	280	1600	3100	2500	11.3	9.0	0.8	45	130
15–18 years	1000	775	300	1600	3500	2500	11.3	9.5	1.0	70	140
19–50 years	700	550	300	1600	3500	2500	8.7	9.5	1.2	75	140
50+ years	700	550	300	1600	3500	2500	8.7	9.5	1.2	75	140
Females											
11–14 years	800	625	280	1600	3100	2500	14.8[5]	9.0	0.8	45	130
15–18 years	800	625	300	1600	3500	2500	14.8[5]	7.0	1.0	60	140
19–50 years	700	550	270	1600	3500	2500	14.8[5]	7.0	1.2	60	140
50+ years	700	550	270	1600	3500	2500	8.7	7.0	1.2	60	140
Pregnancy	—[6]	—[6]	—[6]	—[6]	—[6]	—[6]	—[6]	—[6]	—[6]	—[6]	—[6]
Lactation											
0–4 months	+550	+440	+50	—[6]	—[6]	—[6]	—[6]	+6.0	+0.3	+15	—[6]
4+ months	+550	+440	+50								

Source: Gandy 2014. Tab A3.5, p. 933. Reproduced with permission from Wiley Blackwell.

[1] Phosphorus (P) RNI is set to equal to calcium (Ca) in mmol values; 1 mmol Ca = 40 mg, 1 mmol P = 30.9.

[2] 1 mmol = 23 mg sodium (Na): 1 g salt (NaCl) contains 17.1 mmol, Na.

[3] 1 mmol = 39.1 mg.

[4] Intakes of dietary chloride should equal sodium intakes in molar terms. 1 mmol chloride = 35.5 mg.

[5] Supplements may be required if menstrual losses are high.

[6] No increment.

References

Department of Health (1991) *Dietary Reference Values for Food and Nutrients for the United Kingdom*. HMSO, London.

Scientific Advisory Committee on Nutrition (SACN) (2011) *Dietary Reference Values for Energy*. The Stationery Office, London.

APPENDIX A2

Weights and measures

Height/length

1 inch = 2.54 cm
1 foot (12 inches) = 30.48 cm (0.305 m)
1 yard (36 inches) = 91.44 cm
1 centimetre = 0.394 inch
1 metre = 39.37 inches

Table A2.1 Inches and centimetres conversion table.

Inches to centimetres		Centimetres to inches	
Inches	**Centimetres**	**Centimetres**	**Inches**
1	2.54	1	0.39
2	5.08	2	0.79
3	7.62	3	1.18
4	10.16	4	1.57
5	12.70	5	1.97
6	15.25	6	2.36
7	17.78	7	2.76
8	20.32	8	3.15
9	22.86	9	3.54
10	25.40	10	3.94
20	50.8	20	7.87
30	76.2	30	11.81
40	101.6	40	15.75
50	127.0	50	19.69
60	152.4	60	23.62
70	177.8	70	27.56
80	203.2	80	31.50
90	228.6	90	35.43
100	254.0	100	39.37

Source: Gandy (2014). Reproduced with permission from Wiley Blackwell.

Dietetic and Nutrition Case Studies, First Edition.
Edited by Judy Lawrence, Pauline Douglas, and Joan Gandy.

Companion Website: http://www.manualofdieteticpractice.com/

Table A2.2 **Height conversion table.**

Feet	Inches	Metres
4	0	1.22
4	0.5	1.23
4	1	1.24
4	1.5	1.26
4	2	1.27
4	2.5	1.28
4	3	1.29
4	3.5	1.31
4	4	1.32
4	4.5	1.33
4	5	1.35
4	5.5	1.36
4	6	1.37
4	6.5	1.38
4	7	1.40
4	7.5	1.41
4	8	1.42
4	8.5	1.43
4	9	1.45
4	9.5	1.46
4	10	1.47
4	10.5	1.49
4	11	1.50
4	11.5	1.51
5	0	1.52
5	0.5	1.54
5	1	1.55
5	1.5	1.56
5	2	1.57
5	2.5	1.59
5	3	1.60
5	3.5	1.61
5	4	1.63
5	4.5	1.64
5	5	1.65
5	5.5	1.66
5	6	1.68
5	6.5	1.69
5	7	1.70
5	7.5	1.71
5	8	1.73
5	8.5	1.74
5	9	1.75
5	9.5	1.76
5	10	1.78

Table A2.2 (*continued*)

Feet	Inches	Metres
5	10.5	1.79
5	11	1.80
5	11.5	1.82
6	0	1.83
6	0.5	1.84
6	1	1.85
6	1.5	1.87
6	2	1.88
6	2.5	1.89
6	3	1.90
6	3.5	1.92
6	4	1.93
6	4.5	1.94
6	5	1.96
6	5.5	1.97
6	6	1.98

Source: Gandy (2014). Reproduced with permission from Wiley Blackwell.

Weight

1 ounce = 28.35 g
1 pound (16 oz) = 454 g (0.45 kg)
1 stone (14 lb) = 6.35 kg
1 kilogram (1000 g) = 2.2 lb

Volume

1 fluid oz = 28.41 mL
1 pint (20 fluid oz) = 568.3 mL (or 0.568 L)
1 Litre (1000 mL) = 1.76 pints

Table A2.3 Ounces and grams conversion table (approximate rounded figures).

Ounces to grams			Grams to ounces	
Ounce	Gram	(approximate conversion)	Gram	Ounce (approximate conversion)
1	28	(25–30)	10	0.35 (0.33 oz)
2	57	(50–60)	15	0.53 (0.5 oz)
3	85	(75–90)	20	0.71 (0.75 oz)
4 (0.25 lb)	113	(100–120)	30	1.06 (1 oz)
5	142	(150)	40	1.41
6	170	(175)	50	1.76 (1.75 oz)
7	198	(200)	60	2.12 (2 oz)
8 (0.5 lb)	227	(225)	70	2.47
9	255	(250)	80	2.82
10	284	(300)	90	3.17
11	312	(325)	100	3.53 (3.5 oz)
12 (0.75 lb)	340	(350)	110	3.88
13	368	(375)	120	4.23
14	397	(400)	130	4.58
15	425	(425)	140	4.94
16 (1 lb)	454	(450)	150	5.29
			175	6.31
			200	7.05
			225	7.94 (8 oz/0.5 lb)
			250	8.82
			300	10.58
			350	12.34 (12 oz/0.75 lb)
			400	14.1
			450	15.9 (16 oz/1 lb)
			500	17.6
			1000	35.27 (2.2 lb)

Source: Gandy (2014). Reproduced with permission from Wiley Blackwell.

Table A2.4 Body weight conversion table (stones and lb to kg).

Stone	Pound	Kilogram	Stone	Pound	Kilogram	Stone	Pound	Kilogram	Stone	Pound	Kilogram	Stone	Pound	Kilogram
0	1	0.45	6	5	40.37	9	13	63.05	13	7	85.73	17	1	108.41
	2	0.90		6	40.82	10	0	63.50		8	86.18		2	108.86
	3	1.36		7	41.28		1	63.96		9	86.64		3	109.32
	4	1.81		8	41.73		2	64.41		10	87.09		4	109.77
	5	2.27		9	42.18		3	64.86		11	87.54		5	110.22
	6	2.72		10	42.64		4	65.32		12	88.00		6	110.68
	7	3.17		11	43.09		5	65.77		13	88.45		7	111.13
	8	3.63		12	43.55		6	66.23	14	0	88.91		8	111.59
	9	4.08		13	44.00		7	66.68		1	89.36		9	112.04
	10	4.54	7	0	44.45		8	67.13		2	89.81		10	112.49
	11	4.99		1	44.91		9	67.59		3	90.27		11	112.95
	12	5.44		2	45.36		10	68.04		4	90.72		12	113.40
	13	5.90		3	45.81		11	68.49		5	91.17		13	113.85
				4	46.27		12	68.95		6	91.63	18	0	114.31
1	0	6.35		5	46.72		13	69.40		7	92.08		1	114.76
2	0	12.70		6	47.17	11	0	69.85		8	92.53		2	115.21
3	0	19.05		7	47.63		1	70.31		9	92.98		3	115.67
4	0	25.40		8	48.08		2	70.76		10	93.44		4	116.12
	1	25.86		9	48.54		3	71.22		11	93.90		5	116.58
	2	26.31		10	48.99		4	71.67		12	94.35		6	117.03
	3	26.76		11	49.44		5	72.12		13	94.80		7	117.48
	4	27.22		12	49.90		6	72.58	15	0	95.26		8	117.94
	5	27.67		13	50.35		7	73.03		1	95.71		9	118.39
	6	28.12	8	0	50.80		8	73.48		2	96.16		10	118.84
	7	28.57		1	51.26		9	73.94		3	96.62		11	119.30

	8	29.03		2	51.71		10	74.39		4	97.07		12	119.75
	9	29.48		3	52.16		11	74.84		5	97.52		13	120.20
	10	29.93		4	52.62		12	75.30		6	97.98	19	0	120.66
	11	30.39		5	53.07		13	75.75		7	98.43		1	121.11
	12	30.84		6	53.52	12	0	76.20		8	98.88		2	121.56
	13	31.30		7	53.98		1	76.66		9	99.34		3	122.02
5	0	31.75		8	54.43		2	77.11		10	99.79		4	122.47
	1	32.21		9	54.89		3	77.57		11	100.24		5	122.93
	2	32.66		10	55.34		4	78.02		12	100.70		6	123.38
	3	33.11		11	55.79		5	78.47		13	101.15		7	123.83
	4	33.57		12	56.25		6	78.93	16	0	101.61		8	124.29
	5	34.02		13	56.70		7	79.38		1	102.06		9	124.74
	6	34.47	9	0	57.15		8	79.83		2	102.51		10	125.19
	7	34.93		1	57.61		9	80.29		3	102.97		11	125.65
	8	35.38		2	58.06		10	80.74		4	103.42		12	126.10
	9	35.83		3	58.51		11	81.19		5	103.87		13	126.55
	10	36.29		4	58.97		12	81.65		6	104.33	20	0	127.27
	11	36.74		5	59.42		13	82.10		7	104.79		7	130.45
	12	37.19		6	59.88	13	0	82.55		8	105.24	21	0	133.64
	13	37.65		7	60.33		1	83.01		9	105.69		7	136.82
6	0	38.10		8	60.78		2	83.46		10	106.14	22	0	140.00
	1	38.56		9	61.24		3	83.92		11	106.60		7	143.18
	2	39.01		10	61.69		4	84.37		12	107.04	23	0	146.36
	3	39.46		11	62.14		5	84.82		13	107.50	24	0	152.73
	4	39.92		12	62.60		6	85.28	17	0	107.96	25	0	159.09

Source: Gandy (2014). Reproduced with permission from Wiley Blackwell.

Table A2.5 Pints and litres conversion table.

Fluid ounce/pint	Millilitre per litre	Millilitre per litre	Fluid ounce/pint
1 fl oz	28	50 mL	1.75 fl oz
0.25 pint (5 fl oz)	142	100 mL	3.5 fl oz
0.5 pint (10 fl oz)	284	200 mL	7 fl oz
0.75 pint (15 fl oz)	426	250 mL	8.8 fl oz
1 pint	568	500 mL	17.6 fl oz
2 pints	1.1 L	750 mL	26.4 fl oz
3 pints	1.7 L	1000 mL	1.76 pints (1.75 pints)
4 pints	2.3 L		
5 pints	2.8 L		

Source: Gandy (2014). Reproduced with permission from Wiley Blackwell.

Reference

Gandy, J. (2014) *Manual of Dietetic Practice*, 5th edn. Wiley Blackwell, Oxford.

APPENDIX A3
Dietary data

Conversion factors

Energy

Table A3.1 Nutrient energy yields.

Nutrient	kcal/g	kJ/g
Protein	4	17
Fat	9	37
Carbohydrate	3.75	16
Sugar alcohols	2.4	10
Ethyl alcohol	7	29
Glycerol	4.31	18
Medium chaintriglyceride (MCT)	8.4	35

Source: Gandy (2014). Reproduced with permission from Wiley Blackwell.

Units used in energy balance
1000 J = 1 kJ
1000 kJ = 1 MJ
1 kcal = 4.184 kJ (The Royal Society (London) recommended conversion factor)
1 kJ = 0.239 kcal
1 W = 1 J/s
0.06 W = 1 kJ/min
86.4 W = 1 kJ/24 h

Protein and nitrogen

Dietary protein (g) = dietary nitrogen (g) × 6.25
Dietary nitrogen (g) = dietary protein (g) ÷ 6.25

This conversion factor is only appropriate for a mixture of foods. For milk or cereals alone, the factors 6.4 or 5.7 should be used.

Dietetic and Nutrition Case Studies, First Edition.
Edited by Judy Lawrence, Pauline Douglas, and Joan Gandy.

Companion Website: http://www.manualofdieteticpractice.com/

Vitamins

Vitamin A

The active vitamin A content of a diet is usually expressed in retinol equivalents.

1 μg retinol equivalent = 1 μg retinol or 6 μg β-carotene

1 IU vitamin A = 0.3 μg retinol or 0.6 μg β-carotene

Vitamin D

1 μg vitamin D = 40 IU

1 IU = 0.025 μg vitamin D

Nicotinic acid/tryptophan

1 mg nicotinic acid = 60 mg tryptophan

Nicotinic acid content mg equivalents = Nicotinic acid (mg) + tryptophan (mg)/60

Vitamin E

Vitamin E activity is expressed as D-α-tocopherol equivalents. Activity is expressed as international units (IU):

1 IU is equivalent to 0.67 mg D-α-tocopherol

Table A3.2 Mineral content of compounds and solutions.

Solution/compound	Mineral content	
1 g sodium chloride	393 mg Na	17 mmol Na
1 g sodium bicarbonate	273 mg Na	12 mmol Na
1 g potassium bicarbonate	524 mg K	13.4 mmol K
1 g calcium chloride (hydrated)	273 mg Ca	7 mmol Ca
1 g calcium carbonate	400m g Ca	10 mmol Ca
1 g calcium gluconate	93 mg Ca	2.3 mmol Ca
1 L normal saline	3450 mg Na	150 mmol Na

Source: Gandy (2014). Reproduced with permission from Wiley Blackwell.

Food exchange lists

Carbohydrate

Table A3.3 Food portions containing approximately 10 g carbohydrate.

Food	Weight (g)	Description
Wholemeal bread	25	1 thin slice/large loaf
White bread	20	1 thin slice/small loaf
Potatoes – boiled	60	1 size of hen's egg

Table A3.3 (*continued*)

Food	Weight (g)	Description
Potatoes – mashed	60	1 scoop
Potatoes – roast	40	1 very small
Sweet potato – boiled	50	1 size of hen's egg
Rice – boiled, brown, white	30	¾ tablespoon
Pasta – boiled, for example, spaghetti, macaroni	50	1 tablespoon
Pulses, for example, lentils	60	2 tablespoons
Peas – frozen	100	3 tablespoons
Parsnip – boiled	80	1 medium
Sweet corn – boiled	50	2 tablespoons
Thick soup, for example, tinned vegetable	100	1 small tin
Thin soup, for example, minestrone	250	1 standard mug
Sausages	100	2 large sausages
Beef burger, economy	100	1 economy burger
Beef burger, 100% meat = no CHO	—	—
Fish fingers	60	2 fish fingers
Breakfast cereals, for example, bran flakes	15	2 tablespoons
Breakfast cereals, for example, wheat bisk type	20	1 bisk
Muesli, no added sugar	15	¾ tablespoon
Porridge – made with water	125	Small average portion
Biscuits – plain digestive	15	1 digestive
Apple, pear	100	1 medium
Orange	120	1 small
Banana	45	½ small banana
Melon – galia, honeydew	200	1 medium slice
Pineapple, fresh	100	1 large slice
Grapes	70	15 large grapes
Orange juice – no added sugar	110	½ average glass
Apple juice – no added sugar	100	½ average glass
Cranberry juice	70	⅓ average glass
Milk – full fat, semi or skimmed	200	1 average glass
Yoghurt – low fat, fruit	70	½ small pot
Yoghurt – low fat, plain	135	1 small pot
Ice cream – plain dairy, vanilla	50	1 small scoop
Lemonade	170	1 small glass
Lucozade®	60	⅓ average glass
Cola	90	½ average glass
Beer – best bitter	450	¾ pint glass
Lager – premium	400	¾ pint glass
Wine – medium white	330	2½ small wine glasses
Wine – red contains 0.2 g CHO/100 mL	—	—
Crisps	20	¾ small packet
Peanuts – dry roasted	100	1 large packet

Source: Gandy (2014). Reproduced with permission from Wiley Blackwell.

Protein

Table A3.4 Food portions containing approximately 6 g or 2 g protein.

Food	Portion size	Protein per portion (g)	Approximate energy per portion (kcal)
Milk	180 mL	6	115 (full-fat) 85 (semi-skimmed) 60 (skimmed)
Cheddar cheese	25 g	6	100
Yoghurt	125 g	6	125
Egg	50 g (one average hen's egg)	6	70
Meat/poultry lean cooked	25 g	6	40
White fish	35 g	6	30
Baked beans	120 g	6	100
Peas	100 g	6	70
Bread (1 large thin slice)	25 g	2	50
Pasta (boiled)	50 g	2	50
Rice (boiled)	100 g	2	140
Most breakfast cereals	25 g	2	90
Digestive biscuits	15 g (one biscuit)	2	70
Potatoes	140 g	2	100
Crisps	30 g	2	160

Source: Gandy (2014). Reproduced with permission from Wiley Blackwell.

Potassium

Table A3.5 Food portions containing approximately 4 mmol potassium.

Food	Portion size providing approximately 4 mmol potassium
Milk	100 mL
Yoghurt	60 g
Cheddar cheese	130 g
Egg	100 g (2 small eggs)
Meat/fish	50 g
White flour	120 g
Wholemeal flour	45 g
White bread	160 g
Wholemeal bread	70 g
Apple	125 g
Orange with skin	100 g
Grapes/orange without skin	50 g
Potato boiled	50 g
Orange juice	100 mL
Tomato juice	60 mL

Source: Gandy (2014). Reproduced with permission from Wiley Blackwell.

Sodium

Table A3.6 No added salt and 40 mmol sodium diets.

No added salt	40 mmol sodium diet
This restricts sodium intake to less than 100 mmol Na^+/day A pinch of salt may be used in cooking, but none should be added to food at the table The following foods must be avoided: • Bacon, ham, sausages, paté • Tinned fish and meat • Smoked fish and meat • Fish and meat pastes • Tinned and packet soups • Sauce mixes • Tinned vegetables • Bottled sauces and chutneys • Meat and vegetable extracts, stock cubes • Salted nuts and crisps • Soya sauce • Monosodium glutamate • Cheese – up to 100 g/week • Bread – up to 4 slices per day	In addition to the above-listed foods, the following restrictions apply: • No salt to be used in cooking or at table • Salt-free butter or margarine must be used • Milk should be restricted to 300 mL/day • Breakfast cereals must be salt free

Source: Gandy (2014). Reproduced with permission from Wiley Blackwell.

E number classification system

Summary of E number classification
E100–180: Colours
E200–283: Preservatives
E300–321: Antioxidants
E322–495: Emulsifiers, stabilisers, acidity regulators, thickeners
E950–969: Artificial sweeteners

Table A3.7 Commonly used additives.

Type of additive	E number	Chemical name
Colours		
Natural and nature identical colours	E101	Riboflavin (yellow)
	E100	Curcumin (yellow)
	E120	Cochineal (red)
	E140	Chlorophyll (green)
	E150a	Plain caramel (brown/black)
	E153	Carbon (black)
	E160a	Alpha, beta and gamma carotene (yellow/orange)
	E160b	Annatto (yellow/red)
	E160c	Capsanthin (paprika extract) (red/orange)
	E160d	Lycopene (red extract from tomatoes)
	E162	Beetroot red (betanin) (purple/red)
	E163	Anthocyanins (red/blue/violet)
Synthetic colours	E102	Tartrazine[1] (yellow)
	E104	Quinoline yellow[1]
	E110	Sunset yellow FCF[1]
	E122	Carmoisine (Azorubine)[1] (red)
	E123	Amaranth[1] (purple red)
	E124	Ponceau 4R[1] (red)
	E127	Erythrosine[1] (pink/red)
	E128	Red 2 G[1]
	E129	Allura red AC[1]
	E132	Indigo carmine (Indigotine)[1] (blue)
	E142	Green S[1]
	E150b–d	Caustic sulphite caramel; ammonia caramel; sulphite ammonia caramel (brown/black)
	E151	Black PN[1]
	E154	Brown FK[1]
	E155	Brown HT[1]
	E180	Lithol Rubine BK (Pigment Rubine; Rubine)[1]
Preservatives		
Sorbic acid and its derivatives	E200	Sorbic acid
	E201–203	Sodium, potassium and calcium sorbates
Benzoic acid and derivatives	E210	Benzoic acid
	E211–213	Sodium, potassium and calcium benzoates
	E214–219	Ethyl, methyl or propyl hydroxybenzoates
Sulphur dioxide and derivatives	E220	Sulphur dioxide
	E221	Sodium sulfite
	E222	Sodium hydrogen sulfite (sodium bisulfite)
	E223	Sodium metabisulfite
	E224	Potassium metabisulfite
	E226	Calcium sulfite
	E227	Calcium hydro gen sulfite (calcium bisulfite)

Table A3.7 (*continued*)

Type of additive	E number	Chemical name
Nitrites and nitrates	E249	Potassium nitrite
	E250	Sodium nitrite
	E251	Sodium nitrate
	E252	Potassium nitrate
Acetic, lactic and propionic acid derivatives	E260–263	Acetic acid and acetates
	E270	Lactic acid
	E280–283	Propionic acid and propionates
Antioxidants		
Ascorbic acid and derivatives	E300	Ascorbic acid (vitamin C)
	E301–304	Ascorbates and ascorbyl palmitate
Tocopherols	E306	Vitamin E
	E307–309	Synthetic tocopherols
Gallates	E310–312	Propyl, octyl and dodecyl gallates
BHA/BHT	E320	Butylated hydroxyanisole (BHA)
	E321	Butylated hydroxytoluene (BHT)
Emulsifiers and stabilisers		
Emulsifier	E322	Lecithins
Acidity regulators, buffers, stabilisers	E325–327	Sodium, potassium and calcium lactate
	E330–333	Citric acid; sodium, potassium and calcium citrates
	E334–337	Tartaric acid; sodium and potassium tartrates
	E338–341	Phosphoric acid; sodium, potassium and calcium phosphates and orthophosphates
	E350–352	Sodium, potassium and calcium malates
Gelling agents	E401–405	Sodium, ammonium, potassium and calcium alginates
	E406	Agar
	E407	Carrageenan
Gums	E410	Locust bean gum
	E412	Guar gum
	E413	Tragacanth
	E414	Gum arabic
	E415	Xanthan gum
Emulsifiers/stabilisers	E471–477	Esters and glycerides of fatty acids (e g mono and diglycerides of fatty acids or glyceryl monostearate and distearate)

[1] Azo dye.

Reference

Gandy, J. (2014) *Manual of Dietetic Practice*, 5th edn. Wiley Blackwell, Oxford.

APPENDIX A4

Body mass index

Dietetic and Nutrition Case Studies, First Edition.
Edited by Judy Lawrence, Pauline Douglas, and Joan Gandy.

Companion Website: http://www.manualofdieteticpractice.com/

Table A4.1 BMI ready reference table.

BMI	Weight (kg)																							
Morbidly obese (BMI > 40)	45	102	104	107	110	113	116	119	121	124	127	131	134	137	140	143	146	150	153	156	159	163	170	173
	44	99	102	105	108	110	113	116	119	122	125	128	131	134	137	140	143	146	149	153	156	159	166	169
	43	97	100	102	105	108	111	113	116	119	122	125	128	131	134	137	140	143	146	149	152	156	162	166
	42	95	97	100	103	105	108	111	113	116	119	122	125	128	131	134	137	140	143	146	149	152	159	162
	41	93	95	98	100	103	105	108	111	113	116	119	122	125	127	130	133	136	139	142	145	148	155	158
Obese (BMI 31–40)	40	90	93	95	98	100	103	105	108	111	113	116	119	122	124	127	130	133	136	139	142	145	151	154
	39	88	91	93	95	98	100	103	105	108	111	113	116	119	121	124	127	130	132	135	138	141	147	150
	38	86	88	91	93	95	98	100	103	105	108	110	113	115	118	121	124	126	129	132	135	138	143	146
	37	84	86	88	90	93	95	98	100	102	105	107	110	112	115	118	120	123	126	128	131	134	140	143
	36	81	84	86	88	90	93	95	97	100	102	104	107	109	112	115	117	120	122	125	128	130	136	139
	35	79	81	83	86	88	90	92	95	97	99	102	104	106	109	111	114	116	119	122	124	127	132	135
	34	77	79	81	83	85	87	90	92	94	96	99	101	103	106	108	111	113	116	118	121	123	128	131
	33	75	77	79	81	83	85	87	89	91	94	96	98	100	103	105	107	110	112	115	117	120	125	127
	32	72	74	76	78	80	82	84	87	89	91	93	95	97	100	102	104	106	109	111	114	116	121	123
	31	70	72	74	76	78	80	82	84	86	88	90	92	94	96	99	101	103	105	108	110	112	117	120
Overweight (BMI 26–30)	30	68	70	72	73	75	77	79	81	83	85	87	89	91	93	96	98	100	102	104	106	109	113	116
	29	66	67	69	71	73	75	77	78	80	82	84	86	88	90	92	94	97	99	101	103	105	110	112
	28	63	65	67	69	70	72	74	76	78	79	81	83	85	87	89	91	93	95	97	99	102	106	108
	27	61	63	64	66	68	70	71	73	75	77	78	80	82	84	86	88	90	92	94	96	98	102	104
	26	59	61	62	64	65	67	69	70	72	74	76	77	79	81	83	85	87	88	90	92	94	98	100

(continued overleaf)

Table A4.1 *(continued)*

BMI	Weight (kg)																							
Normal weight (BMI 20–25)	25	57	58	60	61	63	64	66	68	69	71	73	74	76	78	80	81	83	85	87	89	91	95	96
	24	54	56	57	59	60	62	63	65	67	68	70	71	73	75	76	78	80	82	83	85	87	91	93
	23	52	54	55	56	58	59	61	62	64	65	67	68	70	72	73	75	77	78	80	82	83	87	89
	22	50	51	53	54	55	57	58	60	61	63	64	66	67	69	70	72	73	75	77	78	80	83	85
	21	48	49	50	52	53	54	56	57	58	60	61	63	64	65	67	68	70	72	73	75	76	79	81
	20	45	47	48	49	50	52	53	54	56	57	58	60	61	62	64	65	67	68	70	71	73	76	77
Underweight (BMI 16–19)	19	43	44	46	47	48	49	50	52	53	54	55	57	58	59	61	62	63	65	66	68	69	72	73
	18	41	42	43	44	45	47	48	49	50	51	52	54	55	56	57	59	60	61	63	64	65	68	70
	17	39	40	41	42	43	44	45	46	47	48	50	51	52	53	54	56	57	58	59	61	62	64	66
	16	36	37	38	39	40	41	42	43	45	46	47	48	49	50	51	52	53	55	56	57	58	61	62
Severely underweight (BMI < 16)	15	34	35	36	37	38	39	40	41	42	43	44	45	46	47	48	49	50	51	52	53	55	57	58
	14	32	33	34	35	35	36	37	38	39	40	41	42	43	44	45	46	47	48	49	50	51	53	54
	13	30	30	31	32	33	34	35	35	36	37	38	39	40	41	42	43	44	44	45	46	47	49	50
	12	27	28	29	30	30	31	32	33	34	34	35	36	37	38	38	39	40	41	42	43	44	46	47
	11	25	26	27	27	28	29	29	30	31	31	32	33	34	35	35	36	37	38	39	39	40	42	43
	10	23	24	24	25	25	26	27	27	28	29	29	30	31	31	32	33	34	34	35	36	37	38	39
Height (m)		1.5	1.52	1.54	1.56	1.58	1.6	1.62	1.64	1.66	1.68	1.7	1.72	1.74	1.76	1.78	1.8	1.82	1.84	1.86	1.88	1.9	1.94	1.96
Height (feet inches)		411	50	51	51½	52¼	53	53¼	54½	55½	56	57	57¼	58½	59¼	510	511	511¾	60½	61¼	62	63	64½	65½

Source: Gandy (2014). Reproduced with permission from Wiley Blackwell.

Reference

Gandy, J. (2014) *Manual of Dietetic Practice*, 5th edn. Wiley Blackwell, Oxford.

APPENDIX A5
Anthropometric and functional data

Demiquet and mindex

$$\text{Demiquet} = \frac{\text{Weight (kg)}}{\text{Demispan (m)}^2}$$

$$\text{Mindex} = \frac{\text{Weight (kg)}}{\text{Demispan (m)}}$$

Table A5.1 Distribution of demiquet and mindex in a normal population over the age 65 years.

	Percentiles				
	10th	30th	50th	70th	90th
Men (Demiquet, kg/m^2)					
64–74 years	87.6	99.6	106.7	117.1	130.7
75+ years	84.5	98.9	106.3	113.4	125.0
Women (Mindex, kg/m)					
64–74 years	68.3	77.8	84.8	92.3	110.6
75+ years	63.1	73.6	81.7	88.4	102.2

Source: Gandy 2014. Reproduced with permission from Wiley Blackwell.

Dietetic and Nutrition Case Studies, First Edition.
Edited by Judy Lawrence, Pauline Douglas, and Joan Gandy.

Companion Website: http://www.manualofdieteticpractice.com/

Upper arm anthropometry

Table A5.2 Triceps skinfold thickness (TSF).

		Centiles						
	Mean (mm)	5th	10th	25th	50th	75th	90th	95th
				Men				
18–74 years	12.0	4.5	6.0	8.0	11.0	15.0	20.0	23.0
18–24 years	11.2	4.0	5.0	7.0	9.5	14.0	20.0	23.0
25–34 years	12.6	4.5	5.5	8.0	12.0	16.0	21.5	24.0
35–44 years	12.4	5.0	6.0	8.5	12.0	15.5	20.0	23.0
45–54 years	12.4	5.0	6.0	8.0	11.0	15.0	20.0	25.5
55–64 years	11.6	5.0	6.0	8.0	11.0	14.0	18.0	21.5
65–74 years	11.8	4.5	5.5	8.0	11.0	15.0	19.0	22.0
				Women				
18–74 years	23.0	11.0	13.0	17.0	22.0	28.0	34.0	37.5
18–24 years	19.4	9.4	11.0	14.0	18.0	24.0	30.0	34.0
25–34 years	21.9	10.5	12.0	16.0	21.0	26.5	33.5	37.0
35–44 years	24.0	12.0	14.0	18.0	23.0	29.5	35.5	39.0
45–54 years	25.4	13.0	15.0	20.0	25.0	30.0	36.0	40.0
55–64 years	24.9	11.0	14.0	19.0	25.0	30.5	35.0	39.0
65–74 years	23.3	11.5	14.0	18.0	23.0	28.0	33.0	36.0

Source: Gandy 2014. Reproduced with permission from Wiley Blackwell.

Table A5.3 Mid-arm circumference (MAC).

		Centiles						
	Mean (cm)	5th	10th	25th	50th	75th	90th	95th
				Men				
18–74 years	31.8	2A5	27.6	29.6	31.7	33.9	36.0	37.3
18–24 years	30.9	25.7	27.1	28.7	30.7	32.9	35.5	37.4
25–34 years	30.5	25.3	26.5	28.5	30.7	32.4	34.4	35.5
35–44 years	32.3	27.0	28.2	30.0	32.0	34.4	36.5	37.6
45–54 years	32.7	27.8	28.7	30.7	32.7	34.8	36.3	37.1
55–64 years	32.1	26.7	27.8	30.0	32.0	34.2	36.2	37.6
65–74 years	31.5	25.6	27.3	29.6	31.7	33.4	35.2	36.6
				Women				
18–74 years	29.4	23.2	24.3	26.2	28.7	31.9	35.2	37.8
18–24 years	27.0	22.1	23.0	24.5	2A5	28.8	31.7	34.3
25–34 years	28.6	23.3	24.2	25.7	27.8	30.4	34.1	37.2
35–44 years	30.0	24.1	25.2	26.8	29.2	32.2	36.2	38.5
45–54 years	30.7	24.3	25.7	27.5	30.3	32.9	36.8	39.3
55–64 years	30.7	23.9	25.1	27.7	30.2	33.3	36.3	38.2
65–74 years	30.1	23.8	25.2	27.4	29.9	32.5	35.3	37.2

Source: Gandy 2014. Reproduced with permission from Wiley Blackwell.

Table A5.4 Mid-arm muscle circumference (MAMC) – MAMC (cm) = MAC (cm) – (TSF (mm) × 0.314).

		Centiles						
	Mean (cm)	**5th**	**10th**	**25th**	**50th**	**75th**	**90th**	**95th**
			Men					
18–74 years	28.0	23.8	24.8	26.3	27.9	29.6	31.4	32.5
18–24 years	27.4	23.5	24.4	25.8	27.2	28.9	30.8	32.3
25–34 years	28.3	24.2	25.3	26.5	28.0	30.0	31.7	32.9
35–44 years	28.8	25.0	25.6	27.1	28.7	30.3	32.1	33.0
45–54 years	28.2	24.0	24.9	26.5	28.1	29.8	31.5	32.6
55–64 years	27.8	22.8	24.4	26.2	27.9	29.6	31.0	31,8
65–74 years	26.8	22.5	23.7	25.3	26.9	28.5	29.9	30.7
			Women					
18–74 years	22.2	18.4	19.0	20.2	21.8	23.6	25.8	27.4
18–24 years	20.9	17.7	18.5	19.4	20.6	22.1	23.6	24.9
25–34 years	21.7	18.3	18.9	20.0	21.4	22.9	24.9	26.6
35–44 years	22.5	18.5	19.2	20.6	22.0	24.0	26.1	27.4
45–54 years	22.7	18.8	19.5	20.7	22.2	24.3	26.6	27.8
55–64 years	22.8	18.6	19.5	20.8	22.6	24.4	26.3	28.1
65–74 years	22.8	18.6	19.5	20,8	22.5	24.4	26.5	28.1

Source: Gandy 2014. Reproduced with permission from Wiley Blackwell.

Estimating height from ulna length

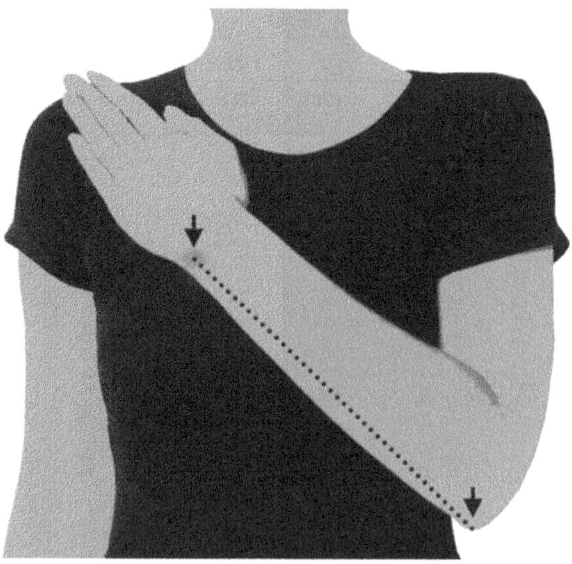

Figure A5.1 How to measure ulna length. (Gandy (2014). Reproduced with permission from Wiley Blackwell.)

Table A5.5 **Estimates of height from ulna length.**[1]

Men Height (m)		Ulna length (cm)	Women Height (m)	
<65 years	>65 years		<65 years	>65 years
1.94	1.87	32.0	1.84	1.84
1.93	1.86	31.5	1.83	1.83
1.91	1.84	31.0	1.81	1.81
1.89	1.82	30.5	1.80	1.79
1.87	1.81	30.0	1.79	1.78
1.85	1.79	29.5	1.77	1.76
1.84	1.78	29.0	1.76	1.75
1.82	1.76	28.5	1.75	1.73
1.80	1.75	28.0	1.73	1.71
1.78	1.73	27.5	1.72	1.70
1.76	1.71	27.0	1.70	1.68
1.75	1.70	26.5	1.69	1.66
1.73	1.68	26.0	1.68	1.65
1.71	1.67	25.5	1.66	1.63
1.69	1.65	25.0	1.65	1.61
1.67	1.63	24.5	1.63	1.60
1.66	1.62	24.0	1.62	1.58
1.64	1.60	23.5	1.61	1.56
1.62	1.59	23.0	1.59	1.55
1.60	1.57	22.5	1.58	1.53
1.58	1.56	22.0	1.56	1.52
1.57	1.54	21.5	1.55	1.50
1.55	1.52	21.0	1.54	1.48
1.53	1.51	20.5	1.52	1.47
1.51	1.49	20.0	1.51	1.45
1.49	1.48	19.5	1.50	1.44
1.48	1.46	19.0	1.48	1.42
1.46	1.45	18.5	1.47	1.40

[1]See Figure A5.1.

Source: Gandy 2014. Reproduced with permission from Wiley Blackwell.

Measure between the point of the elbow (olecranon process) and the midpoint of the prominent bone of the wrist (styloid process) (left side if possible).

Table A5.6 Classification of body mass index and risk of comorbidities in adults.

Classification	BMI (kg/m²)	BMI (kg/m²) Asian origin	Risk of comorbidities
Underweight	<18.5	<18.5	Low (but risk of other clinical problems increased)
Normal range	18.5–24.9	18.5–22.9	Average
Overweight	25.0–29.9	23–27.4	Increased risk
Obese Class I	30.0–34.9	27.5–32.4	Moderate
Obese Class II	35.0–39.9	32.5–37.4	Severe
Obese Class III	>40.0	>37.5	Morbid obesity

Source: Gandy 2014. Reproduced with permission from Wiley Blackwell.

Table A5.7 Waist measurements in adults as a predictor of health risk.

	Men	Asian men	Women	Asian women
Waist circumference				
Increased risk	≥94 cm		≥80 cm	
Substantially increased risk	≥102 cm	≥90 cm	≥88 cm	≥80 cm
Waist to hip ratio				
Increased risk	≥0.9		≥0.85	

Source: Gandy 2014. Reproduced with permission from Wiley Blackwell.

Table A5.8 Weight adjustments for amputations.

Body part	Percentage of body weight
Upper limb	5.0
Forearm	1.6
Hand	0.7
Lower limb	16.0
Lower leg	4.4
Foot	1.5

Source: Gandy 2014. Reproduced with permission from Wiley Blackwell.

Table A5.9 Dynamometry (grip strength).

	Normal values (kg)	85% of normal (values at or below this level are indicative of protein malnutrition) (kg)
Men		
18–69 years	40.0	34.0
70–79 years	32.5	27.5
80+ years	22.5	19.0
Women		
18–69 years	27.5	23.0
70–79 years	25.0	21.0
80+ years	20.0	17.0

Source: Gandy 2014. Tab 2.2.3, p. 49. Reproduced with permission from Wiley Blackwell.

References

Bishop, C.W., Bowen, P.E. & Ritchey, S.J. (1981) Norms for nutritional assessment of American adults by upper arm anthropometry. *American Journal of Clinical Nutrition,* **34**, 2530–2539.

Elia M. (2003) *Development and use of the Malnutrition Universal Screening Tool ('MUST') for adults.* BAPEN.

Gandy, J. (2014) *Manual of Dietetic Practice,* 5th edn. Wiley Blackwell, Oxford.

Griffith, C.D.M. & Clark, R.G. (1984) A comparison of the 'Sheffield' prognostic index with forearm muscle dynamometry in patients from Sheffield undergoing major abdominal and urological surgery. *Clinical Nutrition,* **3**, 147–151.

Klidjian, A.M., Foster, K.J., Kammerling, R.M., Cooper, A. & Karran, S.J. (1980) Relation of anthropometric and dynamometric variables to serious post-operative complications. *British Medical Journal,* **281**, 899–901.

Lehmann, A.B., Bassey, E.J., Morgan, K. & Dallosso, H.M. (1991) Normal values for weight, skeletal size and body mass indices in 890 men and women aged over 65 years. *Clinical Nutrition,* **10**, 18–22.

World Health Organization (2008). *Waist circumference and waist-hip ratio.* Report of a WHO expert consultation. www.who.int [last accessed on 16 February 2013].

World Health Organization (WHO) (1998). *Obesity: preventing and managing the global epidemic.* Report of a WHO consultation on obesity, Geneva: WHO.

World Health Organization Expert Consultation (2004) Appropriate body mass index for Asian Populations and its implications for policy and intervention strategies. *Lancet,* **363**, 157–164.

APPENDIX A6

Predicting energy requirements

Table A6.1 **Basal metabolic rate (BMR).**

	Age (years)	BMR prediction equation (MJ/d)
Males	<3	0.255 (w) − 0.141
	3–10	0.0937 (w) + 2.15
	10–18	0.0769 (w) + 2.43
	18–30	0.0669 (w) + 2.28
	30–60	0.0592 (w) + 2.48
	>60	0.0563 (w) + 2.15
Females	<3	0.246 (w) − 0.0965
	3–10	0.0842 (w) + 2.12
	10–18	0.0465 (w) + 3.18
	18–30	0.0546 (w) + 2.33
	30–60	0.0407 (w) + 2.90
	>60	0.0424 (w) + 2.38

Source: Gandy 2014. Tab A8.1, p. 948. Reproduced with permission from Wiley Blackwell.

References

Henry, C.J. (2005) Basal metabolic rate studies in humans: measurement and development of new equations. *Public Health Nutrition*, **8**, 1133–1152.

Scientific Advisory Committee on Nutrition (2011) *Dietary recommendations for energy*. Working Group Report. www.sacn.gov.uk/pdfs/sacn_energy_report_author_date_10th_oct_fin.pdf [accessed on online 22 March 2012].

Dietetic and Nutrition Case Studies, First Edition.
Edited by Judy Lawrence, Pauline Douglas, and Joan Gandy.

Companion Website: http://www.manualofdieteticpractice.com/

APPENDIX A7

Clinical chemistry

Conversion calculations

mg to mmol: $\dfrac{\text{mg}}{\text{atomic weight}}$

mmol to mg: mmol × atomic weight

Milliequivalents (mEq)

$$1\,\text{mEq} = \frac{\text{atomic weight (mg)}}{\text{valency}}$$

To convert
mg to mEq: (mg × valency)/atomic weight
mEq to mg: (mEq × atomic weight)/valency

For minerals with a valency of 1, mEq = mmol
For minerals with a valency of 2, mEq = mmol × 2

Table A7.1 Atomic weights and valencies.

Mineral	Atomic weight	Valency
Sodium	23.0	1
Potassium	39.0	1
Phosphorus	31.0	2
Calcium	40.0	2
Magnesium	24.3	2
Chlorine	35.4	1
Sulphur	32.0	2
Zinc	65.4	2

Source: Gandy (2014). Reproduced with permission from Wiley Blackwell.

Dietetic and Nutrition Case Studies, First Edition.
Edited by Judy Lawrence, Pauline Douglas, and Joan Gandy.

Companion Website: http://www.manualofdieteticpractice.com/

Table A7.2 Mineral content of compounds and solutions.

Solution/compound	Mineral content	
1 g sodium chloride	393 mg Na	(17.1 mmol Na^+)
1 g sodium bicarbonate	274 mg Na	(12 mmol Na^+)
1 g potassium bicarbonate	390 mg K	(10 mmol K^+)
1 g calcium chloride (dihydrate)	273 mg Ca	(6.8 mmol Ca^{2+})
1 g calcium carbonate	400 mg Ca	(10 mmol Ca^{2+})
1 g calcium gluconate	89 mg Ca	(2.2 mmol Ca^{2+})
1 L normal saline	3450 mg Na	(150 mmol Na^+)

Source: Gandy (2014). Reproduced with permission from Wiley Blackwell.

Table A7.3 Conversion factors for mmol/mg/mEq.

Mineral	mg/mmol		mg/mEq		mmol/mEq	
	mg=	mmol=	mg=	mEq=	mmol=	mEq=
Sodium	mmol × 23	mg ÷ 23	mEq × 23	mg ÷ 23	mEq	mmol
Potassium	mmol × 39	mg ÷ 39	mEq × 39	mg ÷ 39	mEq	mmol
Phosphorus	mmol × 31	mg ÷ 31	mEq × 15.5	mg ÷ 15.5	mEq ÷ 2	mmol × 2
Calcium	mmol × 40	mg ÷ 40	mEq × 20	mg ÷ 20	mEq ÷ 2	mmol × 2
Magnesium	mmol × 24.3	mg ÷ 24.3	mEq × 12.15	mg ÷ 12.15	mEq ÷ 2	mmol × 2
Chlorine	mmol × 35.4	mg ÷ 35.4	mEq × 35.4	mg ÷ 35.4	mEq	mmol
Sulphur	mmol × 32	mg ÷ 32	mEq × 16	mg ÷ 16	mEq ÷ 2	mmol × 2
Zinc	mmol × 65.4	mg ÷ 65.4	mEq × 32.7	mg ÷ 32.7	mEq ÷ 2	mmol × 2

Source: Gandy (2014). Reproduced with permission from Wiley Blackwell.

Osmolarity and osmolality

Osmolality is the number of osmotically active particles (milliosmoles) in a kilogram of solvent. Osmolarity is the number of osmotically active particles in a litre of solution (i.e. solvent + solute).

In body fluids, there is only a small difference between the two. However, in commercially prepared feeds, osmolality is always much higher than osmolarity. Osmolality is therefore the preferred term for comparing the potential hypertonic effect of liquid diets (although, in practice, it is often osmolarity which is stated).

The osmolality of a liquid feed is considerably influenced by the content of amino acids and electrolytes such as sodium and potassium. Carbohydrates with a small particle size (e.g. simple sugars) increase osmolality more than complex carbohydrates with a higher molecular weight. Fats do not increase the osmolality of solutions because of their insolubility in water.

The osmolality of plasma is normally in the range of 280–300 mosmol/kg and the body attempts to keep the osmolality of the contents of the stomach and intestine at an isotonic level. It does this by producing intestinal secretions, which dilute a concentrated meal or drink. If enteral feeds with a high osmolality are administered, large quantities of intestinal secretions will be produced rapidly in order to reduce the osmolality. In order to avoid diarrhoea, it is, therefore, important to administer such feeds slowly; the number of mosmoles given per unit of time is more important than the number of mosmoles per unit of volume.

Biochemical and haematological reference ranges

The results of laboratory tests are interpreted by comparison with reference or normal ranges. These are usually defined as the mean ± 2SD (standard deviation), which assumes a Gaussian or normal (symmetrical) type distribution (Figure A7.1). Unfortunately, most biological data have a skewed rather than a symmetrical distribution and more complex statistical calculations are required to define the reference ranges.

The reference ranges as defined usually include approximately 95% of the normal 'healthy' population; consequently, 5% of this population will have values outside the reference range but cannot be said to be abnormal. The use of reference ranges may be illustrated by taking the reference range of blood urea as 3.3–6.7 mmol/L. Approximately 95% of the normal 'healthy' population would come within these limits. However, it would be wrong to interpret a value of 6.4 mmol/L as normal

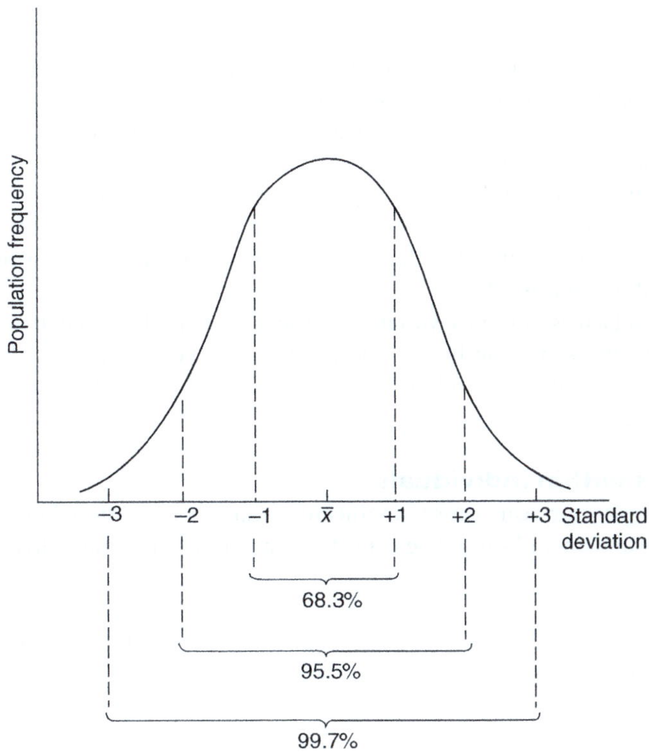

Figure A7.1 Normal distribution curve. (Gandy (2014). Reproduced with permission from Wiley Blackwell.)

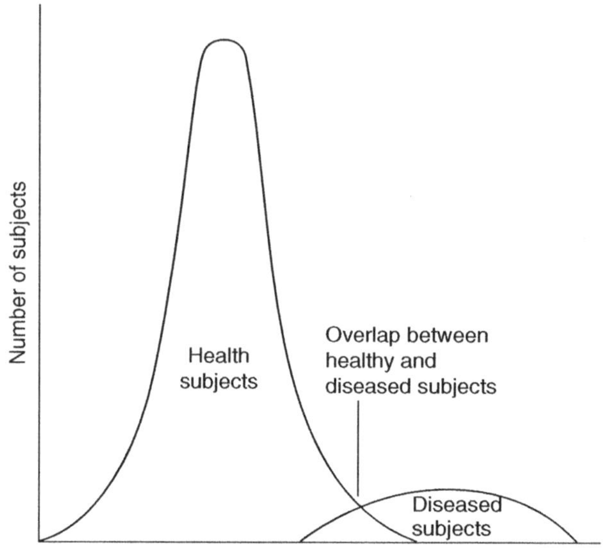

Figure A7.2 Theoretical distribution of values for in health and disease. (Gandy (2014). Reproduced with permission from Wiley Blackwell.)

while assuming a value of 7.0 mmol/L to be abnormal. Nature 'abhors abrupt transitions', so there is no clear-cut division between 'normal' and 'abnormal'. This applies equally well to body weight and height and also to measurements undertaken in the laboratory.

The majority of the normal 'healthy' population will have results close to the mean value for the population as a whole, and all values will be distributed around that mean. Therefore, the probability that a value is abnormal increases further it is from the mean value (Figure A7.2).

A variety of factors can cause variation in the biochemical and haematological constituents present within the blood. These can be conveniently divided into factors causing variation within an individual and those causing variation between groups of individuals.

Variations within individuals

The following factors can cause significant variation in clinical biochemical and haematological data and should be considered when interpreting individual results.

Diet

Variation in diet can affect the levels of triglycerides, cholesterol, glucose, urea and other blood constituents.

Drugs

These can have significant effects on a number of biochemical determinations, often resulting from secondary effects on sensitive organs, for example, liver, kidney and endocrine glands. Steroids, including oral contraceptives, can cause variations in a number of biochemical and haematological parameters, including a reduction in albumin, increases in several carrier proteins, for example, transcortin, thyroxine-binding globulin, caeruloplasmin and transferrin, and also increases in coagulation factors, for example, fibrinogen, factor VII and factor X.

Menstrual cycle

Several biochemical constituents show marked variations with the phase of the cycle; these include the pituitary gonadotrophins, ovarian steroids and their metabolites. There is also a marked fall in plasma iron just before and during menstruation. This is probably caused by hormonal changes rather than blood loss.

Muscular exercise

Moderate exercise can cause increases in levels of potassium, together with a number of enzymes including aspartate transferase, lactate dehydrogenase, creatine kinase and hydroxybutyrate dehydrogenase.

Posture

Significant differences in the concentration of many blood constituents may be obtained by collecting blood samples from ambulant compared with recumbent individuals. The red cell and white cell counts, together with the concentration of proteins (e.g. albumin, immunoglobulins) and protein-bound substances (e.g. calcium, cholesterol, T4, cortisol), may decrease by up to 15% following 30 min of recumbency. This is probably due to fluid redistribution within the body. Hospitalised patients usually have their blood samples collected early in the morning following overnight recumbency and, consequently, have significantly lower values than the normal ambulant (outpatient) population.

Stress

Both emotional and physical stress can alter circulating biochemical constituents, causing increases in the levels of pituitary hormones [e.g. adrenocorticotropic hormone (ACTH), prolactin, growth hormone] and adrenal steroids (cortisol).

Time of day

Some substances exhibit a marked circadian (diurnal) variation, which is independent of meals or other activities, for example, serum cortisol, iron and the amino acids tyrosine, phenylalanine and tryptophan. Cortisol levels are at their highest in the morning (9 am) and at their lowest levels at midnight, while iron concentration may decrease by 50% between the morning and evening. Plasma phenylalanine levels are at their lowest after midnight and reach their highest concentrations between 8.30 and 10.30 am.

Variations between groups of individuals

Several factors influence the reference values quoted for individuals. These include age, sex and race.

Age

The blood levels of many biochemical and haematological constituents are age related; these include haemoglobin, total leucocyte count, creatinine, urea, inorganic phosphate and many enzymes, for example, alkaline phosphatase, creatine kinase and γ-glutamyl transferase. Haemoglobin levels and total leucocyte counts are highest in newborns and gradually decrease through childhood, reaching the adult reference range at puberty. As creatinine is related to muscle mass, paediatric reference ranges are lower than those of adults. Urea levels rise slightly with age, but this may well indicate impaired renal function. Alkaline phosphatase activity and inorganic phosphate levels are at their highest during childhood, reaching peak levels at puberty.

Gender

Many biochemical and haematological parameters show concentration differences that are sex dependent, including creatinine, iron, urea, urea and the various sex hormones. Ferritin, haemoglobin and red cell counts are slightly higher in men than in women. Creatinine and urea levels are 15–20% lower in pre-menopausal females than in males. Pre-menopausal women also have lower serum iron levels than men, but after the menopause iron levels are similar in both sexes.

Race

Racial differences have been reported in some biochemical constituents, including cholesterol and protein. The reference ranges for cholesterol are higher in Europeans than in similar groups of Japanese. Similarly, the Bantu Africans have higher serum globulins than corresponding Europeans. African and Middle-Eastern individuals have lower total leucocyte and neutrophil counts than other races. Some of these racial differences are probably genetic in origin although the environment and diet may also be contributory factors.

Laboratory variations

Methods of analysis and standardisations vary considerably from laboratory to laboratory. These differences will influence the quoted reference ranges, and therefore, readers are advised to use only those quoted by their local laboratory. Local reference ranges may be at variance with the levels quoted in the following tables.

Correction of serum calcium for low albumin

$$\text{corrected serum calcium level (mmol/L)}$$
$$= \text{measured serum calcium (mmol/L)} + \left(\frac{40 - \text{measured albumin}}{40}\right)$$

An alternative (and possibly more accurate) equation is

$$\text{corrected serum calcium level (mmol/L)}$$
$$= \text{measured serum calcium (mmol/L)} + [(40 - \text{measured albumin}) \times 0.02]$$

Table A7.4 Adult normal values.

Substance	Value	Substance	Value
Albumin	32–50 g/L	Red cell count	
Bicarbonate	20–29 mmol/L	Males	$4.5–6.5 \times 10^{12}$/L
Bilirubin	<17 µmol/L	Females	$3.8–5.8 \times 10^{12}$/L
Calcium	2.15–2.55 mmol/L	Mean cell haemoglobin (MCH)	27–32 pg
Chloride	97–107 mmol/L	Mean cell volume (MCV)	77–95 fl
Total cholesterol	<5 mmol/L	Mean cell haemoglobin concentration	32–36 g/dL
Creatinine	60–125 mmol/L	White blood count (WBC)	$4.0–11.0 \times 10^{9}$/L
Glucose (fasting)	<6.1 mmol/L	Neutrophils	$2.0–7.5 \times 10^{9}$/L
Phosphate	0.7–1.5 mmol/L	Eosinophils	$0.04–0.4 \times 10^{9}$/L
Magnesium	0.7–1.0 mmol/L	Monocytes	$0.2–0.8 \times 10^{9}$/L
Osmolality	278–305 mOsmol/kg	Basophils	$0.0–0.1 \times 10^{9}$/L
Potassium	3.5–5.0 mmol/L	Lymphocytes	$1.5–4.5 \times 10^{9}$/L
Sodium	135–150 mmol/L	Platelets	$150–400 \times 10^{9}$/L
Total protein	63–80 g/L	Erythrocyte sedimentation rate	2–12 mm/1st h
Triglycerides	0.55–1.90 mmol/L	Ferritin (varies with age)	14–200 µg/L
Urate	0.14–0.46 mmol/L	Pre-menopausal women	14–148 µg/L
Urea	3.0–6.5 mmol/	Serum B_{12}	150–700 ng/L
Haemoglobin		Serum folate	2.0–11.0 µg/L
Male	13.0–18.0 g/dL	Red cell folate	150–700 µg/L
Female	11.5–16.5 g/dL	Prothrombin time (PT)	12–14 s
Haematocrit (PCV)			
Male	0.40–0.52	Activated partial thromboplastin time (APTT)	26.0–33.5 s
Female	0.36–0.47	Thrombin time (TT)	9 3 s of control

Source: Gandy 2014. Reproduced with permission from Wiley Blackwell.

Table A7.5 Normal adult urine values.

Substance	Value
Albumin	< 20 mg/24 h
Calcium	<7.5 mmol/24 h
Creatinine	9–15 mmol/24 h
Phosphate	15–50 mmol/24 h
Osmolality	50–1500 mOsmol/24 h
Potassium	14–120 mmol/24 h
Protein	<150 mg/24 h
Sodium	100–250 mmol/24 h
Urate	<3.0 mmol/24 h
Urea	250–600 mmol/24 h

Source: Gandy (2014). Reproduced with permission from Wiley Blackwell.

Table A7.6 Normal adult faecal values.

Substance	Value
Faecal fat	<18 mmol/24 h
Nitrogen	70–140 mmol/24

Source: Gandy (2014). Reproduced with permission from Wiley Blackwell.

Table A7.7 Conversion chart for HbA1c from % to IFCC mmol/mol.

%	mmol/mol	%	mmol/mol	%	mmol/mol	%	mmol/mol	%	mmol/mol	%	mmol/mol	%	mmol/mol	%	mmol/mol	%	mmol/mol	%	mmol/mol
4.0	20	5.0	31	6.0	42	7.0	53	8.0	64	9.0	75	10.0	86	11.0	97	12.0	108	13.0	119
4.1	21	5.1	32	6.1	43	7.1	54	8.1	65	9.1	76	10.1	87	11.1	98	12.1	109	13.1	120
4.2	22	5.2	33	6.2	44	7.2	55	8.2	66	9.2	77	10.2	88	11.2	99	12.2	110	13.2	121
4.3	23	5.3	34	6.3	45	7.3	56	8.3	67	9.3	78	10.3	89	11.3	100	12.3	111	13.3	122
4.4	25	5.4	36	6.4	46	7.4	57	8.4	68	9.4	79	10.4	90	11.4	101	12.4	112	13.4	123
4.5	26	5.5	37	6.5	48	7.5	58	8.5	69	9.5	80	10.5	91	11.5	102	12.5	113	13.5	124
4.6	27	5.6	38	6.6	49	7.6	60	8.6	70	9.6	81	10.6	92	11.6	103	12.6	114	13.6	125
4.7	28	5.7	39	6.7	50	7.7	61	8.7	72	9.7	83	10.7	93	11.7	104	12.7	115	13.7	126
4.8	29	5.8	40	6.8	51	7.8	62	8.8	73	9.8	84	10.8	95	11.8	105	12.8	116	13.8	127

Source: Gandy (2014). Reproduced with permission from Wiley Blackwell.

To be even more accurate, the serum protein level should also be considered:

$$\text{corrected serum calcium level (mmol/L)} = \text{measured serum calcium (mmol/L)} + [(72 - \text{measured protein}) \times 0.02]$$

This corrected calcium value should be added to that obtained from the correction for low albumin, and a mean of the two levels obtained, calculated to two decimal places.

References

Provan, J. (2005) *Oxford Handbook of Clinical and Laboratory Investigation*, 2nd edn. Oxford University Press, Oxford.

Gandy, J. (2014) *Manual of Dietetic Practice*, 5th edn. Wiley Blackwell, Oxford.

Index

Page numbers in *italics* denote figures, those in **bold** denote tables.

Dietetic and Nutrition Case Studies, First Edition.
Edited by Judy Lawrence, Pauline Douglas, and Joan Gandy.

Companion Website: http://www.manualofdieteticpractice.com/

Printed and bound by CPI Group (UK) Ltd, Croydon, CR0 4YY
10/09/2025
14733082-0001